SPORTS INJURIES

Their Prevention and Treatment

Third Edition

Lars Peterson MD, PhD
Professor, Department of Orthopaedics,
University of Gothenburg
Clinical Director, Gothenburg Medical Center
Gothenburg

and

Per Renström MD, PhD
Professor, Karolinska Institutet
Director, Section of Sports Medicine, Department of
Orthopaedics, Karolinska Hospital
Consultant, Tipskliniken, St Göran's Hospital
Stockholm

Martin Dunitz

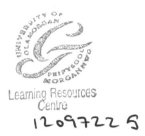

© **Martin Dunitz Ltd 2001**

Although every effort has been made to ensure that all owners of copyright material have been acknowledged in this publication, we would be glad to acknowledge in subsequent reprints or editions any omissions brought to our attention.

First edition originally published in Sweden in 1977 in cooperation with the Swedish Sports Federation and Folksam Insurance Company.

Second edition (English-language edition) first published in the United Kingdom in 1986 by Martin Dunitz Ltd, The Livery House, 7—9 Pratt Street, London NW1 0AE.

Although every effort has been made to ensure that drug doses and other information are presented accurately in this publication, the ultimate responsibility rests with the prescribing physician. Neither the publishers nor the authors can be held responsible for errors or for any consequences arising from the use of information contained herein. For detailed prescribing information or instructions on the use of any product or procedure discussed herein, please consult the prescribing information or instructional material issued by the manufacturer.

A CIP record for this book is available from the British Library.

ISBN: (book) 1 85317 119 0
(book + CD-ROM of selected illustrations) 1 85317 984 1

Composition by Scribe Design, Gillingham, Kent, UK

Printed and bound in Singapore by Kyodo Printing Pte. Ltd.

Contents

Contributors

The authors are very grateful to the following for their work and assistance on portions of the text:

Scott Lynch, MD   Department of Orthopaedics
                            Penn State University
                            Hershey, Pennsylvania, USA

Denise Alosa, ATC   University of Vermont
                            Burlington, Vermont, USA.

The following artists contributed to the book:

Lennart Molin
Tommy Berglund
Tommy Bolic Eriksson
Marian Tasker.

The excellent studio photographs were taken by:

Ole Roos   Svensk Sportfoto & Bildmedia
                            Mölndal, Sweden.

Authors' acknowledgments

The first edition of this book was published in 1977. The second edition was published in 1983 and in the English language in 1986: the book was later translated into ten other languages and we have been told that ours is the most widely diffused book available on sports injuries. This third edition is the result of several years of work, continuously not only updating and rewriting the text but also initiating the artwork and the photographs. There are, however, several people who have been very helpful and contributed to this book in their own way, and for this we are very grateful.

Great illustrations are of the greatest importance. Illustrations for the first edition were mainly down by Tommy Bolic Eriksson, for the second by Tommy Berglund, and for the third by Lennart Molin. These excellent illustrators have fulfilled our intentions skillfully and with great imagination. Our friend Ole Roos has given us his support and professional help with the photographs in the book. His professional skills are gratefully acknowledged.

Scott Lynch has helped us a lot with the work for this book and contributed with his expertise, especially in the hand and wrist chapters. Scott is a great orthopedic surgeon and we really appreciate his collaboration. Denise Alosa has worked out the rehabilitation program and we are very grateful for the skillful work she has put in. Anna Frohm-Grönqvist, RPT, from Bosön, and Dane Thomas, from the Karolinska Institutet, have critically shared their expertise by reviewing the rehabilitation chapter. We are furthermore grateful to other people who have given constructive criticism to the manuscript, such as Margaret Olmedo, MD, Louisiana State University, and Professor Bengt Saltin, Copenhagen. Magnus Tengvar, Radiologist, from Sophiahemmet, Stockholm, has generously provided us with most of the MRI pictures.

We would like to thank our secretaries Carrie Plunkett, Burlington, Vermont, and Louise von Essen, Section of Sports Medicine, Karolinska Hospital, Stockholm, for their invaluable help in typing out the manuscripts for this book. We would also like to thank Robert Peden of Martin Dunitz Publishers for his excellent scrutiny of the language and work on the editorial details. Robert has put much effort into the whole production process of this book, continually meeting with us and applying the necessary pressure. We would like to thank Martin Dunitz also for his great support and for taking on the publication of this book.

We are happy that this book has caught the interest of so many people. This book is based on and colored by our own philosophy and our personal experiences. We really do hope that you, as a reader, will enjoy it.

Publishers' acknowledgments

The publishers are very grateful to the All Sport picture agency for permission to reproduce the following Figures by their photographers:

front cover (Karl Weatherly); 2.1 (Shaun Botterill); 2.3 (Mike Powell); 2.18 (left, Todd Warshaw; right, Dan Smith); 2.29 (Alvin Chung); 2.30 (Alvin Chung); 3.2 (left, Mike Powell; right, Alvin Chung); 3.3 (Gary M Prior); 3.4 (left, Otto Greule; right, Jim Commentucct); 3.5 (Stu Forster); 3.6 (Chris Cole); 3.7 (Clive Brunskill); 3.8 (Trevor Jones); 4.7 (Simon Bruty); 5.2 (Mike Powell); 6.5 (right, Mike Powell); 6.7; 7.13 (left; middle, Doug Pensinger); 8.4; 8.10 (Mike Powell); 8.14 (Gary Prior); 8.19 (Mike Powell); 9.2 (Stu Forster); 9.3 (inset: David Cannon); 9.4; 9.6 (top, Simon Bruty; middle, Mike Powell; bottom, Gray Mortimore); 9.9 (Gray Mortimore); 9.16 (Tony Duffy); 9.21 (Yann Guichaoua); 10.4 (Mike Powell); 10.6 (left); 10.19 (Gray Mortimore); 10.25 (Mike Powell); 11.22 (Stephen Dunn); 11.45 (Jim De Frisco); 11.47 (Doug Pensinger); 12.11 (above, Pascal Rondeau); 12.13A (Gray Mortimore); 13.4 (Stephen Munday); 14.12 (Gray Mortimore); 17.1 (Didier Givois); 17.2 (David Leah); 18.2 (Clive Brunskill); 18.3 (Adam Pretty); 20.1 (Gray Mortimore);

to Blackwell Scientific Publishers for permission to reproduce Figures 3.11 and 3.12 from Johnson R and Renström P, in Renström PA (ed.) *Clinical Practice of Sports Injury: Prevention and Care* (1994) p. 676;

to Fotograf Roland Rygin for permission to reproduce Figure 12.5 (right);

to the International Society of Biorheology and IOS Press for permission to reproduce Figure 20.2 from Woo SL et al in *Biorheology* 19 (1982) 397;

and to Prisma Forlag for permission to reproduce Figure 2.15 from Eriksson BO, Mellstrand T, Peterson L et al, *Sjukdomar, läkemedel och idrott* (1990) p. 251.

Preface

Millions of people of all ages participate in sports or are physically active in other ways. Around the world every day sports give a feeling of togetherness and social interaction as well as of well-being.

Physical activity is also very important for one's overall health. Regular physical activity, exercise, training and sports can increase cardiovascular, metabolic and muscular functional capacity and help efforts to reduce risk factors for diseases: they thus play a favorable role in both primary and secondary prevention, as well as in therapy and rehabilitation. Physical activity is beneficial for all the tissues in the body and can help reduce the risks of injury, especially for overuse injuries. According to the US Surgeon General's Report on Physical Activity and Health, regular physical activity performed on most days of the week reduces the risk of developing or dying of something that causes illness and death. Physical activity improves health in the following ways: it reduces the risks of dying from heart disease, or of developing diabetes, high blood pressure, or colon cancer; it also helps those who already have high blood pressure to reduce it, helps control weight, helps build and maintain healthy bones, muscles and joints, helps older adults become stronger and better able to move without falling, and promotes psychological well-being.

Being physically active is thus beneficial and essential for good health, which is of great value for the active individual as well as for society. Some contend that sports injuries and problems are very costly for society, so it should be pointed out that *the cost to society of injuries in sports is very small compared to the health and social benefits generated by sports and physical activity.*

There are, however, potential risks for injuries and other medical problems. With increased information about the value of physical activities and about how injuries can best be treated and prevented, the costs to society will decrease. There is therefore a great need for sports medicine expertise and information. Hopefully, this book will fill an important role in spreading information about how most correctly to manage and prevent injuries in sports and physical activity.

Introduction

Sports medicine encompasses the following elements: preparation and training; prevention of injuries and illnesses; diagnosis and treatment of injuries and illnesses; and rehabilitation and return to physical activity and participation in sports. This book deals mainly with the part of sports medicine focused on injuries, their prevention, diagnosis, treatment and rehabilitation (i.e. orthopedic sports medicine).

Preparation and training includes instruction in training methods, technique, dietary requirements, the abusive effects of drugs, alcohol and doping as a whole, as well as psychological preparations for competition. This part is only briefly discussed in this book.

The *prevention* of injuries in sports depends on being well prepared, but also on appropriate clothing and protection, good equipment, sensible rules, adequate facilities, regular health controls, and so on.

Diagnosis and treatment of injuries are the main bulk of orthopedic sports medicine. A correct diagnosis is a requirement for successful treatment. Serious acute injuries are generally treated adequately in the emergency departments. The subacute and chronic injuries present more of a problem to the coach, the trainer, or the physician. Injuries such as those from overuse of the tendons and bones, as well as articular cartilage injuries, are often difficult to diagnose and treat, and they are not always well understood.

Rehabilitation and return to sport often require teamwork involving the physician, the physical therapist, the trainer, and the athlete. Injuries heal at varying paces depending on what type of tissue is involved, but also on the severity and location. If the rehabilitation is to be successful, it is essential that the person in charge of treatment have a thorough knowledge of the healing process in the different tissues and also be familiar with the demands of the sports concerned.

Finally, sports medicine is a discipline involving many different medical specialties. The sports medicine doctor can be an orthopedic surgeon, a rehabilitation specialist, a family physician, a rheumatologist, or one of many other specialists. In a few countries there are special education programs to become a sports medicine specialist. Every country has its own slightly different system, but it is to be hoped that in the long term there will be some kind of consensus in this area. Whatever the training, a good sports medicine doctor will be one familiar with the principles of sports medicine as outlined above, as well as with the demands of the different sports.

Glossary

Note: Illustrations of anatomic terms are listed in *italic* in the Index.

abduct: to move a part of the body away from the midline of the body.
adduct: to move a part of the body toward the midline of the body.
avulsion fracture: tearing off of an attachment to a bone.
bursa: a small sac of fibrous tissue, lined with a synovial membrane and filled with synovia.
cartilage: dense connective tissue composed of a matrix produced by specialized cells (chondroblasts).
chondral: describing cartilage.
concentric work: muscle contraction during shortening of the muscle.
crepitation: creaking or crackling sound.
cutting: a sudden sharp turn (e.g. as performed by the knee in running sports).
debridement: excision of devitalized material.
distal: situated away from the origin or point of attachment or the median line in the body.
dorsiflexion: backward flexion of the foot or hand or their digits, i.e. bending towards the upper surface.
eccentric work: muscle contraction during lengthening of the muscle.
epiphysis: the end of a long bone, initially separated by cartilage from the shaft of the bone.
evert: turn outwards.
exostosis: bony outgrowth.
hallux: the big toe.
hypertrophy: increase in the size of tissue or an organ brought about by the enlargement of its cells rather than by an increase in their numbers.
hypotrophy: decrease in the size of tissue or an organ brought about by the shrinking of its cells rather than by a decrease in their numbers.
invert: turn inwards.
isokinetic training: a form of muscle traning performed at a constant speed and against a variable resistance.
isometric training: a form of muscle training performed at a constant position (without a change in the length of the muscle) and variable load.
isotonic training: a form of muscle training performed at variable load.
-itis: inflammation of an organ, tissue, etc.
kinetic chain: multi-segmental motion involving one or more joints: (closed) when the distal segment is stable and the proximal is free; (open) when the proximal segment is stable and the distal segment is free.
lateral: relating to or situated at the side of an organ or organism.

ligament: a tough band of white fibrous connective tissue that links two bones together.

luxation: complete dislocation of a joint: opposing articular surfaces are no longer in contact.

medial: relating to or situated in the central region of an organ, tissue or the body.

multiplane exercises: limbs are exercised in a variety of different planes of motion (frontal, sagittal).

osteochondral: describing bone and cartilage.

osteophytes: bony deposits.

periosteum: a layer of dense connective tissue that covers the surface of a bone, except at the articular surfaces.

plantar: relating to the sole of the foot.

pronation: the act of turning the hand or foot so that the palm or sole faces downwards.

proprioception: the ability to apprehend positional changes of parts of the body or degrees of muscular activity without the aid of sight.

proximal: situated close to the origin or point of attachment or close to the median line in the body.

rotator cuff: the area of mergence of the tendons of subscapularis, supraspinatus, infraspinatus and teres minor muscles.

subluxation: partial dislocation of a joint: opposing articular surfaces are no longer correctly aligned.

supination: the act of turning the hand or foot inward so that the palm or sole faces as far upwards as possible.

synovia: thick colorless lubricating fluid that surrounds a joint or bursa and fills a tendon sheath, secreted by the synovial membrane.

trabecular: porous (cancellous) bone.

valgus: describing any deformity that displaces a joint towards the midline.

varus: describing any deformity that displaces a joint away from the midline.

1 General principles

Sports injuries are caused by trauma of different degree. For simplification we divide injuries into traumatic injuries, caused by large forces (macrotrauma), and overuse syndromes, caused by repetitive microtrauma.

Traumatic injuries

Acute traumatic injuries are common in athletics and attract the most publicity and research. This is because the cause of the injury can be pinpointed, making it easier to define the injury and search for an appropriate treatment.

The frequency of traumatic injuries varies greatly between sports. Contact sports, such as soccer, ice hockey, team handball, wrestling, American football, and rugby, tend to have higher rates of traumatic injuries.

The cause and severity of a traumatic injury are usually obvious. The athlete will usually experience rapid onset of pain, and swelling will begin to develop but typically requires several hours to reach its maximum. For this reason, the best time to examine a traumatic injury is immediately after it has occurred, before the swelling makes the athlete unable to tolerate the pain associated with exploration of the injured area.

Initial control of swelling can contribute greatly to a quicker return to sport. Treatment principles are described in Chapter 5. Once these early interventions have been completed, an assessment is made as to whether further advice is needed from a doctor and appropriate action is taken.

Overuse syndromes

Overuse syndromes are difficult to diagnose and treat. These injuries are becoming increasingly common as both participation in sport in general and the intensity and duration of training increase.

Although overuse injuries (stress fractures) were first documented as early as 1855, little research has been done since, and today's knowledge is based mainly on practical, clinical experience. Overuse injuries are generally caused by repetitive overloading, resulting in microscopic injuries to the musculoskeletal system. Tissues can withstand great loads

1

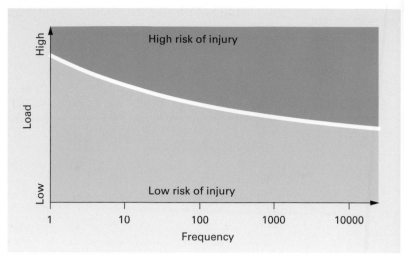

Figure 1.1 The relationship between load and frequency in injury.

but there is a critical limit to this capacity, which varies greatly between individuals and according to the frequency of load (Figure 1.1). Tissues may be made more susceptible to injury by *intrinsic* factors such as malalignment of the leg, muscle imbalance, and other anatomical problems, and *extrinsic* factors such as training errors, faulty technique, incorrect equipment and surfaces and poor conditions.

The actual frequency of injury due to overuse is unknown, but it is estimated that 25–50% of athletes visiting sports medicine clinics have sustained an overuse injury. The age of occurrence of overuse injuries also varies: they are most common in top-level athletes aged 20–29 years, but are also seen in noncompetitive athletes aged 30–49 years. In adults, overuse injuries are more prevalent after 2 years of regular daily training. Some sports carry a greater risk: 80% of overuse injuries are reported to occur in endurance sports such as long-distance running, or in individual sports requiring skilled technique and repetitive movements, such as tennis, gymnastics, and weightlifting; of these injuries, 80% occurred in the lower extremities of the body, most frequently at the knee (28%) and at the ankle, foot, and heel (21%). For most overuse injuries, the under-lying problem is an inflammatory response. Overuse injuries in tendons are often secondary to degeneration (p. 43).

Inflammation

Inflammation is the body's response to tissue injury caused by pressure, friction, repeated load or overload, and external trauma. Trauma is associated with bleeding, which causes swelling and increased pressure. Both extrinsic and intrinsic factors (see above) contribute to the inflam-matory reaction in tendon sheaths, tendon and muscle attachments, bursae, and the periosteum. Overuse injuries can result from various combinations of frequency and loading, such as:

- normal load at high frequency/many repetitions;
- heavy load at normal frequency;
- heavy load at high frequency.

Inflammation also occurs in response to bacterial infections. It both confines and combats such infections as well as stimulating healing. Whatever the nature of the underlying cause, the inflammatory response leads to impaired and painful mobility of the affected part and thus enforces rest. If it affects gliding surfaces, such as those of tendons and their sheaths, crepitus or 'creaking' may develop. If inflammation goes unchecked, scar tissue will develop, and early intensive treatment is therefore recommended.

The most important step in the management of inflammation is the removal or reversal of its cause. Next in importance is the reduction of swelling so as to relieve pain, improve mobility, and encourage healing. Symptoms typical of inflammation include the following:
- swelling caused by accumulation of fluid;
- redness caused by increased blood flow;
- local rise of temperature, caused by increased blood flow around the injured area;
- tenderness on touching the affected area;
- impaired function of the affected part due to swelling and tenderness.

Inflammation often begins insidiously, and initially pain and stiffness may decrease or even disappear after warm-up. Usually, however, the pain returns and intensifies during continued activity and unless a rest break is taken, there is a great danger of entering the 'pain cycle' where continued activity leads to further injury, inflammation and pain. Unless the cycle is interrupted, chronic pain results and can be extremely difficult to treat.

Pain

The sensation of pain originates in free nerve endings which end blindly between the tissue cells. These pain receptors are present in most tissues, but are especially numerous in the skin. Pain is a mechanism to alert us to injury so that we can react appropriately.

Different types of pain that may be experienced include acute pain caused by a fracture, aching pain caused by chronic inflammation, continuous pain such as heartburn, pounding pain such as vascular compromise, referred pain caused by nerve entrapment, and burning pain. The type of pain can be a pointer to the correct diagnosis. The most common types encountered in sports injuries are acute pain, and the chronic, dull ache experienced following activity or during the night due to chronic inflammatory problems. Pain can often be effectively treated with medication, but it will not go away until its cause has been removed.

Pain should be interpreted as a warning sign of tissue injury and should lead to modification of activity or resting the injured tissue.

3

2 Injuries in musculoskeletal tissues

Injuries to bone

Skeletal injuries are common in sport, especially in contact sports such as football (Figure 2.1), and in individual sports such as skiing, gymnastics, and riding.

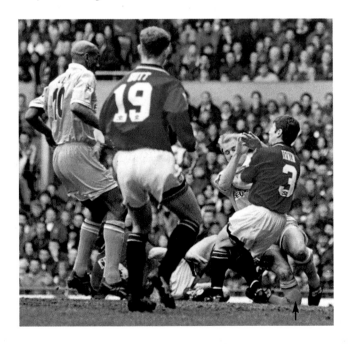

Figure 2.1 One of the players here has suffered a fracture of the lower leg (arrow) (by courtesy of All Sport: photographer, Shaun Botterill).

Functional anatomy

The bones of the skeleton primarily serve three purposes. The first is to provide a rigid weightbearing structure, enabling the body to stand: this is the primary function of the pelvis, spine and lower extremities. The second is to provide rigid attachment sites for the muscles, tendons and ligaments, to allow efficient movement. The third is to protect vulnerable soft tissues.

Bones are living material and can remodel themselves in response to changes in the local environment (Wolff's law). Activity causes the bones to become strong; inactivity weakens them (see p. 481). Pounding activities such as running cause thickening and strengthening of the weightbearing bones. Bones are also able to react to other stressors, such as fractures: the cells within the bone are able to remove the dead bone of the fracture and replace it with new, healthy bone. Some stress on the bone promotes the healing process, but too much will damage the healing structures, so a 'happy medium' must be attained. Disruption of the healing process can result in a non union.

Bones are better at resisting compression rather than tension and/or torsion. That is why most fractures occur when a bone is twisted or bent. The bending motion puts tensile stress (pulling apart) on the opposite side of the bone, where the fracture begins. The repetitive tensile stresses on the bone can result in stress fractures.

Fractures

A fracture is a potentially serious injury, damaging not only bone but also the soft tissues in the surrounding area—tendons, ligaments, muscles, nerves, blood vessels, and skin. Fractures may be the result of direct trauma, e.g. an impact to the leg, or indirect trauma, e.g. when the foot is trapped, causing the athlete to fall awkwardly and break the leg.

Types of injury

Skeletal fractures may be transverse, oblique, spiral, or comminuted (Figure 2.2). When the fractured ends of the bone pierce the skin the injury is an open or compound fracture (Figure 2.3); when the skin remains undamaged, it is a closed or simple fracture. With compound fractures there is a great risk of infection to the bone, and special treatment is required. If the fracture involves an adjacent articular joint surface it is called an articular surface fracture. An avulsion fracture means that a bone attached to a muscle or ligament has been torn away.

The different types of fracture displacement are angulation, rotation, and shortening. The aim of any treatment should be to return the

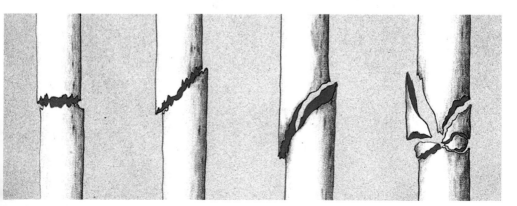

Figure 2.2 Different types of fractures (**from left**) transverse fracture, oblique fracture, spiral fracture and comminuted fracture.

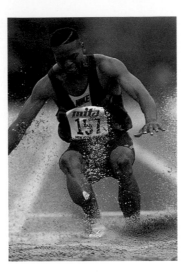

Figure 2.3 The fractured tibia is here seen piercing the skin (by courtesy of All Sport: photographer, Mike Powell).

fractured ends as precisely as possible into their correct position, that is, to reduce displacement and return the bone to its normal alignment by manipulation. For fractures in children and adolescents, see p. 444.

Associated soft tissue injuries

The soft tissues around the fracture are often damaged by sharp fragments of bone, and the more violent the impact the greater the risk of extensive soft tissue injury (Figure 2.4). Such injuries can increase hemorrhage and delay healing, and may even cause more problems than

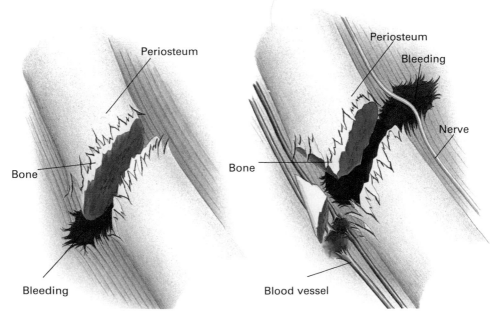

Figure 2.4 (**Left**) Fracture with bleeding and rupture of the periosteum. (**Right**) Fracture with bleeding and rupture of the periosteum, also affecting nerves and blood vessels.

the fracture itself. It is rare for major blood vessels and nerves to be damaged when a fracture occurs, but this may be a complication of fractures of the humerus just above the elbow, and fractures of the wrist.

Location

Certain sports lead to characteristic injuries: fractures of the lower leg predominate among soccer players; fractures of the forearm are common in gymnasts; and fractures of the clavicle in horseback riders.

Symptoms and diagnosis

The following features suggest that a fracture has occurred:
- swelling and progressive bruising in the injured area;
- tenderness and pain around the site of injury caused by both movement and loading of the limb;
- deformity and abnormal mobility of the fractured bone.

Sometimes fractures may cause few or none of these signs and symptoms. This can be true of fractures of the neck of the femur or of the humerus when the fractured surfaces of the bone are driven into each other, becoming firmly impacted and giving the fracture stability.

Treatment

When a fracture is suspected, the *athlete* or *trainer* should:
- cover an open injury with a sterile compress, a clean bandage or cloth;
- immobilize the limb by splinting or bracing;
- elevate the injured limb;
- arrange transport to hospital for treatment and X-ray examination as soon as possible. If bandages or splints are unavailable, improvisation is necessary: clean handkerchiefs, belts, straps, items of clothing, and sporting equipment can all be used. Elegance is not important, but effective immobilization is essential if pain and further injury are to be prevented. It is usual for an injured arm to be supported by strapping it to the body, and for an injured leg to be strapped to the other leg. Immobilization should include the joints on either side of the fracture. The injured athlete should avoid food and drink if surgery may be indicated.

It is the *doctor's* function to correct any significant displacement as soon as possible in order to control bleeding, reduce pain and improve blood supply.
- In cases of fracture without displacement, the injured part is immobilized and supported by the application of a cast, boot, or brace. After a cast is applied the athlete must be alert for increased pain, swelling, or a tingling sensation distal to the cast, and seek medical advice if it occurs; the cast may need to be removed and changed. Ambulatory treatment and early protected motion can be important in many fractures and may allow an early return to training and competition. This can be achieved by use of fracture bracing, orthotics and, in some cases, by external fixation (using a frame system).
- In cases of fracture with displacement, the fractured ends are realigned by manipulation (reduced) either without surgery (a *closed* procedure), or with surgery (an *open* procedure). In the latter case, internal fixation of the fracture is achieved by the use of cerclage (steel wire), plates,

screws, rods, pins, or nails. Internal fixation usually also requires the application of a cast or brace, which can be removed after a short time; some cases allow early immobilization without a cast. External fixation may be used for open fractures.

Aftercare

Active muscular exercises such as flexing and lifting (Chapter 20) must involve all parts of the body not in a cast to maintain general cardiovascular fitness and avoid muscle hypotrophy. Muscles inside the cast can be exercised isometrically; where movement is possible dynamic exercises can be included.

The length of time spent in a cast or brace depends on the location of the fracture, its severity, and the rate of progression through the healing process. A fracture of the wrist may be immobilized for 4–6 weeks, whereas a fracture of the lower leg is likely to be in a cast or brace for at least 3 months, and an equal period needs to be spent undergoing rehabilitation following removal of the cast.

Stress fractures

Stress fractures (also called fatigue or insufficiency fractures) occur most frequently as a result of repeated loading of the skeleton over a long period and are probably preceded by periostitis.

Causes

Stress fractures can appear following the application of a normal load at high frequency (e.g. long-distance running); of a heavy load at normal frequency (e.g. repeatedly running 100 m (or 100 yards) carrying a second person); or of a heavy load at high frequency (e.g. intensive weight training). The last is the most dangerous, as it is likely not only to cause stress fractures but also to overload other tissues. There is an increased incidence of stress fractures in athletes because of an increase in bone width and hip rotation. Athletes with leg-length discrepancy, or excessively high or low foot arches, also have increased incidence of stress fractures. Running more than 100 km (60 miles) per week and playing basketball are associated with stress fractures, and these injuries are more common in young people and in women. There is also a greater incidence in women with menstrual disturbances and eating disorders, and in women taking oral contraceptive medication.

There are two theories about the origin of stress fractures. The *fatigue theory* states that during repeated protracted effort, such as running, the muscles pass their peak of endurance and are no longer able to support the skeleton during impact as the foot strikes the ground. The load is therefore transferred directly to the skeleton; its tolerance is eventually exceeded and a fracture occurs (in the same way that a paperclip breaks after repeated bending).,

The *overload theory* is based on the fact that certain muscle groups contract in such a way that they cause the bones to which they are attached to bend. The contraction of the calf muscles, for example, causes the tibia to bend forward like a drawn bow. After repeated contractions the innate strength of the tibia is exceeded and it breaks.

Stress fractures occur in healthy individuals at all ages from 7 years upwards. They follow normal activity and affect healthy bones which have not been subjected to impact. The inadequately trained are more likely than others to suffer these fractures, which should be suspected in any athlete who complains of bone pain, particularly pain in the legs during exercise.

Stress fractures occur in the tibia in 44–50% of cases (p. 341), in the fibula in 12–16%, in the metatarsal bones in 16–20%, and in the femur in 6–8%. The calcaneus, navicular bone, humerus, pelvis, and vertebrae are also affected, but less frequently. Stress fractures are bilateral in 25% and multiple in 8–12%. They do not occur in the same site twice. Almost every bone in the body can suffer from stress fractures. Runners typically sustain stress fractures in the lower third of the fibula, usually 5–7 cm (2–3 in) above the lateral malleolus. High-jumpers may sustain stress fractures in the upper third of the fibula.

Stress fractures can occur in the metatarsal bones of the foot (p. 412), and should be suspected if pain has been present for 6–8 weeks or more. (This injury is known as the 'march fracture' because it used to be common in the army.) Other stress fractures in the foot include the Jones fracture of the proximal fifth metatarsal (p. 412), which often requires surgery or immobilization with avoidance of weightbearing, and the navicular stress fracture of the midfoot (p. 410), which can be difficult to diagnose. An early bone scan is the key to detecting this stress fracture and its nature can then be evaluated by CT scan. A potentially serious location of stress fractures is the neck of the femur; such fractures often need surgical treatment to ensure healing and to prevent dislocation and vascular necrosis of the head of the femur. Groin pain in athletes should not be neglected, as this fracture must be excluded.

| **Symptoms and diagnosis** | The following suggest a diagnosis of stress fracture. |

The following suggest a diagnosis of stress fracture.
- Symptoms begin insidiously in 50% of the cases, and acutely without apparent injury in the remaining 50%.
- The pain is activity-related. In the first week of symptoms pain is felt during activity, but not at rest. When training is hard, the pain increases in intensity and eventually a dull ache may persist after exercise. Pain can often be felt at night.
- Local swelling and tenderness can be felt over the fracture area.

Plain radiography has poor sensitivity but high specificity in the diagnosis of stress fractures. The typical radiographic picture of a stress fracture shows new periosteal bone formation, a visible area of sclerosis (harder bone), and the presence of a callus or a visible fracture line. However, these abnormalities may not be seen unless the symptoms have been present for at least 2–3 weeks, as these findings may be signs of healing; only 40–50% of the X-rays show changes initially (Figure 2.5). This emphasizes the importance of repeating X-ray examination if the first X-ray is negative but symptoms persist. If the plain radiograph is positive, there is no need for further examinations.
- A bone scan is required where there is a strong suspicion of a stress fracture (Figure 2.6). A triple-phase bone scan is 100% sensitive. Changes on bone scan may be seen as early as 48–72 hours after the

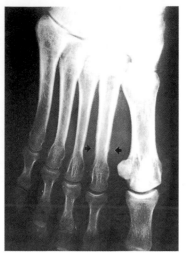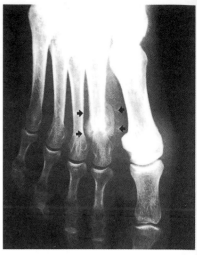

Figure 2.5 (**Left**) X-ray of the foot showing a stress fracture of the second metatarsal bone at an early stage (see arrows). (**Right**) X-ray of the same stress fracture six weeks after the first symptom. The ossification around the bone is a sign of healing.

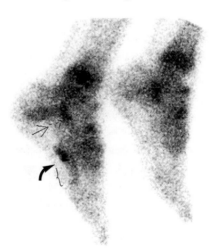

Figure 2.6 Bone scan (right foot): dark area (curved arrow) shows increased uptake of radioactive substance, which indicates a stress fracture of the proximal fifth metatarsal bone. (Left foot) Normal uptake.

beginning of the symptoms. The greatest disadvantage of a bone scan is its lack of specificity, as the fracture itself is not visualized; and other lesions such as tumor or infection can also cause localized increased signal intensity.

– In stress fractures all three phases of the triple-phase bone scan can be positive. Another bony problem such as medial tibial syndrome (shin splints) is only positive on delayed images. The diagnosis of a stress fracture is defined as a localized increase in signal intensity.

– In some cases other imaging may be valuable. A computed tomographic (CT) scan can be helpful in evaluating a bone stress fracture. Magnetic resonance imaging (MRI) performed 3 weeks after the onset of symptoms can be valuable in separating stress fractures from a suspected bone tumor or infection.

Treatment	When a stress fracture occurs, the *athlete* should: – rest the injured area for 2–8 weeks depending on the type of injury until the pain has resolved and healing can be seen on X-ray; – keep up conditioning in the swimming pool or by cycling; – gradually return to activity when activities of daily living are pain-free, and when there is no local tenderness.

The *doctor* may:
– prescribe crutches to relieve the injured part, especially in a femoral neck fracture;
– apply a walking boot or a plaster cast for 2–6 weeks if the pain is severe, or if the fracture is located on the tibia, navicular bone or the proximal fifth metatarsal;
– check the progress of healing with X-ray examinations;
– pay particular attention to stress fractures in the femoral neck, the anterior aspect of the medial tibia, proximal fifth metatarsal, and navicular bone.

These fractures often need surgery in order to heal and in order to allow the athlete to return to activities within reasonable time without risking complications.

Prevention

Stress fractures are to be avoided, and risk factors must be analyzed and eliminated. Athletes should assess their training methods with the coach, trainer, physical therapist, and physician, and pay particular attention to footwear and equipment. The time it takes tissue to adapt is important. Other risk factors include the 'female triad' of menstrual disturbances, low bone density, and dietary problems (p. 470). Bone geometry and biomechanical abnormalities should also be analyzed.

Bibliography
Brukner P, Benal K (1997) Stress fractures in female athletes. Diagnosis, management and rehabilitation. Injury Clinic. *Sports Medicine* December, 24/6: 419–429.

Medial tibial stress syndrome (periostitis, 'shin splints')

Pain syndrome in the lower leg is caused by a periosteal reaction of the posteromedial border of the tibia. Biopsy studies demonstrate chronic inflammation. This condition is probably a preliminary stage to stress reaction or stress fracture of the tibia. This syndrome has many names, as there is still confusion over the term 'shin splints'; the term 'medial stress syndrome' has been coined, as the pain and tenderness are located along the inner distal two-thirds of the tibia shaft. Chronic inflammation at the muscular attachment along the posterior medial tibia and bony changes (the stages before stress fracture) are considered to be the most likely cause of medial tibial stress syndrome. Diagnosis and treatment are discussed on p. 339. Another cause of lower leg pain is compartment syndrome (p. 334).

Diseases of bone

Osteoporosis

Osteoporosis is the world's most common bone disease, being almost universal in older women owing to postmenopausal hormonal changes and a decrease in activity. Half of all women over 45 years old have some X-ray evidence of osteoporosis, and by age 75 years that proportion increases to 90%. Osteoporosis also occurs in younger women as part of the 'female triad' (p. 470).

Osteoporosis is a reduction in bone mineral density due to an imbalance between resorption and formation. The bone most frequently affected is the trabecular bone at the distal end of the radius in the wrist, the vertebral bodies of the spine, and the neck of the femur. Risks for primary osteoporosis may be genetic, hormonal, nutritional, or related to lifestyle, such as exercise. Secondary osteoporosis may be caused by underlying disease or drugs.

Bone consists of collagen and a mineral structure of calcium and phosphorus which gives the bone its hardness. Inactivity, aging, hormonal and nutritional problems may cause the bone to lose its calcium to varying degrees, making it more susceptible to injury. As well as major fractures, microfractures (fractures that are not immediately visible) are more likely to occur as the bone weakens.

Physical activity increases bone density in most people and should be recommended to all. Regular exercise maintains bone mass in post-menopausal women and improves the overall health. Calcium supplements may be used for prevention, but only under medical advice. Good diet is a necessity. When osteoporosis causes pain, the person should keep as active as possible, perhaps with the aid of painkillers, to prevent further deterioration and muscle weakness.

The International Sports Medicine Federation (FIMS) has developed the following recommendations on osteoporosis and exercise, included here with permission:

1. Weightbearing physical activity is essential for normal development and maintenance of a healthy skeleton. Activities that focus on increasing muscle strength may also be beneficial, particularly for non-weightbearing bones.
2. Recent evidence demonstrating that growing bone is more responsive to mechanical loading and physical activity than mature bone suggests that regular exercise during early life may be an important factor in the prevention of osteoporosis in later life.
3. Excessive endurance training may induce hormonal changes and menstrual disturbances, and even adversely affect bone structure.
4. Exercise cannot be recommended as a substitute for hormone replacement therapy during menopause.

5. Activities that improve strength, flexibility and coordination may indirectly but effectively decrease the incidence of osteoporotic fractures by reducing the likelihood of falling. These should be included in an optimal exercise program for older people.

Joint injuries

A joint is formed by two adjacent bones covered by articular cartilage surfaces. Joints vary in structure, but in general one articular surface is convex (the ball) and the other is concave (the socket). The two fit together to a varying degree in different joints: in the hip the ball is almost entirely surrounded by the 'socket', whereas the knee, shoulder, and finger joints are very shallow.

The opposing ends of the bones are joined by a capsule of connective tissue which surrounds the joint. The joint capsule is lined by a membrane which produces synovial fluid. At points where the strain imposed on the joint is greatest, it is strengthened and protected by ligaments—bands of connective tissue limiting abnormal movement. The entire joint is surrounded by muscles and tendons.

The stability of a joint is influenced by both active and passive factors. Active stability is maintained by muscle activity under the control of the individual. The passive stability is maintained by the ligaments. Without adequate passive stability a joint is unable to function normally.

Ligament injuries

Ligament injuries in athletes are common, particularly around the knee and the ankle. They also occur in the shoulder, elbow, and thumb.

Functional anatomy

Ligaments are attached to the two bones that compose the joint (Figure 2.7). Ligaments provide stability to the joint, while still allowing motion. They cannot actively resist motion, but provide a 'check rein' against instability at the extreme range of motion of the joints. Because of their microstructure ligaments resist tensile forces (pulling apart) well, but are of little value for compressive forces.

Ligaments are injured when forces exceed the ligament's ability to resist a load, which may depend on the rate of injury. Ligaments provide more strength when a load is applied slowly: this is why relatively slow injuries may cause an avulsion fracture (where a small piece of bone breaks off at the ligament attachment) rather than tearing the ligament itself. Fast injuries will cause the ligament to fail before the bone, and resulting in a tear in the midsubstance of the ligament. When the athlete

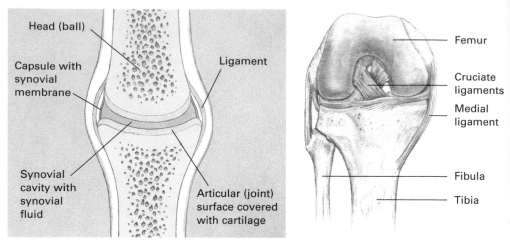

Figure 2.7 (**Left**) Example of the structure of a joint. (**Right**) Knee joint: anterior view.

sprains an ankle the two bones of the ankle joint, the tibia and talus, are rapidly forced apart, causing rupture of the ligaments holding the tibia and talus together.

Types of ligament injury

A ligament tear may affect only a few fibers or the entire ligament (Figure 2.8). In clinical practice it is practical to distinguish between partial and complete tears because the treatment and prognosis are different.

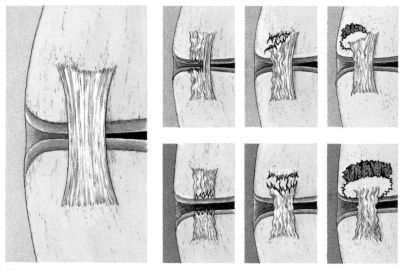

Figure 2.8 (**Left**) Normal ligament. (**Top right**) Part of the ligament is torn while the rest is undamaged; part is torn away without bone; part is torn away with bone. (**Bottom right**) Complete separation of ends; complete detachment from bone; complete detachment of fragment of bone attached to ligament.

1. A *partial tear* involves only some of the ligament fibers and may on occasion affect stability.
   - Part of the ligament may be torn while the rest is undamaged.
   - Part of the ligament attachment may be torn away from its insertion, with or without a fragment of bone.
2. A *complete tear* involves most or all of the ligament fibers and the affected joint is unstable.
   - The ligament may be completely torn and the ends separated from each other.
   - The entire ligament attachment may become detached from the bone.
   - The fragment of bone to which the ligament is attached may be torn away from the rest of the bone.

A partial tear may be classified as a grade I tear (disruption of a few fibers) or a minor grade II tear (disruption of less than half the fibers); in both cases the joint is stable. A major grade II tear corresponds to disruption of more than 50% of the fibers; a grade III tear corresponds to disruption of all the fibers as a complete tear; in both cases the joint is unstable to a varying degree.

A disruption of the fibers of the ligament is often accompanied by bleeding which spreads into surrounding tissue and is frequently seen as bruising. An injury to a ligament within the joint or to the joint capsule may cause hemorrhage into the joint space. Injuries to ligaments can also be accompanied by damage to the articular cartilage surface.

Symptoms and diagnosis

The following symptoms suggest that a ligament injury has occurred:
- bruising, swelling and tenderness around the affected joint caused by bleeding;
- pain when the limb is moved or loaded; there can also be pain on palpation;
- instability of the joint depending on the type of joint and the extent of the injury.

An MRI scan can often show the extent of the ligament injury if the diagnosis is unclear. In all cases of suspected ligament injuries the joint should be tested for stability.

Treatment

In cases of suspected acute ligament injury the *athlete* or *trainer* should:
- support the joint by elastic bandage or a brace;
- apply compression if there is bleeding;
- cool the joint;
- rest and avoid loading of the area (the use of crutches is often valuable);
- elevate the limb.

The *doctor's* function is:
- to determine the stability of the joint (sometimes it is necessary to perform a stability test under anesthesia if the pain is severe);
- to exclude the possibility of a fracture by taking X-rays;
- if the joint is stable, to prescribe early mobilization exercises. A supportive adhesive tape or an orthosis may be valuable depending on the nature and location of the injury. Early motion is important;

– if the joint is unstable, to decide whether the treatment should be nonoperative with early protective motion exercises or application of a supportive adhesive strapping, tape, brace, or cast, or whether surgical treatment is required.

Rehabilitation

Active muscular exercise and mobility training is of the greatest importance during the rehabilitation phase and should be carried out with cooperation between the athlete, coach, doctor, athletic trainer and physical therapist.

The healing of a ligament after an injury can take a long time, usually more than 6 weeks. If the ligament is part of a capsule, like the medial collateral ligament of the knee, early motion is usually allowed in combination with orthotic support. If the ligament is intra-articular, like the anterior cruciate ligament of the knee, the joint is subjected to early motion and/or to later surgery. Early motion exercises for the joint as a whole are usually desirable but should not create a dilemma for the doctor applying treatment. The exercises must not affect the healing of the injured ligament.

In the absence of a fracture or dislocation, all injuries that cause swelling in or around joints and all sprains causing bleeding, swelling, and tenderness should be treated as ligament injuries.

Healing and repair

Ligaments heal by the same response as other tissues. Initially, an influx of inflammatory cells brings repair cells to the region; the cells clean up dead tissue and prepare the region for new tissue. Following this, new blood vessels develop in the area, eventually leading to new cell formation and finally production of new structural tissue between the living cells. The initial tissue is immature, so a period of maturation must take place before healing is complete. This entire process takes many months. However, for most ligament injuries sufficient strength is achieved by about 6–12 weeks to begin strengthening exercises around the joint. This process can begin much earlier for cases of partial tears.

Dislocations

All joints are surrounded by a joint capsule and ligaments. For a dislocation to occur, at least part of the capsule and its ligaments must be torn; therefore any dislocation involves injuries to these structures and sometimes to the articular cartilage. Rehabilitation will depend upon how quickly these damaged tissues heal.

Complete dislocation (luxation) of a joint indicates that the opposing articular surfaces have become separated and are no longer in contact with each other. *Partial dislocation* (subluxation) of a joint indicates that the articular surfaces remain in partial contact with each other but are no longer correctly aligned. Again, there may be capsule, ligament, and cartilage injuries.

Location

Complete dislocations most frequently affect the shoulder, elbow, finger joints, and patella, while partial dislocations usually affect the knee and ankle joints. The acromioclavicular joint can be subject to a complete or a partial separation (see below).

Symptoms and diagnosis

The following symptoms suggest a dislocation:
- pain on movement;
- abnormal contour of the joint;
- swelling and tenderness;
- instability of the joint of varying degree;
- An X-ray will determine whether a fracture has occurred and may also determine the degree of dislocation, whether it is partial or complete.

Treatment

The doctor's function is to reduce the joint, i.e. to manipulate the articular surfaces of the bones back to their normal positions, with the help of local or sometimes general anesthesia. Further treatment is aimed at restoring the stability and function of the joint. Depending upon the degree of instability present, the doctor will suggest the most suitable treatment for the joint involved. This can include early mobilization with strength training or immobilization for a varying period (1–6 weeks) followed by exercises or surgical treatment. Injuries may recur in the shoulder joint and the patella; young athletes are particularly susceptible, especially after inadequate treatment or rehabilitation. Dislocations may be complicated by damage to nerves and blood vessels.

Separations

The term 'separation' is most commonly applied to injuries of the acromioclavicular joint—the joint on top of the shoulder between the clavicle (collar bone) and acromion (the extension of the shoulder blade). Injury to the ligaments holding the clavicle in position allows upward displacement of the clavicle (p. 118).

Meniscus and disk injuries

Meniscus injuries of the knee are described on page 294. A small meniscus-like structure is sometimes present in the acromioclavicular and sternoclavicular joints on the shoulder (p. 118). A small disk is present in the radioulnar joint of the wrist.

Articular cartilage injury

The smooth, white, shiny covering of the bones of the joints is known as articular cartilage. Damage to this articular cartilage can occur through trauma, but more commonly is a result of repetitive small injuries from pounding activities—popularly called 'wear and tear arthritis' or osteoarthritis, although it should be called osteoarthrosis or arthrosis.

Articular cartilage injuries are recognized as a common problem in athletes. Owing to more active treatment of ligament injuries and the use of arthroscopy and MRI, the frequency of articular cartilage injuries has been found to be much higher than previously thought. In acute and chronic injuries to the knee joint treated surgically, more than 40% of the patients were found to have articular cartilage injuries down to the subchondral bone (the bone underlying the cartilage).

In patients with chronic anterior cruciate ligament rupture, articular cartilage injuries have been found in 20–70%. Articular cartilage injuries are serious, especially in young athletes, and continued activity may ruin the joint function along with the career of the athlete.

Functional anatomy

Articular cartilage covers the ends of joining bones and optimizes joint function by reducing friction and increasing shock absorption. Cartilage consists of cells called chondrocytes and the surrounding supportive tissue, the matrix. The chondrocytes comprise only 5% of the total volume of the cartilage and are organized in columns; the cells are round in the deep layer and flattened towards the surface (Figure 2.9). The chondrocytes produce the matrix, consisting of protein cores (collagen), which armour the cartilage and give the tensile strength to the tissue, and also produce proteoglycans, a compound of protein and carbohydrates, which attract water and keep the water content in the cartilage to about 70% of the total volume. The proteoglycans bind water and contribute to the shock-absorbing function of cartilage. In the absence of weightbearing the water originating from the synovial fluid is sucked into the matrix by the action of proteoglycans. During weightbearing the water content of the cartilage is reduced by compressing the water back into the joint. All nutrients and oxygen are supplied to the cartilage from the synovial fluid produced by the synovial joint capsule. The synovial fluid (joint fluid) also lubricates the articular cartilage surfaces, reducing the friction between them.

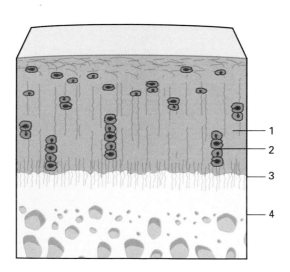

Figure 2.9 Structure of cartilage: 1, cartilage matrix; 2, chondrocytes (cartilage cells); 3, tidemark; 4, bone below the cartilage (subchondral and trabecular)

Articular cartilage is a unique tissue in that it lacks a vascular, nerve, and lymphatic supply. The lack of a vascular supply means that cartilage cannot heal by inflammatory tissue repair and is dependent on the exchange of synovial fluid for nutrients and oxygen. The metabolic turnover is slow. The lack of nerve supply means that injuries to the cartilage will not cause pain, unless surrounding tissues such as the synovial lining, the subchondral bone, or the periosteum are affected by the injury.

Mechanism of injury

Injuries to the articular cartilage can be caused by distortion, dislocation, or contusion of the joint. Cartilage injuries are often associated with ligament injuries or subluxation of the joint. Articular cartilage injuries may also be caused by repetitive microtrauma. Fractures running into the articular cartilage surface may leave articular defects. Malalignment of a joint may be a contributory factor for repeated microtrauma and unfavorable loading to the articular surface, resulting in wearing down of the cartilage over time.

Grading of articular cartilage injuries

Articular cartilage damage may be superficial (partial), deep (complete, full), or osteochondral.
– Superficial articular cartilage injuries extend into the upper 50% of the depth of the cartilage; these injuries will not heal, and will not progress unless located in weightbearing areas.
– Deep or full-thickness articular cartilage injuries extend down to the subchondral bone but not through it; they will not heal, but will progress to osteoarthritis.
– Osteochondral (bone and cartilage) injuries extend down through the subchondral bone into the trabecular bone and may heal by inflammation, allowing vascular (blood) ingrowth with fibroblast (fibrous cell) invasion that will produce a fibrous tissue repair.

Articular cartilage injuries may be graded clinically according to the Outerbridge classification (Figure 2.10):
– grade I: fissures extending only into the superficial cartilage;

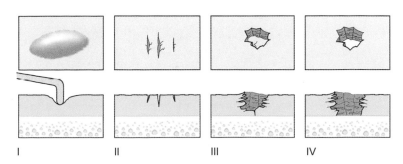

Figure 2.10 Surface and cross-sectional views of articular cartilage injuries I–IV.

- grade II: increased fibrillation of the surface and multiple fissures extending to half the depth of the cartilage;
- grade III: increased fissures and cracks extending down to the subchondral bone, but no denuded bone;
- grade IV: complete loss of cartilage and exposure of the subchondral bone.

Articular cartilage injuries may fragment into loose bodies that interfere with the joint function.

Healing and repair

Injuries limited to the articular cartilage have a low capacity for healing or repair. Both superficial and full-thickness cartilage injuries may progress owing to mechanical wear and breakdown of the matrix by enzymes released from the injured chondrocytes. For 10–14 days after cartilage injury the chondrocytes actively produce repair tissue, but this repair activity ends for unknown reasons.

The breakdown of the matrix will finally cause osteoarthritis (p. 25), which is a very severe condition when both articulating surfaces are injured. With continued high activity levels, especially with ligamentous instability or joint malalignment, articular cartilage injuries will progress rapidly to traumatic osteoarthritis.

The inability of cartilage to repair itself is partly because the chondrocytes are encapsulated in the matrix and cannot migrate into the damaged area to create repair tissue. An osteochondral injury may heal by migration of fibroblasts from the subchondral bone marrow into the defect. However, the resultant fibrous repair tissue provides little resistance to wear and has lower shock-absorptive properties; osteoarthritis may ensue.

Location

Articular cartilage injuries are most frequent in the knee but also occur in the ankle, elbow, shoulder, and hip joints. Ligament injuries or malalignment of a joint are often associated with the articular cartilage injury.

Acute articular cartilage injuries

Articular cartilage injuries may be diagnosed in the acute or chronic phase.

/mptoms
.nd diagnosis

- There may be a history of distortion, dislocation, or contusion of the joint.
- Swelling may occur due to effusion or bleeding.
- Pain occurs when the joint is moved or loaded.
- 'Catching' or 'locking' occur on joint motion or weightbearing.
- Crepitation (creaking) is noted on joint motion.

Treatment

The athlete may:
- cool the joint with an ice pack;
- support the joint with elastic bandaging;
- encourage rest and unloading of the injured area;
- elevate the limb;
- consult a doctor;
- carry out unloading and nonpounding exercise.

The doctor may:
- perform a clinical examination with stability testing;
- request an X-ray or MRI to exclude fractures or cartilage avulsions;
- aspirate the joint if swelling is causing pain;
- perform arthroscopy for the definite diagnosis of articular cartilage injury and removal of loose cartilage;
- fix or remove osteochondral fragments a few days after the injury;
- treat the patient with early range-of-motion exercise and partial weightbearing for 6–8 weeks.

Chronic articular cartilage injuries

If the athlete is still symptomatic after 2–3 months, further diagnostic and therapeutic measures are needed.

Symptoms and diagnosis
- There is pain and swelling during and after activity.
- 'Locking' or 'catching' symptoms occur on activity.
- Tenderness over the affected joint lines, swelling due to effusion, and pain on weightbearing are characteristic.
- An X-ray, MRI, and bone scan could be of value.
- Arthroscopy is useful to evaluate the size, depth, and location of the injury (Figure 2.11).

Nonsurgical treatment

Conservative treatment includes reducing or changing activity, exercise to improve muscle strength, endurance and proprioception, and anti-inflammatory medication.

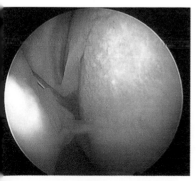 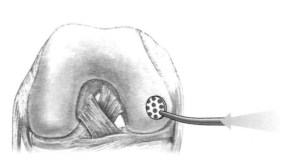

Figure 2.11 (Left) Arthroscopic view of medial femoral condyle: chronic articular cartilage injury, extending to subchondral bone. (**Right**) Microfracturing creates small openings through the subchondral bone, to allow vascular and stem cell growth from the bone marrow.

Surgical treatment involving bone	– Debridement of lost cartilage and flaps of cartilage interfering with joint function is necessary. This may be followed by drilling, microfracturing (picking), or abrasion to create vascular ingrowth and fibroblast invasion for fibrous repair of the defect (see Figure 2.11). The treatment is almost always performed arthroscopically.
	– *Drilling* creates multiple drill holes through the subchondral bone of the defect into the trabecular bone.
	– *Microfracturing* or 'picking' is the creation of small fractures in the subchondral bone to encourage bleeding into the defect, creating fibrous repair.
	– *Abrasion arthroplasty* is the superficial abrading of the subchondral bone surface to create bleeding from capillaries in the subchondral bone allowing fibrous repair of the defect.
Surgical treatment involving tissue engineering	– *Perichondral and periosteal grafting* is the implantation of tissue with chondroid (cartilage-like) potential, such as perichondrium and periosteum, to an abraded surface of the subchondral bone. Long-term results are unclear.
	– *Autologous chondrocyte transplantation* is suitable for localized cartilage injuries to the femoral articular surface of the knee (Figure 2.12). At the

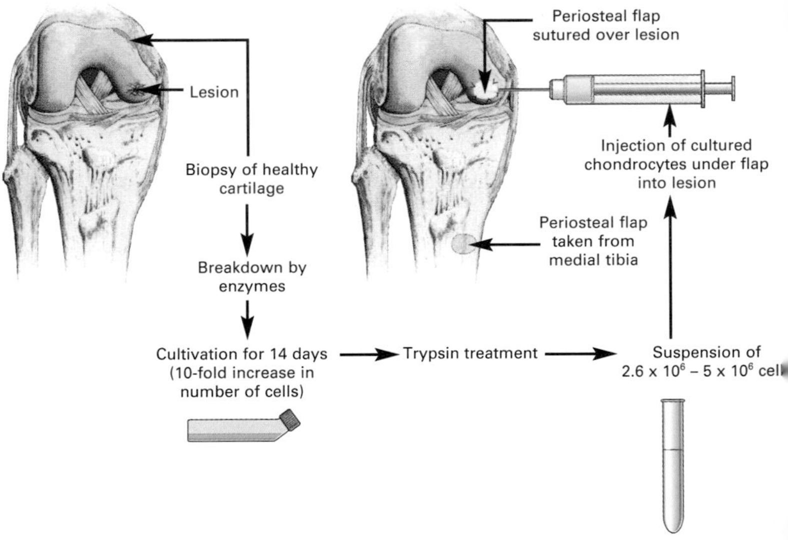

Figure 2.12
Autologous chondrocyte transplantation: cartilage cells are cultured and then re-introduced.

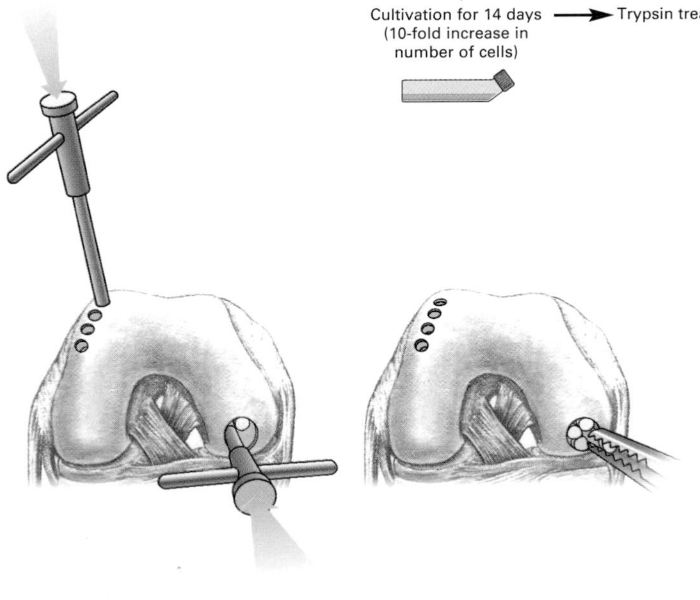

Periosteal flap sutured over lesion

Lesion

Biopsy of healthy cartilage

Breakdown by enzymes

Injection of cultured chondrocytes under flap into lesion

Periosteal flap taken from medial tibia

Cultivation for 14 days (10-fold increase in number of cells) ⟶ Trypsin treatment ⟶ Suspension of 2.6 x 10⁶ – 5 x 10⁶ cell

Figure 2.13
Osteochondral grafting: bone and cartilage cylinders harvested from minor weightbearing areas of the joint are transplanted into drilled holes in the damaged area.

arthroscopic evaluation of the injury, cartilage slices are harvested for cell culturing. Two weeks later, the patient is operated on with excision of the chondral injury; the cultured cells are injected into the defect, which has been covered with periosteum. Long-term results are promising.

– *Osteochondral grafting* of cylinders of bone and overlying cartilage has been used for minor injuries with promising results (Figure 2.13).

Rehabilitation Early range-of-motion exercise is of greatest importance for restoring the joint function. It should be carried out in cooperation with the athletic trainer, coach, doctor, and physiotherapist. Muscle strength training, progressive loading of the joint, subsequent return to athletic training and competitive sport, and weightbearing, should be judged on an individual basis.

Prognosis Untreated articular cartilage injuries may progress to osteoarthritis by mechanical and enzymatic breakdown, resulting in permanent dysfunction of the joint. Early diagnosis and optimal treatment of articular cartilage injuries in athletes are important for a good prognosis.

Osteochondritis dissecans

Osteochondritis dissecans (OCD) is a localized separation of a segment of bone and cartilage from the surrounding, normal bone and cartilage. If the bony part of the fragment becomes necrotic (dead), there will be no healing and there will be a complete separation of the fragment from the surrounding tissue (Figure 2.14).

In 75% of cases the lesion is localized to the medial femoral condyle of the knee. It can also occur in the ankle, the elbow, the shoulder, and the hip joints. It can start from the age of 5–10 years, up to 40 years, but is more common at 10–20 years of age. It is 2–3 times more common in males. OCD can be divided into a juvenile form and an adult form. The juvenile form affects children and adolescents up to the closure of the epiphyses (growth zones); the adult form also affects adolescents after

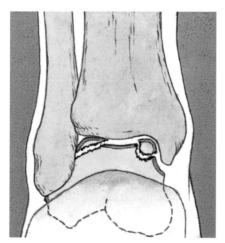

Figure 2.14 Osteochrondritis dissecans in the talar bone of the ankle.

23

closure of the epiphyses. The younger the patient and the earlier the detection of OCD, the better are the results of treatment and the prognosis.

Mechanism of injury

Many etiologies have been proposed for OCD. Trauma or repetitive microtrauma with impingement of the tibial spine against the lateral aspect of the medial femoral condyle has been proposed as a cause in the knee joint. Distortions of a joint may be common, as well as repetitive overload as in the ankle and elbow (compare 'Thrower's elbow' on p. 169). Even a vascular cause, with circulatory disturbances in the bone, has been discussed. The appearance of OCD has been shown to be sports-related in young, active patients.

It is important to distinguish between a stable fragment and an unstable fragment. A total detachment of the fragment will leave an empty bed and a defect in the articular surface.

Symptoms and diagnosis
- Pain is diffuse over the joint.
- 'Catching', and 'locking' and 'giving way' are often present.
- There is recurrent effusion of the joint.
- An X-ray examination and MRI confirm the diagnosis.
- Arthroscopic examination will help in deciding upon appropriate treatment. Any loose bodies can be removed and loose flaps debrided.
- Bone scans can support the diagnosis and the healing.

Treatment
The *doctor* may:
- prescribe rest along with muscle strength training;
- immobilize with a brace and no sports activities for 3–4 months in juvenile athletes;
- operate in symptomatic cases where conservative treatment has failed:
  • in acute cases with a loose fragment or partly avulsed fragment, especially in a juvenile athlete, fix the fragment using resorbable pins or screws;
  • remove all loose bodies;
  • in small defects try drilling, microfracturing and abrasion (p. 22) or osteochondral cylinder grafts;
  • in both small and large defects try autologous chondrocyte transplantation (p. 22) or other appropriate techniques.

Healing and return to sport
In the juvenile form after conservative treatment, an evaluation with MRI or bone scan, or arthroscopy should be performed before sport is resumed. Regaining muscle strength and mobility of the joint is important.

In the adult form and/or after surgery, an MRI or arthroscopy should be performed before any return to sporting activities.

Prognosis
The prognosis is better in the juvenile form, especially if it is treated early. An OCD in a weightbearing condyle will, within 20–30 years, progress to osteoarthritis of the knee in 80% of cases.

Diseases of joints

The articular surfaces of joints are covered with cartilage which has no blood supply and, therefore, does not heal well when injured. Articular cartilage reduces friction and increases shock absorption between bones. The membrane lining the joint capsule secretes synovial fluid, which supplies the nutrients required by the cartilage and also serves to reduce friction during joint movements.

Osteoarthritis (osteoarthrosis)

The term 'osteoarthritis' applies particularly to the degeneration and excessive wear of articular cartilage, although gradual changes in underlying bone tissue (subchondral bone) also occur. The condition is one which develops and progresses with increasing age. It may be 'primary' or 'secondary'.

- Primary osteoarthritis, the cause of which is unknown, occurs most frequently in women and in people with diabetes. Obesity is probably of no significance so far as onset of the disease is concerned, but it does accelerate the degenerative process once it has begun.
- Secondary osteoarthritis may follow either injury or joint disease. Fractures of articular surfaces, including damaged cartilage, ligament injuries, and dislocations are all possible causes, as are infections and rheumatoid arthritis. Persistent inappropriate loading of joints, for example in joggers who run on a camber, may in rare cases also result in osteoarthritis.

Pathological changes

Whether osteoarthritis is primary or secondary, the changes that occur in the joints are similar (Figure 2.15). Initially the articular cartilage softens. Subsequently the surface becomes uneven, and the cartilage 'frays' and develops cracks which may extend down to the bone beneath. Ultimately the cartilage is worn away to reveal the bone which then has

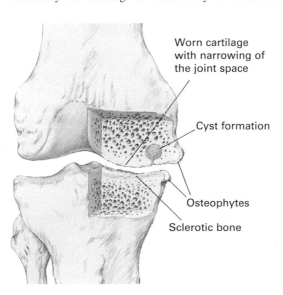

Worn cartilage with narrowing of the joint space

Cyst formation

Osteophytes

Sclerotic bone

Figure 2.15
Changes in osteoarthritic bone (by permission of Prisma Forlag).

to serve as the loadbearing surface of the joint. Simultaneously the bone hardens (sclerosis) and areas of low density (cysts) begin to form. New cartilage cells laid down around the worn cartilage become ossified, and bony projections (osteophytes) are formed as a result of thickening of the joint capsule. The changes are seen most frequently in the hip and knee joints, and less frequently in the ankle, and are clearly visible on X-ray examination carried out with the joint under load.

Symptoms and diagnosis

- *Pain*. Some pain is usually present. Even when it is absent during normal daily activities, it can often be precipitated by increasing the load on the affected joint. Initially pain develops gradually, and in athletes it may disappear during warm-up only to return once training or competition is over. Pain at rest occurs when osteoarthritis has reached an advanced stage and at this point sleep may be disturbed.
- *Joint abnormalities*. A variety of changes may be found around an osteoarthritic joint on clinical examination. They include swelling, impaired range of movement, muscle hypotrophy (loss of mass), tenderness, crepitus, local increased temperature, and instability and/or abnormal joint movements resulting from ligament laxity.
- *Stiffness*. Stiffness typically occurs after a period of inactivity, and a limp may also be present. It is most common in the morning.
- *X-ray changes*. These include narrowing of the joint space, cysts, osteophytes, and sclerosis. There may also be evidence of increased production of synovial fluid.

Treatment

The changes of osteoarthritis cannot be reversed, but a variety of approaches may be adopted to relieve symptoms and to delay further degeneration.
- The load on the affected joint should be reduced. It may be necessary to discontinue pounding and weightbearing sporting activity if a hip or knee is affected, in which case physical fitness can be maintained by cycling or swimming.
- Active mobility and muscle-strengthening exercises should be carried out under the direction of a physical therapist (and possibly in a pool). Passive exercises—those that involve no effort on the part of the patient, whose joints are manipulated—should be avoided.
- Ultrasound, shortwave therapy and hot packs can have a beneficial psychological effect, and a heat retainer may be used.
- A walking-stick, used on the healthy side when one hip or knee is affected, or lightweight shock-absorbing hiking poles, can be used.
- Bandages or braces of various sorts may be used to relieve the load on joints.
- Anti-inflammatory and pain-relieving medication may be prescribed.
- Surgery may be necessary when the degenerative changes are severe.

Osteoarthritis and sport

Athletes who suffer from osteoarthritis should take the advice of their doctors with regard to continuing sporting activities. Each case has to be considered on its own merits. In the early stages there is usually no reason to cease participation in sport, although there may need to be a change in the type of exercise. Cycling and swimming may be recommended rather than running in order to eliminate or at least reduce load on an affected joint. Active mobility and muscle-strengthening exercises should be encouraged to prevent or delay deterioration. Once a damaged hip or knee has been replaced surgically by a prosthetic joint, sporting activity should only be resumed after consultation with the doctor in charge.

Rheumatoid arthritis

Rheumatoid arthritis, which is classified as an autoimmune disease (a disease of the body's own immune system) although its precise cause is not known, is a chronic inflammatory condition which affects joints, tendons, tendon sheaths (fascia), muscles, and bursae, as well as other tissues throughout the body. It is three times more common in women than in men and usually begins in the age ranges 20–30 years or 45–55 years; however, it can begin in childhood.

Pathological changes

The first stage in rheumatoid arthritis is inflammation of the synovial (joint lining) membrane (synovitis) associated with the deposition of protein (fibrin). As a result of the inflammation, fluid is secreted into the joint, causing swelling. The inflammatory tissue grows towards the center of the joint space and coats the articular surfaces and the surrounding ligaments and tendons. At the same time, the articular cartilage is destroyed systematically from its surface inwards to the underlying bone, and cysts form in the adjacent bone. As the inflammatory tissue begins to be replaced by scar tissue, the joint capsule becomes thickened and can consequently impede the mobility of the joint and increase the swelling.

Symptoms and diagnosis

The following symptoms suggest a diagnosis of rheumatoid arthritis:
– pain and swelling of joints;
– joint stiffness which is particularly pronounced in the mornings and after activity;
– joint deformities, muscular hypotrophy, and tendon abnormalities;
– periods of relapse and remission in the course of the condition.

For practical purposes, rheumatoid arthritis is considered to be present if three or four of the following criteria are fulfilled:
1. Morning stiffness.
2. Pain and tenderness in at least one joint.
3. Soft tissue swelling or excessive fluid in at least one joint.
4. When (2) or (3) is present, swelling in at least one other joint.
5. Symmetrical joint swelling.
6. Nodules on tendons at sites typical of rheumatoid arthritis.
7. X-ray changes typical of rheumatoid arthritis.
8. Blood tests showing changes typical of rheumatoid arthritis.

| Treatment | As with osteoarthritis, there is no cure for rheumatoid arthritis. However, its manifestations and progress can temporarily be controlled and symptoms relieved by: |

As with osteoarthritis, there is no cure for rheumatoid arthritis. However, its manifestations and progress can temporarily be controlled and symptoms relieved by:

- physiotherapy and maintenance of general physical fitness;
- anti-inflammatory medication;
- steroid medication;
- current medication to treat the cause of the disease;
- local treatment with steroids or gold in advanced cases;
- surgery, in severe cases.

Rheumatoid arthritis and sport

Rheumatoid arthritis does not have to exclude sport. Physical activities that are known to have a beneficial effect should be encouraged. Above all, athletes with arthritis should indulge in active exercises requiring muscular effort. Hiking, swimming, and crosscountry skiing are beneficial.

Other diseases of the joints

Joint infections

Infection may reach a joint either via the blood circulation (from the urinary tract, respiratory tract, sinuses, mouth and so on), directly through an open wound, or following a surgical procedure. Medical advice is essential if a joint infection is suspected.

Gout

Gout is caused by accumulation of uric acid crystals in joints, and 95% of the victims are middle-aged men. The first metatarsophalangeal joint (at the base of the big toe) is most frequently affected, and during an acute attack—which usually lasts 2–7 days—becomes red, hot, swollen, and exquisitely painful. Chronic gout may affect more than one joint, in which case it may mimic other generalized joint diseases.

Medical examination and advice are recommended for the athlete with gout; treatment may include anti-inflammatory and other medicines, dietary modifications, and rest.

Injuries to muscle

Muscle injuries are among the most common, most misunderstood, and inadequately treated conditions in sports medicine. Their significance is often underestimated because most patients can continue their daily activities soon after injury. According to some studies, muscle injuries account for 10–30% of all injuries in sport. Furthermore, it has been found that 30% of all soccer injuries are muscle injuries.

Muscles can be damaged both by direct trauma (impact) and by indirect trauma (overloading). The resultant injuries can be divided into ruptures and hematomas:

– *ruptures* can be complete or partial, and may be subdivided into strains and compression injuries;
– *hematomas* are the result of the injury and may be either inter- or intramuscular (there are major differences in the treatment and diagnosis of the two types).

Muscle injuries are usually benign but often annoying for the athlete because inadequate treatment can cause long absences from sporting activity. Some knowledge of the normal structure and function of muscles is necessary in order to understand how injuries may best be prevented and treated.

Muscle structure

The human body possesses more than 300 clearly defined muscles, comprising about 40% of the total body weight. Each muscle has an upper origin (head) and a lower insertion, with the bulky part between them (the belly) forming the actively contracting portion. The muscle is attached to bone by tendons. A skeletal muscle is composed of thousands of long, narrow muscle cells or fibers containing contractile elements, and is surrounded by a membrane or sheath. The muscle fibers are bound

Muscle belly   Muscle bundle (fasciculus)   Muscle fiber   Myofibril

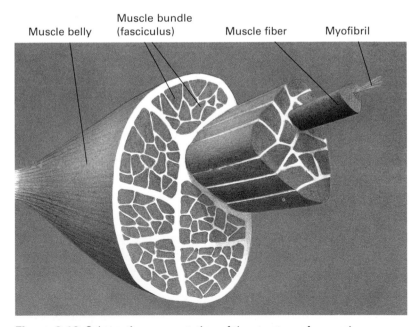

Figure 2.16 Schematic representation of the structure of a muscle.

together in bundles (fasculi), which are combined to form the muscle belly (Figure 2.16). In some muscles, the belly is divided into several parts. Each belly has its own origin or head, a muscle with two heads being known as a biceps, three heads a triceps, and four heads a quadriceps.

There are two basic types of muscle fiber—*slow* (type I or red) and *fast* (type II or white). Slow fibers obtain their energy from glucose derived from glycogen in the presence of oxygen via the blood circulation (aerobically), while fast fibers obtain theirs from glucose stored in muscular glycogen and converted into energy without the use of oxygen (anaerobically). Slow fibers, in comparison with fast fibers, are smaller, have a lower anaerobic glycolytic capacity, and a slower speed of contraction; they are supplied with a greater network of capillaries, have fewer nerves and have a lower level of endurance. The slow fibers respond very well to static and low dynamic exercise, while the fast fibers respond better to dynamic exercise, especially of high intensity. The fast fibers are subdivided into type IIa, characterized by great strength lasting over a long period, and type IIb, having similar strength over a short period. When a muscle is contracted, the different fibers are activated sequentially–type I, followed by type IIa, and finally type IIb. There are considerable variations in the composition of individual muscles. The most usual combination is that of equal numbers of fast and slow fibers, but in an athlete who excels in endurance sports (e.g. marathon running) there will be a preponderance of slow fibers, while in a sprinter there will be more fast fibers. A knowledge of fiber distribution in muscles is important when training for specific sports.

Muscle tissue is invested with an extensive network of small blood vessels (the capillaries) averaging about 3000 per mm^2 on cross-section. When the muscle is at rest, 95% of the capillaries are closed, but when physical activity is undertaken they open progressively to ensure an ample blood flow to the working tissue.

Training can result in the following effects on muscle:
- muscle enzyme levels increase;
- the number of subcellular units in which energy conversion takes place (mitochondria) increases with aerobic training;
- storage of fuel for the production of energy increases;
- the capillary network increases;
- muscular volume increases (hypertrophy) with strength training.

This combination of effects increases muscle strength, stability, stamina, and a capacity for rapid contraction. Various types of muscle training are described on p. 488.

Types of injury to the muscle–tendon complex

Muscles and tendons function together as units. In principle, injuries can affect the muscle origin, the muscle belly, the point at which muscle and tendon merge (the muscle–tendon junction), the tendon itself, and the

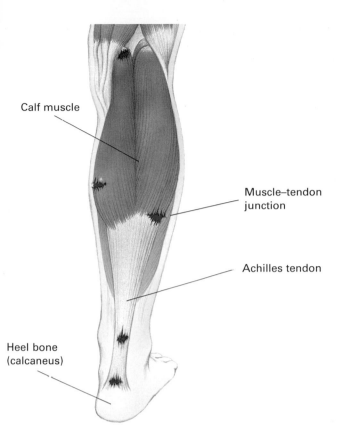

Calf muscle

Muscle–tendon
junction

Achilles tendon

Heel bone
(calcaneus)

Figure 2.17 Locations of injuries in the muscle/tendon complex: the junction of muscle and tendon is the most common.

insertion of the tendon into bone and periosteum. In practice, injuries to the muscles usually occur at the muscle–tendon junction regardless of the strain rate (Figure 2.17). More force and energy absorption occurs before failure in contracting muscles than in nonstimulated muscles, and isometrically preconditioned muscles require greater forces and an increase in length before failure occurs than non-preconditioned muscle. Maintaining strength and a proper warm-up can therefore protect a muscle–tendon unit from injury.

Muscle ruptures

Muscle fibers respond and adapt quickly to change. Damaged muscle can heal quickly with fibers regenerated in about 3 weeks. When injury occurs, however, there is almost inevitably some degree of bleeding, and this can affect the healing process mechanically by reducing contact between the ruptured ends of the muscle fibers. If bleeding can be controlled, healing is more likely to be quick and complete.

Sporting activities can cause a number of different types of muscle rupture.

1. *Strains.* These are caused by overstretching or eccentric overload, and are located in the muscle–tendon junction. These ruptures occur as a result of the intrinsic force generated in the athlete's muscles, often in the change between eccentric and concentric traction.

2. *Contusions*. These occur as a result of direct impact (trauma). The muscle is pressed against the underlying bone, e.g. when a player's knee hits another's thigh during a soccer game. A muscle tear and heavy bleeding deep within the muscle may result.

A distinction should be made between *complete* ruptures, in which all the muscle fibers are torn and function is lost, and *partial* ruptures, which involve only some fibers, with preserved continuity and some function. A number of factors contribute towards the occurrence of muscle ruptures:
– the muscle may have been poorly prepared because of inadequate training or lack of warm-up;
– the muscle may have been weakened by previous injury followed by inadequate rehabilitation;
– the muscle may previously have been extensively injured with resultant scar tissue formation (scar tissue is less elastic than muscle and therefore more susceptible to recurrent injury);
– a muscle that is overstrained or fatigued is injured more easily;
– tense muscles that do not allow a full range of joint movement may be injured in sports demanding flexibility;
– muscles subjected to prolonged exposure to cold are less contractile than normal.

Strains

Strains frequently occur in sports that require explosive muscular effort over a short period of time, for example in baseball, sprinting, jumping, American football, and soccer (Figure 2.18). When the demand made upon a muscle exceeds its innate strength, rupture may occur; for example, in overload during eccentric muscle traction. Other examples in sport include sudden stopping, deceleration (eccentric work), rapid

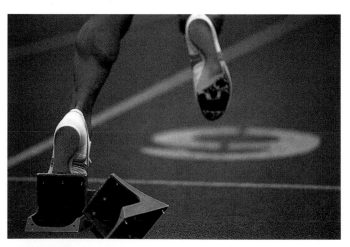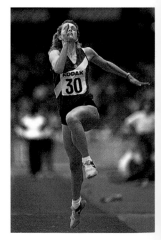

Figure 2.18 An explosive effort is required in (**left**) sprinting and (**right**) jumping (by courtesy of All Sport: photographers, Todd Warshaw and Dan Smith.)

acceleration (concentric work) or a dangerous combination of deceleration and acceleration when turning, cutting, jumping and so on.

Strains often occur in muscles that move two joints, for example, the hamstring muscles which flex the knee and extend the hip joint. These muscles cannot perform the two functions at the same time during running, so they are strictly governed by a sensitive neuromuscular system. Failure of this system will potentiate injuries. Other examples of muscles susceptible to distraction ruptures are the quadriceps muscle in the front of the thigh, the gastrocnemius muscle in the calf, and the biceps muscle in the upper arm.

Strains can be classified by the degree of rupture: first- and second-degree strains are partial ruptures, and third-degree strains are complete ruptures or disruptions.

– A *first-degree* or *mild strain* describes an overstretching of the muscle with a rupture of less than 5% of the muscle fibers. There is no great loss of strength or restriction of movement. Active movement or passive stretching will, however, cause pain around the area of damage and there will be some discomfort. It should be remembered that a small rupture or mild strain can be just as distressing to the athlete as a more serious injury.

– A *second-degree* or *moderate strain* involves a more significant but less than complete tear of the muscle. The pain will be aggravated by any attempt to contract the muscle.

– A *third-degree* or *severe strain* involves complete disruption of the muscle.

Symptoms and diagnosis

The following features suggest that a strain has occurred.

– A sharp or stabbing pain is felt at the moment of injury and reproduced by contracting the muscle concerned. Usually there is little pain if the muscle is rested.

– In a partial rupture the resulting pain can inhibit muscle contraction. In complete ruptures, the muscles are unable to contract for mechanical reasons.

– In partial ruptures it is sometimes possible to feel a defect in part of the muscle on examination. In a completely ruptured muscle the defect can be felt across the entire muscle belly. The muscle may 'bunch up' and form a lump resembling a tumor.

– There is often localized tenderness and swelling over the damaged area.

– After about 24 hours, bruising and discoloration may be seen, often below the site of injury; these are signs of bleeding within the damaged muscle. Muscle spasm may occur.

Clinical examination by local inspection and palpation is initially carried out to analyze the degree of trauma. The most effective diagnostic test is often a test of function, with or without resistance.

Healing

When a muscle is overstretched, the muscle fibers and blood vessels will tear. The torn ends will retract from the injured area, leaving it filled with blood. Initially there will be inflammation and thereafter resorption of the bleeding. The repair of a muscle injury involves two 'competitive' events: *formation of new muscle fibers* (regeneration) and the simultaneous *production of scar tissue* (granulation tissue).

Skeletal muscle has a great capacity to regenerate but the new muscle fibers will be shorter and incorporate inelastic scar tissue. If the scar covers a large area, function will be impaired because contraction is restricted. Areas of different elasticity may be formed in the muscle which increase the risk of recurrence of rupture. It is therefore important to follow a muscle injury with a long-lasting rehabilitation program.

Contusion ruptures

When direct impact is the cause of injury, deep rupture and bleeding can occur as the contracted muscle is compressed against the underlying bone. Contusion ruptures can also occur in superficial muscles, in which case the symptoms are similar to those caused by strains (see above).

Muscular hematoma

During physical activity there is a substantial redistribution of blood flow. In the muscles, it increases from about 0.8 litres per minute (1.7 US pints/min) (15% of cardiac output) at rest to at least 18 l/min (38 pt/min) (72% of cardiac output) during strenuous effort. It follows that the blood supply to the muscles during sporting activity is enormous; the extent of bleeding when the muscle is damaged is directly proportional to muscle blood flow and inversely proportional to muscle tension at the time of injury. The effect of an injury depends upon its location and extent rather than upon its cause, and in the following paragraphs no distinction is made between contusion and distraction ruptures. Treatment, healing, and rehabilitation also vary according to the type, location, and extent of hemorrhage and ruptured tissue.

Intramuscular hematoma

Bleeding within a muscle may be caused by rupture or impact (Figure 2.19). It begins within the muscle sheath (fascia) and causes an increase in intramuscular pressure which counteracts any tendency to further bleeding by compressing the blood vessels. The resultant swelling persists beyond the first 48 hours and is accompanied by tenderness, pain, and impaired mobility. Swelling may increase as the bleeding draws fluid from the surrounding tissue (osmosis), and muscle function may be completely absent. If the muscle sheath is damaged, blood may spread into the space between the muscles (see below) or out into the surrounding tissues. Intramuscular hematomas may create an acute compartment syndrome (p. 336) due to increased intracompartmental pressure, but this is rare.

Intermuscular hematoma

Bleeding may occur between muscles when a muscle fascia and its adjacent blood vessels are damaged. After an initial increase, causing the bleeding to spread, the pressure falls quickly. Typically, bruising and swelling, caused by a collection of blood, appear distally to the damaged area 24–48 hours after the injury, due to gravity. Because there is no sustained increase in pressure, the swelling is temporary and muscle function returns rapidly. Provided immediate treatment is available, recovery can be expected to be speedy and complete.

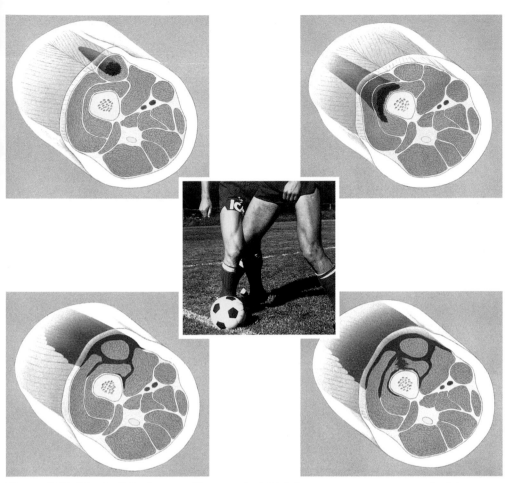

Figure 2.19 (**Center**) The impact of knee against thigh in soccer can cause muscular injury. (**Top left**) Example of a superficial intramuscular hematoma. (**Top right**) Example of a deep intramuscular hematoma. (**Bottom left**) Example of an intermuscular hematoma. (**Bottom right**) Example of a deep intramuscular hematoma with an intermuscular spread.

Treatment of acute injury	The *athlete* or *trainer* should stop or control muscle bleeding in the acute phase irrespective of its cause, by use of the following measures:

- encouraging rest;
- bandaging the injured part—compression is the most effective way to limit bleeding;
- cooling the affected area to limit pain;
- elevating the limb;
- relieving load on the limb. If the injury affects the leg, crutches should be used until a definite diagnosis has been made. When an arm is involved, splinting may help during the acute phase.

The body's defense against bleeding (coagulation or clotting) comes into action as soon as the injury occurs and continues to function for several hours. The repair mechanism, however, is unstable during the first 24–36 hours, so that further bleeding may occur as a result of another impact, vigorous muscular contraction or unprotected weightbearing.

Massage–which can cause repeated minor trauma to the site of injury–should not be used within 48–72 hours of a muscular injury.

If there is any suspicion of a major muscle rupture or significant bleeding, a doctor should be consulted as soon as possible.

The *doctor's* action will depend upon the extent of the injury. If the injury is severe, admission to hospital for observation may be indicated as the bleeding and swelling may increase, impairing the blood supply and raising the intramuscular pressure; this can be dangerous if left unmonitored. If the bleeding is not extensive, or if there is any uncertainty about the nature or extent of the injury, 48–72 hours' rest may be prescribed. Precise diagnosis can be difficult in the acute phase and for the first 2–3 days an injury should be considered as potentially serious.

Early and repeated examinations of the injured area are necessary in order to distinguish between intermuscular and intramuscular bleeding. Decreasing swelling and rapid recovery of function suggest the former, and persistent or increasing swelling with poor function the latter.

After 48–72 hours the following questions should be answered:
1. Has the swelling resolved? If not, intramuscular hematoma is probably present.
2. Has the bleeding spread and caused bruising at some distance from the injury? If not, hematoma is probably intramuscular.
3. Has the contractile ability of the injured muscle returned or improved? If not, the injury probably involves an intramuscular hematoma.
4. Is the hematoma a symptom of a total or partial muscle rupture?

It is important that an accurate diagnosis be made, because premature exercise of a muscle affected by extensive intramuscular hematoma or a complete rupture can cause complications in the form of further bleeding and sometimes increased scar tissue formation. This in turn is likely to lead to a more protracted healing process and possibly even permanent disability. Treatment beyond the first 72 hours depends upon the diagnosis.

Treatment after 72 hours

After initial acute treatment, minor partial ruptures, intermuscular hematomas and minor intramuscular hematomas should be managed by the following measures:
– support with an elastic bandage;
– local application of heat; contrast treatment using heat and cold may sometimes be of value.

For an optimal result, muscle exercises should commence after 2–5 days of rest, depending on the character of the injury.

Exercises should adhere to specific principles (see Chapters 20 and 21) and be carried out in the following order:

1. Static exercises without load.
2. Static exercises with light load.
3. Limited dynamic muscle training with exercises within the active range of motion to the pain threshold.
4. Dynamic exercises with increasing load. Ice treatment can be applied after the exercise program to limit pain and swelling.
5. Stretching exercises to improve range of movement. It is important not to neglect exercising the muscles that act in the opposite direction (antagonists) to the one that has been injured.
6. Functional and proprioceptive training.
7. Gradually increasing activity and load to the injured muscle. If a lower limb is affected, it may be advisable to replace running by cycling and swimming and other types of water training.
8. Sport-specific training.

If the symptoms caused by the injured muscle are serious initially or fail to improve, it is important to exclude intramuscular hematoma and tissue damage. To elucidate the situation, the *doctor* may take one or more of the following steps:

– carry out a further local examination;
– measure intramuscular (intracompartmental) pressure;
– puncture and aspirate the injured area with a needle if fluctuation is present;
– carry out an ultrasound or MRI examination; ultrasound examination is the most accurate way to evaluate a muscle injury and to follow healing;
– undertake surgery.

When the diagnosis is established, there are a number of options:

– an elastic support bandage, a program of muscle exercises as outlined above, and anti-inflammatory medication;
– surgery may be considered in cases of extensive bleeding, especially when it is intramuscular and involves complete or partial rupture affecting more than half the muscle belly. It is particularly important when the damaged muscle is unique in the function it performs or is without agonists (muscles with similar function), e.g. pectoralis major. The aim of surgery is to remove any intervening blood clots and repair the torn muscle fibers by suturing them together; this procedure minimizes scar tissue formation. A period of immobilization in a brace is usually necessary after muscle surgery.

Rehabilitation

Rehabilitation after surgery is planned jointly by the athlete and the treating team, taking into consideration the location and severity of the injury. When rehabilitation is started early, healing is more rapid, with restoration of circulation and improvement in strength. The athlete can begin static muscle exercises and motion with the doctor's agreement, soon after the operation, and later progress to dynamic strength and flexibility training.

Return to sporting activity

A muscle injury can be considered completely healed when there is no pain or tenderness on full contraction of the muscle. Once complete muscle function, full flexibility in adjacent joints, and a normal pattern of movement are regained, a full training program can be resumed.

The time taken for a complete muscle rupture to heal is 3–16 weeks, depending on the location and extent of the injury. In cases of intramuscular hematoma, in which tissue damage is often a feature, the healing time may be 2–8 weeks or even longer, whereas sporting activity can often be resumed only 1–2 weeks after an intermuscular hematoma. Conditioning exercises and gradually progressive muscle exercise against resistance should take priority over explosive training exercises when sporting activity is resumed.

The athlete who has sustained a muscle injury should not participate in competition until no pain is experienced during strenuous training.

Complications of muscle injury

Scar tissue formation

Muscle fibers that have been overloaded with resultant bleeding and rupture become less contractile. The space between ruptured muscle fiber ends fills with blood which clots and is gradually replaced by connective tissue. The formation of scar tissue may leave the muscle with areas of varying elasticity; further injury (rupture or hematoma) may then occur if the muscle is exercised too hard, too soon. If scar tissue causes persistent problems it may be necessary to remove it surgically (Figure 2.20); this, however, is not common.

Traumatic myositis ossificans ('charley horse', heterotopic bone formation)

If immediate treatment is inadequate, a deeply located intramuscular hematoma may gradually become calcified and ossified. Ossification continues as long as healing is disrupted by repeated impact or contraction. This will result in areas of varying strength and elasticity in the affected muscle, and an increased risk of further injury. Ossification is a lengthy inflammatory process for which doctors hesitate to recommend active treatment for a long period. If muscle function and flexibility are significantly impaired for more than 6–10 weeks and X-rays reveal ossification, then surgical removal of the ossification should be considered. Return to sport is possible after 8–10 weeks.

Misdiagnosis of tumor

Complete muscle ruptures can sometimes be misinterpreted and diagnosed as tumors during their later stages. A mass may be found which increases gradually in size. A thorough clinical examination is essential if the correct diagnosis is to be made.

The following sequence of events is typical. The adductor longus muscle is located on the inner (medial) side of the thigh and its function is to draw the leg inwards (adduction); it originates in the pubic bone and is inserted into the femur. Partial rupture usually affects its origin

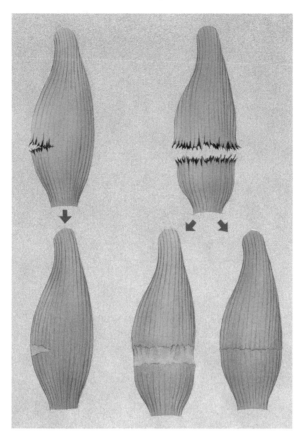

Figure 2.20 Partial and total muscle ruptures and healing results. **(Top left)** Partial muscle rupture. **(Top right)** Total muscle rupture. **(Lower left)** Healed partial muscle rupture which has not been operated on. **(Above middle)** Scar tissue of healed total muscle rupture which has not been operated on. **(Lower right)** Healing of total muscle rupture which has been operated on; the hematoma is removed and the torn muscle ends are sutured together.

and complete rupture its insertion. The latter may occur without pain and without causing any major problems. Gradually, however, an enlarging lump in the thigh becomes more noticeable. It may be mistaken for a tumor, but in fact is caused by an increase in muscle bulk. The original muscle, having shortened following rupture, is forced to work over a shorter distance, and therefore harder than previously, when a new insertion is formed by scar tissue (p. 238). The diagnosis of 'old total rupture of adductor longus' is not difficult to make, provided examination takes place with the muscle in both the relaxed and the contracted states.

Myositis

Myositis or muscle inflammation is rare; it mainly affects the muscles of the thigh, back, shoulder, and calf.

Symptoms and diagnosis

The following may suggest a diagnosis of myositis:
- pain in the affected muscle group on exertion;
- symptoms increasing as effort becomes more intensive and repetitive;
- tender, firm areas felt on examination of the muscle;
- muscle cramp.

Treatment

When myositis occurs, the *athlete* should:
- use anti-inflammatory medication;
- rest the muscle in question or reduce training;
- apply local heat and use a heat retainer.

Muscle cramp

Muscle cramp affects most people at some time in their lives. Athletes may suffer cramp in a muscle during or after strenuous exertion such as a soccer match or a long-distance race. Tennis players competing in very hot conditions frequently suffer from cramp.

Causes

- During protracted exercise, especially when the weather is very hot, vast amounts of fluid can be lost from the body. This dehydration predisposes the muscle to cramp, though the exact connection is not known: glycogen depletion and salt deficiency may contribute.
- The type of cramp that affects soccer players towards the end of a match is probably caused by changes in the musculature resulting from earlier muscular bleeding, small muscle ruptures, or the athlete's general state of health or training.
- The precise causes of muscle cramp are not clear, but any factors that impair the circulation should be considered. These include close-fitting socks, shoes laced too tightly, an accumulation of lactic acid in the muscles, varicose veins, cold weather, and infections.

Prevention and treatment

The *athlete* should:
- prevent muscular cramp by good basic training and warm-up exercises and by using the correct equipment;
- ensure adequate nutrition and intake of fluid, electrolyte reserves, and full glycogen deposits (lost fluid and electrolytes must be replaced, especially in a hot climate);
- stop the sporting activity when acute cramp occurs and contract the muscle that exerts an effect opposite to the one affected by cramp. For example, if cramp in the calf muscle draws the foot downwards, the foot should be raised carefully, with the knee bent, until it is at right angles to the leg. The movement should not be forced and the affected muscle should be massaged (Figure 2.21).

An athlete who suffers persistent cramps, despite preventive measures, would be wise to seek a medical examination to exclude any specific problems.

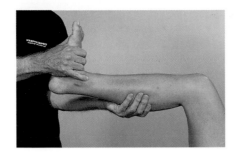

Figure 2.21 To cure cramp in the calf muscle, raise the foot at right angles to the leg with the knee bent and massage the muscle.

Muscle soreness after training

Soreness, with pain, tenderness, and sometimes swelling of the muscles, can appear a few hours after strenuous training. The pain occurs during both active exercise and passive movements, and the muscles may feel weak. Many athletes experience the problem in late autumn (fall) and early spring when they change surfaces and either do not adjust their shoes to the new surface or start training too energetically. The symptoms appear mainly during the kind of exercise in which muscles lengthen and contract simultaneously (eccentric action or negative work).

In untrained individuals who are suddenly subjected to strenuous exertion, muscle changes in the form of tissue damage to the small elements of the muscle fiber have been seen within 2–7 days. These ruptures have been connected with stiffness after training, and disappear after the musculature has been allowed to rest. The fiber elements contain no sensory bodies and do not in themselves cause any pain; when they are ruptured, however, the muscle cell wall is also damaged and there may be ruptures of the muscle capillaries. These alterations cause pressure increases and impaired blood flow; swelling may occur, which is sensed as stiffness and pain. The condition is not dangerous and usually disappears after a few days.

Preventive measures and treatment

The following measures help to minimize the problem.
- The training program should be adjusted according to the level of training achieved and the surface used. Appropriate equipment is important.
- If a minor degree of soreness is felt, training can be continued but should be modified. The intensity of training should always be increased gradually, especially during the initial stages.
- Gentle movements and warm surroundings help to ease the pain.

Bibliography
Garrett W (1990) Muscle strain injuries. *Medicine and Science in Sports and Exercise* 22:436–438.
Järvinen M, Vadimo M (1996) Muscle injuries in sport. In Järvinen H, ed. *Balliere's Clinical Orthopedics: Soft Tissue Injuries in Sport.* London: Balliere Tindall.

Tendon injuries

Tendon injuries constitute a frequent diagnostic and therapeutic problem in sports medicine. If these injuries are not treated well, they result in chronic and long-lasting problems. The basis for successful management is a correct diagnosis.

A muscle is usually attached to bone by a tendon through which the effects of muscle contraction are conveyed. The main function of a tendon is to transfer forces from the muscle to the bone. The muscle produces force only when contracting, and this has a stretching effect on the tendon. Tendons display great anatomic diversity, with variations in shape, length, vascularity, and the extent of synovial lining. There is also variability in biochemical and biomechanical characteristics.

Tendons regularly used in sport are usually very strong. Peak force in the Achilles tendon has been estimated in running to be nearly 9000 N (1 ton-force) or 12.5 times bodyweight. The rate of force application may, however, be more important than the magnitude of the force as a cause of tissue damage. Tendons withstand tensile forces well, but resist shearing forces less effectively, and provide little resistance to compressive forces. Tendons are composed of collagen, which provides great mechanical strength, and elastin, which provides elasticity.

In the normal resting state, a tendon has a wavy configuration, but if it is strained (elongated) by more than 2%, the wavy pattern disappears and the collagen fibers are subjected to stress. At 4–8% strain, the crosslinks joining the collagen molecules together will start to break as the fibers slide past one another. At 8–10% strain, the tendon will begin to fail and the weakest fibers will rupture (Figure 2.22).

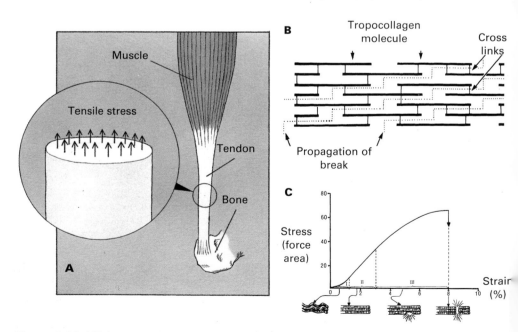

Figure 2.22 (**A**) An example of tensile stress in a tendon. (**B**) Collagen structure of tendon. (**C**) Stress–strain curve.

Tendons are most vulnerable to injury when:
1. Tension is applied quickly and sustained without adequate warm-up.
2. Tension is applied obliquely.
3. The tendon is tensed before the trauma.
4. The attached muscle is maximally innervated and contacted.
5. The muscle group is stretched by external forces.
6. The tendon is weak in comparison to the muscle.

All these factors can apply to athletes of all ages.

Tendon injuries are common in sports because force is focused on the tendon as a part of the muscle unit, thereby increasing the risk of injury. Tendon tissue readily undergoes adaptation to the conditions imposed upon it. A tendon can be subjected to overload (which includes a rapid increase in resistance) or overuse (which is a repetitive motion without increase in resistance). An injury to a tendon represents a failure of the cell matrix (surrounding supportive tissue) to adapt to the load exposure, whether it is a sudden overload or a cumulative overload secondary to cyclic overuse (see Figure 2.22).

Classification of tendon injuries

'Tendinitis' has been the clinical term traditionally applied to virtually all painful tendon structures, including the tendon, the synovial sheath, and the adjacent bursa. It has, however, been established that there is only a limited inflammatory response in the tendon to injury. Injuries are most often associated with a degenerative process, which increases with age as the tendons begin to lose their elasticity. Fatigue ruptures of tendon fibers are probably a contributory cause to tendon problems and may precede degeneration and tendinosis, especially in young athletes.

Degeneration is characterized by disruption of the tendon fibrils, collagen (the protein of which the tendon is built) in the fibril splitting and fragmentation, and loss of collagen orientation. The cell metabolism is altered, and there is a formation of different collagens and proteoglycans, proliferation of capillaries, and minimal inflammatory cell infiltration. Degeneration will result in microtears and disruption of the tissue. The end result is cell hypotrophy (the cells decrease in size).

Contributory causes of tendon degeneration are inadequate oxygen supply, decreased nutrition, hormonal change, chronic inflammation, and aging. The degenerative process is secondary to tensile overuse, fatigue, weakness, and possibly vascular changes. Most spontaneous ruptures of tendons (97%) are preceded by pathologic changes in the tendon.

Injuries to tendons that are associated with degeneration and not inflammation are often located in areas of poor circulation. Achilles tendon injuries, for example, may be located 2–5 cm (1–2 in) proximal to the tendon's attachment to the calcaneus where there is decreased vascularity. Injury to the supraspinatus tendon may occur 1–2 cm (0.5–1 in) from its attachment to the humerus, where blood supply is also poor. Owing to this poor circulation there is also little inflammatory response and repair capacity.

Based on the anatomy of the tendon, it is possible to describe four pathologic conditions. This classification emphasizes the distinction between peritenon, or synovial inflammation, and increasing involvement of the tendon substance as a likely reflection of the failure to adapt to physical load, and emphasizes the variable stress responses in the tendon structure. These categories are:

1. Peritenonitis (paratenonitis, tenosynovitis): inflammation of only the peritenon.
2. Peritenonitis with tendinosis: tendon sheath inflammation associated with intratendinous degeneration.
3. Tendinosis: degeneration in the tendon itself due to cellular hypotrophy.
4. Tendinitis: asymptomatic degeneration (defined above) of the tendon with disruption and inflammatory repair response.

A commonly proposed name for tendon pain problems is *tendinopathy*.

Etiology of tendon injury

Training errors, such as sudden increase in running distance or a change in activity, are the primary etiological factor in most tendon overuse injuries. Errors include increased frequency of training and running on curved trails, hard or slippery roads, or soft beaches. The principle of transition (according to Leadbetter 1992) is that sports injuries are most likely to occur when the athlete experiences any change in mode or use of the involved part. Transition risk is rate-dependent. Examples of transition risk are attempts to increase performance level, improper training, changes in equipment, environmental changes such as new surfaces and different training altitudes, alterations in frequency and intensity or endurance of training, attempts to master new techniques, body growth, and post-injury and post-training recovery.

Changes of lower leg alignment may also cause tendon problems. Excessive foot pronation may result in increased local strain (elongation) on the medial side of the Achilles tendon and increases the risk of overuse injury. Increased pronation also increases the risk of posterior tibial tendon injuries (p. 387).

Diagnostic principles

Acceptable results are most likely to be achieved by correct treatment based upon an accurate diagnosis; this requires a careful history and a thorough clinical examination.

With the development of magnetic resonance imaging (MRI), the evaluation of tendon injuries has improved dramatically. This imaging technique not only gives a correct diagnosis, but also permits assessment of the extent and size of an injury. It provides excellent soft tissue contrast in multiple planes, and permits a detailed assessment of intrinsic abnormalities of ankle joint tendons; it can depict tendinosis, and provides a detailed evaluation of tendon continuation (Figure 2.23). However, MRI is expensive.

Ultrasound is increasingly used (especially in Europe) to evaluate tendon injuries, as it is functional—it can be used during dynamic activities—inexpensive, and can be used to follow the healing process. This technique is valuable, but it depends on a skilled and experienced examiner, and does not show the full extent of the pathological changes

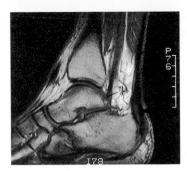

Figure 2.23 MRI of Achilles tendon. Tendinosis is indicated by the arrow.

Treatment principles

The management of tendon injuries depends on the diagnosis. The treatment varies according to the different stages of the healing process.

Tendon strength is a direct function not only of the number and size of collagen fibers, but also of their orientation. These fibers respond favorably to tension and motion and it is therefore important to stimulate protective motion of a tendon as early as possible. Early mobilization should therefore be initiated; it may be limited by protective bracing to decrease tensile loading on the tendon. Motion should start within two weeks of the injury.

Exercises

The pain level is often the guide for the exercise program, and dictates the degree of function in chronic tendon injuries. Pain differs depending on whether it is caused by inflammation or degeneration. Pain can be classified in terms of athletic performance (see Table 2.1).

A period of vulnerability to re-injury exists. In chronic injury it is the history of pain that allows the proper recommendation and adjustment of activity. If an exercise program is carried out correctly, the pain threshold may be reached and surpassed during the last set of 10 repetitions; if there is no pain, the athlete is not working hard enough. As the tendon strengthens, the pain should diminish.

Isometric and concentric exercises have a place in the rehabilitation program, but it is mainly through eccentric exercise that it is possible to have a clear effect on a chronic tendon condition (Figure 2.24). Eccentric exercises can enhance the efficacy of treatment of overuse tendon injuries and stimulate healing (although more research is needed to verify this), and they seem to be effective in the treatment of chronic tendon disorders so that surgery often can be avoided.

The following program was designed to strengthen the tendons to withstand the greater stresses caused by eccentric loading:
1. Stretch—hold stretch statically for 15–30 seconds, and repeat 3–5 times.
2. Eccentric exercise—progress from slow on days 1 and 2, to moderate on days 3–5, and fast on days 6 and 7. Then increase external resistance and repeat the cycle.
3. Stretch statically.
4. Use ice for 5–10 minutes to reduce swelling and moderate pain.

Table 2.1 Classification system for the effect of pain on athletic performance

Level	Description of pain	Sports performance
1	No pain	Normal
2	Pain only with extreme exertion	Normal
3	Pain with extreme exertion and for 1–2 hours afterwards	Normal or slightly decreased
4	Pain during and after vigorous activities	Somewhat decreased
5	Pain during activity severe enough to force termination	Markedly decreased
6	Pain during daily activities	Unable to perform

From Curwin S, Stanish WD (1984) *Tendinitis: Its Etiology and Treatment*, p. 64, Lexington: Health, with permission

Figure 2.24
(**Left**) Concentric contraction; (**Right**) Eccentric action.

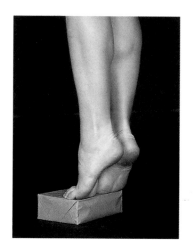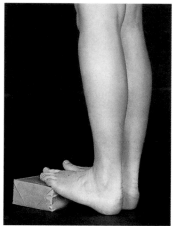

Stretching

Stretching is used extensively and probably has a major role in the treatment of overuse injuries (Figure 2.25). The theoretical basis for stretching is well defined, but the epidemiological and scientific evidence to support it is somewhat scanty. Studies of the biomechanical effects of stretching show that it will result in greater flexibility and increased strength of the muscle–tendon unit. There is, however, a concern as to what stretching techniques or procedures should be used for optimal gains in flexibility. Experimental evaluation of stretching techniques shows that the 'contract, relax, and antagonist contract' method is generally better than 'contract, relax' or 'hold relax' techniques, but the difference is small.

Appropriate exercise promotes healing of tendon injuries.

Figure 2.25
Stretching the
Achilles tendon.

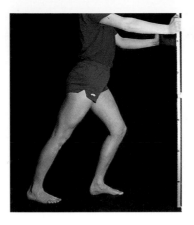 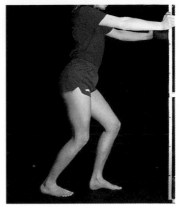

Surgery

The indication for surgery is often persistence of pain and loss of athletic performance. The rationale for surgical treatment of tendon injury is to reactivate the wound repair cycle or remove pathologic tissue. A surgical incision is the most powerful stimulus to local tissue to release the biologic cell mediators of repair. The result is not a regenerated, but a remodeled tendon. There is a lack of scientific evidence about when and how to perform surgery on overuse tendon injuries. The primary reason for operative treatment is still its apparent success in many well-documented cases, and the frequent failure of conservative treatment.

Summary

Treatment of athletes with chronic tendon injuries requires long experience and also cooperation with the physical therapist. Successful treatment of tendon injuries depends on the correct diagnosis. The cause of the injury should be treated. Correction of training errors is often the key to a successful treatment program. Orthotic correction of malalignments is often helpful. Shoes with posterior support in patients with ankle tendon problems may be helpful. Overuse tendon injuries must be carefully managed.

Chronic tendon injuries remain one of the biggest challenges in orthopedic sports medicine.

Complete tendon rupture

Complete tendon rupture (third-degree strain) often occurs in a degenerative tendon and is especially common in older athletes who return to sport after some years' absence from training. These ruptures afflict badminton players in particular, and also participants in tennis, team handball, basketball, rugby, American football, and soccer, as well as long-jumpers, high-jumpers, and runners.

Symptoms and diagnosis	Complete tendon rupture may become apparent as follows.

Symptoms and diagnosis

Complete tendon rupture may become apparent as follows.
- The athlete may be aware of a sudden 'snap' followed by intense pain when the injury occurs.
- The injured athlete is unable to perform movements that require integrity of the affected tendon and its attached muscle.
- A defect, associated with pronounced tenderness, may be felt in the tendon.
- Swelling and bruising, indicating bleeding, occur soon after the injury.
- A thorough clinical examination will confirm the diagnosis.

Location

The tendons most frequently affected by complete rupture are the Achilles, supraspinatus, biceps, quadriceps and patellar tendons.

Treatment

The *athlete* or *trainer* should give immediate treatment according to the guidelines given in Chapter 5.

The *doctor* has a choice of treatment methods depending on the injury location.
- Nonoperative treatment is sometimes tried in recreational and elderly athletes. Complete tears of biceps tendons of the upper arm are, for example, often treated conservatively. There are also reports of successful nonoperative treatment of complete Achilles tendon tears in such patients. Conservative treatment includes functional training, but sometimes immobilization is necessary, e.g. in complete Achilles tendon tears. Mobilization, however, in principle should begin as early as possible.
- Surgery is often recommended as it allows early tension and early mobilization of the tendon. This allows the collagen to become correctly oriented, thereby securing good recovery of strength. The treatment, however, varies from injury to injury.

Partial tendon rupture

In partial tendon rupture (first- and second-degree strains), the tendon is only partly torn. Depending on the extent of the injury, the affected athlete may not always be aware that a rupture has occurred, but believes the tendon to be overused and inflamed. Partial ruptures can be divided into acute and chronic injuries.

Symptoms and diagnosis

Acute partial tendon rupture may become apparent as follows:
- A history of a sudden onset of pain often in combination with a specific event or movement.
- Pain occurs in the injured area on further activity and when movements in adjacent joints are made against resistance.
- A localized distinct tenderness is present in the injured area.
- Swelling, and sometimes a hematoma, may occur.
- A small, tender defect can be felt in the tendon soon after the injury

Chronic partial tendon rupture may become apparent as follows:
- A history of sudden pain is common but often no trauma can be remembered.

- Pain may be experienced during warm-up but may then disappear, only to reappear with greater intensity later.
- Pain may be elicited in the injured area by moving the adjacent joints against resistance.
- A localized distinct tenderness may be present.
- Some swelling may be seen.
- An MRI or an ultrasound examination will show the location and extent of the injury (see Figure 2.23).

Location

The tendon most frequently affected by both acute and chronic partial rupture is the Achilles tendon; the injury may also occur in the patellar tendon, rotator cuff tendons, and the adductor longus tendon.

Treatment

The *athlete* or *trainer* should give immediate treatment to an acute partial tendon rupture as follows:
- treat with ice, compression bandage, rest, and elevation; sometimes crutches can be of value;
- consult a doctor to confirm the diagnosis and thereafter decide upon further treatment.

The *doctor* may:
- apply a plaster cast, a walking boot, or supportive bandage, especially during the acute phase;
- prescribe an exercise program of gradually increasing intensity;
- prescribe anti-inflammatory medication.

If an acute partial tendon rupture is inappropriately treated, inflammatory tissue will form in the injured area and heal only with difficulty. If the healing is prolonged, chronic inflammation may result, giving the same symptoms as chronic tendinitis. It is, therefore, essential that these injuries are treated correctly from the start. When neglected, they can be among the most difficult of all sports injuries to treat.

In cases of chronic rupture (tendinosis) the *athlete* or *trainer* should:
- try an exercise program including a combination of stretching and eccentric exercises;
- try physical treatment methods;
- use a supportive bandage, tape, or brace to unload the injured area;
- use a heat retainer.

The *doctor* may:
- prescribe anti-inflammatory medication;
- operate if the symptoms are prolonged and incapacitating.

Even small partial ruptures should be treated with great concern and respect, otherwise they will heal with scar and granulation tissue. These can cause further problems and lead to a chronic condition which is often very difficult to treat.

The need for surgery seems to increase with the duration of symptoms from the tendon. If a patient has had an Achilles tendon injury for more than 22 months, there is a 38% chance of operative treatment. About 10–20% of athletes with Achilles tendon overuse injuries are operated on sooner or later, and about 70–80% of these athletes make a successful comeback. It takes, however, 6–8 months to full recovery. Repeat surgery is required by 10–20%, and 3–5% are forced to abandon their athletic career.

Peritenonitis (peritendinitis)

Repetitive one-sided movements or persistent mechanical irritation may cause an inflammatory reaction in the tendon sheath, and a minor inflammatory reaction in the tendon itself. The condition frequently becomes chronic and can be difficult to treat.

Location

The Achilles tendon peritenon is mostly affected, along with the sheath and the tendons of the long head of the biceps, the supraspinatus tendon, and the extensor tendons of the wrist and ankle.

Symptoms and diagnosis

- In the acute phase, pain and occasionally crepitus are felt in the affected tendon during and after exercise.
- In chronic conditions, initial pain will often disappear during warm-up.
- There may be diffuse, nonfocal swelling and tenderness.
- Function is impaired.
- Soft tissue X-rays show swelling and sometimes calcification of the affected tissues.

Treatment

When peritendonitis develops the *athlete* or *trainer* should:
- cool the injured area during the acute phase;
- rest the affected part actively until the pain resolves;
- apply local heat and use a heat retainer;
- consult a doctor if the problem persists despite these measures.

The *doctor* has the following treatment options:
- an exercise program which should start as soon as healing permits. In the initial phase, isometric exercises, without load, should be carried out; thereafter, dynamic exercises can begin and should include eccentric exercises, combined with careful stretching. At no time should these exercises exceed the pain threshold;
- supportive strapping and taping;
- anti-inflammatory medication;
- high-voltage galvanic stimulation;
- ultrasound or shortwave therapy;
- surgery.

Insertionitis (tenoperiostitis)

Attachment of a muscle to bone involves a gradual transition from muscle–tendon to cartilage and from mineralized cartilage to bone. Bone–tendon junctions are poorly supplied with blood because the fibro-cartilage creates a 'barrier'; this may explain why these injuries often take a long time to heal and may become chronic.

Inflammation of the muscle–tendon attachment to bone (insertionitis or tenoperiostitis) is caused by repeated strain on the attachment and periosteum. The resultant minor ruptures and bleeding cause irritation and inflammation. Growing individuals rarely suffer from insertionitis because their tendons and muscles are relatively stronger than bone. Instead, they sustain inflammation and fragmentation of bone, for example Osgood–Schlatter disease in the knee and calcaneal apophysitis.

Location

Insertionitis occurs most frequently in the elbow area ('tennis elbow', 'golfer's elbow'), in the groin at the attachment of the adductor longus muscle, in the knee at the proximal and distal attachments of the patellar tendon, in the heel at the Achilles tendon insertion into the calcaneus, and in the attachment of the plantar fascia into the calcaneus (plantar fasciitis).

Symptoms and diagnosis

Insertionitis is characterized by development of the following:
- pain at the attachment site of a muscle or tendon to bone;
- slight swelling and some degree of impaired function;
- a distinct, localized tenderness to pressure over the affected attachment;
- an increase in pain at the site of attachment when the muscle group concerned is contracted.

Treatment

When insertionitis develops the *athlete* or *trainer* should:
- restrict the activity that triggers the pain (crutches may be beneficial);
- cool the injury with ice packs in the acute phase to reduce pain and swelling;
- give support with strapping or taping;
- apply local heat and use a heat retainer after the acute phase.

The *doctor* may:
- give anti-inflammatory medication;
- prescribe an exercise program;
- prescribe a dorsiflexion splint to be used during sleep;
- give local steroid injections at a later stage, combined with rest for 1–2 weeks;
- operate in patients with prolonged pain and chronic conditions.

Prevention

The following measures will reduce the likelihood of insertionitis developing:
- correct training techniques;
- equipment appropriate for the sport concerned (new equipment, especially footwear, should be 'worn in');
- clothing and equipment suitable for the athlete concerned;
- good basic training, and specialized training aimed specifically at vulnerable areas.

Bibliography

Leadbetter WB (1992) Cell matrix response in sports injury. *Clinics in Sports Medicine* July: 533–579.

Fify I, Stannish WD (1992) The use of eccentric training and stretching and the treatment and prevention of tendon injuries. *Clinics in Sports Medicine* July: 601–624.

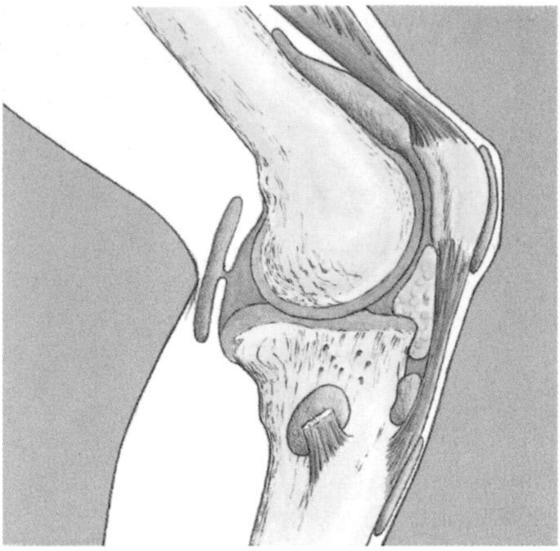

Figure 2.26 Examples of bursae around the knee.

Bursa injuries

Bursae are small, fluid-filled sacs whose function is to reduce friction, distribute stress, and protect the underlying structures. They may be found between a bone and a tendon, between two tendons, or between a bone or tendon and the overlying skin (Figure 2.26). There are a number of permanent bursae around the hips, knees, feet, shoulders, and elbows, and some of these are linked with the adjacent joints. The bursa in the posterior aspect of the knee (popliteal or semimembranosus-gastrocnemius—'Baker'—cyst), for example, is connected with the knee joint, while that located beneath the iliopsoas muscle may be connected with the hip. Acquired bursae are found in areas subject to repeated stress, friction, or pressure, such as those over protruding bones or metallic implants.

Bursitis may be inflammatory, or caused by an impact with subsequent bleeding (hemorrhagic bursitis).

Inflammatory bursitis

Bursitis may be classified as frictional, chemical, or septic, according to its cause. It can occur in isolation or as part of a generalized inflammatory or infectious disease such as rheumatoid arthritis, tuberculosis, or ankylosing spondylitis (Bechterew's disease).

Frictional bursitis

Frictional bursitis occurs when a tendon moves repeatedly over a bursa, often combined with external pressure. Frictional bursitis occurs in athletes who carry out repetitive movements, e.g. tennis players and runners training on one side of the road. It frequently affects bursae in the shoulder, elbow, hip, and knee, and around the heel and the big toe

Symptoms and diagnosis	The mechanical irritation stimulates inflammation which in turn causes fluid to be secreted into the bursa with resultant swelling and tenderness. Fluctuation of the fluid can often be felt when the bursa is examined. If the inflammation is intense, and particularly when it is superficial, the overlying skin is red and hot. Signs and symptoms include: – swelling; – local increase in temperature; – redness; – tenderness; – pain on attempted movement.
Treatment	The *athlete* or *trainer* should: – encourage rest until the pain has resolved completely; – cool the injured area with an ice pack; – apply a bandage to compress the bursa; – relieve any external pressure on the bursa (e.g. by applying a 'dough-nut' of plastic foam with the centre cut out); – use a Neoprene sleeve for compression; – consult a doctor if the swelling is extensive, the skin is red, or the pain is severe and persistent.

The *doctor* may:
– prescribe rest and sometimes a splint for a few days;
– aspirate the fluid from the bursa, sometimes in combination with compression;
– inject steroids locally;
– prescribe anti-inflammatory medication;
– remove the bursa by surgery; removal of an underlying bone spur may sometimes be necessary if it has been a factor in causing the bursitis;
– perform bursoscopy (inspection of the bursa using an arthroscope) and shaving if necessary.

Chemical bursitis

Chemical bursitis is caused by substances formed as a result of inflammatory or degenerative conditions of tendons and should be treated by a doctor at an early stage. The signs and symptoms will resemble those described above. The doctor may initially drain the bursa and inject it with steroids, but if the symptoms persist, surgical excision will become necessary.

Chemical bursitis is generally diagnosed in athletes over 30 years old who have been involved in racket or throwing sports for a number of years. It frequently affects the bursa overlying the supraspinatus tendon in the shoulder and may be associated with calcium deposits from the tendon draining into the bursa (calcific bursitis). In some cases, the bursitis can be secondary and initiate 'pseudogout'.

Septic bursitis

Septic bursitis is caused by bacteria entering a bursa either from the bloodstream or from the environment through damaged skin, for example

<table>
<tr>
<td>Symptoms and diagnosis</td>
<td>where abrasions or blisters have occurred. Superficial bursae, around the elbows and knees, are most frequently affected; athletes and soccer players who are likely to suffer dirty abrasions are most vulnerable. Septic bursitis may rarely occur after aspiration.</td>
</tr>
</table>

Septic bursitis is suggested by:
- pronounced pain and tenderness;
- marked swelling and redness of the affected area;
- considerable impairment of function;
- underlying changes in bone, revealed by X-ray, after protracted infection.

Treatment

When septic bursitis is suspected the *athlete* or *trainer* should:
- rest and relieve pressure on the affected area;
- keep damaged skin clean by washing with soap and water;
- consult a doctor as early as possible.

The *doctor* may:
- treat the underlying cause when bloodstream infection is present;
- possibly apply compression and support for a few days;
- prescribe antibiotics, sometimes intravenous, if there are signs of cellulitis;
- drain the infected bursa;
- resort to surgery if the infection fails to resolve.

Hemorrhagic bursitis

The usual cause of bleeding into a bursa is a direct impact such as a fall. It may also be caused indirectly by tendon rupture or by bleeding within a joint to which the bursa is connected. Blood within the bursa causes chemical irritation, and in severe cases, may clot and cause adhesion of connective tissue and loose bodies (calcifications). Once this has occurred chronic inflammation is likely to ensue.

Location

Hemorrhagic bursitis occurs frequently in players whose sports require them to make repeated contact with a hard surface or object, e.g. team handball and volleyball players. Apart from those in the foot, bursa anterior to the patella, greater trochanter of the femur, the elbow, and above the supraspinatus tendon may be affected.

Symptoms and diagnosis

In cases of acute injury, a hemobursa is suggested by the following signs and symptoms:
- swelling of the bursa as it fills with blood;
- extreme tenderness;
- pain and impaired function of the part in question;
- sometimes redness and damage to the skin.

Treatment

When a hemobursa occurs, the *athlete* or *trainer* should:
- cool the area in order to control bleeding;
- apply a compression bandage;
- rest the affected part.

The *doctor* may:
- drain the bursa by aspiration;
- apply a compression bandage and possibly a plaster splint.

This kind of bursitis may, if not treated properly, cause adhesions and loose bodies; chronic bursitis will result.

Peripheral nerve injuries

Injuries to the peripheral nerves are relatively common, and, if unrecognized can have a devastating effect on the athlete. These nerves can be damaged especially by compression or traction. When nerves such as the common peroneal nerve at the proximal fibula head or the ulnar nerve at the medial epicondyle of the elbow are lying superficially, they can be compressed by excessive pressure (Figure 2.27). A fracture or a dislocation can cause nerve injury when the nerve is overstretched. Damage to the ulnar nerve in the elbow can be caused by stretching during pitching or throwing (p. 171). An inversion injury to the ankle can cause injury to the peroneal nerve. Mechanical failure of a nerve may take place at 30–70% elongation. Uncommon causes for nerve injury are poor circulation which can occur by entrapment, compartment syndrome, or in connection with fracture or dislocation. Laceration and direct injury to the nerve are unusual causes of injury, but can occur in contact sports such as ice hockey, skiing, and American football.

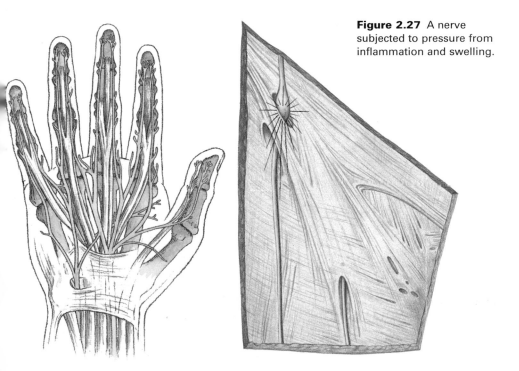

Figure 2.27 A nerve subjected to pressure from inflammation and swelling.

Symptoms and diagnosis

The injury can be difficult to diagnose as the symptoms are sometimes not obvious in the acute phase. They may begin insidiously. The athlete may complain of numbness, tingling, and pain radiating down the extremity.

– Pain or referred pain can sometimes be present. It can limit muscle strength testing. Localized or referred pain can sometimes be temporarily released by an anesthetic injection to allow full assessment of muscle strength.
– Strength testing against resistance is important; nerve injury may cause weakness.
– Hypotrophy (loss of mass) may be seen after 2 weeks and can become extensive.
– Reflex testing is mandatory to look for a peripheral nerve or nerve root injury.
– Sensory abnormalities can produce numbness, tingling or pain.
– Different nerve injuries have special tests. A *Tinel test* (a light tap over the nerve) can be positive, producing radiating tingling or numbness along the nerve segment. There are other specific tests available.
– Electromyographic (EMG) studies allow localization of the peripheral nerve injury and give information about the prognosis. An EMG test consists of two parts: nerve conduction studies (both motor and sensory) and needle electrode examination. These studies should ideally be carried out 3 weeks after the injury. An EMG is performed if a peripheral nerve plexus or nerve root injury is suspected, to confirm the presence of nerve injury, as well as assessing its severity and location. These studies are usually carried out by a neurologist.

Treatment

These syndromes are often self-limiting, but can result in permanent damage. Compression or entrapment injuries can be treated by releasing the pressure in the area. The treatment depends on the mechanism of injury, type of injury, location, and symptoms.

Prognosis and return to sport

In general, proximal nerve injuries have a poor prognosis for neurological recovery. There are many factors affecting the regeneration and recovery of a nerve injury, such as scarring around the area which causes disorganization of the healing tissue. Prolonged injury affects muscle function recovery. There are also other factors to be considered when the prognosis of a nerve injury is predicted. The electromyogram (EMG) studies will help in this evaluation, as well as consultation with an expert.

Peripheral nerve injuries are more common in the upper extremities. One example of peripheral injury is the burner syndrome, which can be seen not only in American football, but also in wrestling, basketball, ice hockey, etc. Other nerves injured in the shoulder are the long thoracic nerve and the suprascapular nerve. The axillary nerve can be injured in 9–18% of anterior shoulder dislocations. In the arm, the median nerve is involved in carpal tunnel syndrome; the ulnar nerve and the radial nerve can also be involved. In the lower extremity, the sciatic nerve is the most important nerve, but is rarely damaged in sports injuries. The common peroneal nerve is a continuation of the sciatic nerve and can be injured when it passes behind the fibular head. This injury can produce pain radiation, numbness, and pain on the dorsum of the foot, as well as weakness. The superficial peroneal nerve entrapment in the distal lateral aspect of the lower leg can cause radiating pain. The tibial nerve can be injured at the tarsal tunnel level. The nerve can be entrapped distal to the tarsal tunnel and can cause problems in the foot. In the groin, the lateral femoral cutaneous nerve, ilioinguinal nerve, genitofemoral nerve, and obturator nerve can be entrapped.

Early detection is important as it allows rehabilitation and modification of the biomechanical causes for the injury before the nerve damage becomes irreversible.

Bibliography
Fineburg J, Nodular S, Kreveckor S (1997) Peripheral nerve injuries in the athlete. *Sports Medicine* 24(6): 385–408.

Miscellaneous injuries

Open wounds

Open wounds are common among athletes, particularly those who play contact sports such as soccer, American football, rugby, and ice hockey. Riders, orienteers, and cyclists, who are likely to sustain falls on to hard surfaces, are also vulnerable. The way in which a wound is inflicted determines its nature and extent, and the possibilities include cuts, contusions, lacerations, gashes, puncture wounds, and abrasions. Some wounds may only affect the outer layers of skin; others may damage tendons, muscles, blood vessels, and nerves.

The healing of a wound is delayed by the presence of dirt and infection, bleeding, gaps between the wound edges, and disturbance of the injured tissue. Treatment aims to eliminate these factors.

Treatment

In order to stop bleeding, the *athlete* or *trainer* should:
- elevate the injured part. In most cases of limb injury, supporting the limb in a raised position with the injured athlete lying supine or on one side is sufficient to stop the bleeding;
- apply direct pressure. With one hand on each side of the wound, press the wound edges together while the injured limb is kept elevated, with the help of a third person if necessary. The risk of contamination of the wound is reduced if the wound surfaces themselves are not touched. If alone, the athlete should stop the bleeding by pressing directly on the wound;
- apply a pressure bandage as soon as first aid supplies have been obtained. The wound edges should be brought into apposition as described above, and a folded pad or clean handkerchief may be

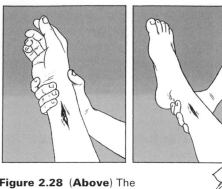

Figure 2.28 (Above) The injured athlete should sit or lie down and keep the injured limb in an elevated position. (**Right**) Example of a pressure bandage used to stop bleeding.

bandaged in place to increase the pressure on the area (Figure 2.28). A tourniquet should never be used, and even a pressure bandage must not be kept in position for more than 10–20 minutes. If a pressure bandage has been necessary to stop the bleeding, a doctor should be consulted.

Cleaning

Superficial wounds that have been contaminated by dirt must be cleaned carefully within 6 hours, otherwise they will become infected as bacteria begin to multiply and penetrate tissues. It is essential that *all dirt is removed*, especially from abrasions on the face, as retained material can cause disfiguring scars. Heavily contaminated abrasions should be cleaned thoroughly for several minutes with soap and water and a soft nail-brush. They should then be rinsed with large amounts of plain water or a saline solution, and covered with a sterile compress, held in place by a bandage. If fluid seeps through the dressing it should be changed daily. A doctor may prescribe medicated dressings to facilitate healing. Small superficial abrasions heal best if cleaned well and left undisturbed.

Deep wounds include skin, underlying connective tissue, and possibly also tendons, muscles, blood vessels, and nerves. The wound edges often gape apart and bleeding can be considerable. Puncture wounds caused by studs or spiked shoes can be treacherous and should always be treated by a doctor. Wounds to the sole of the foot require padding to distribute load when walking. Deep wounds must be cleaned with extreme care, and, when damage is extensive, it is sometimes necessary for the doctor to excise dead tissue (debridement). A sound rule is that wounds that are not treated within 6 hours should be considered to be infected.

Some wounds — those that are deep, those that bleed profusely, and those whose edges do not lie readily in apposition with each other — need to be stitched by a doctor. Stitching should preferably be done within 6 hours of the injury.

Infected wounds are characterized by pain, swelling, redness of the skin and local tenderness. Infection can spread from the wound to the lymph glands via the lymphatic vessels. Infection in the leg, for example, spreads to the glands in the groin. When this happens, the lymphatics appear as red streaks in the skin, and other symptoms, such as fever and general malaise, commonly occur. The affected lymph glands are swollen and tender. The condition should always be treated by a doctor who will prescribe antibiotics in addition to any other treatment. A period of bed rest may be necessary during the acute illness.

Athletes must refrain from training or competition during the course of an infection.

Tetanus prophylaxis

All wounds sustained in an outdoor environment carry some risk of tetanus, and it is common practice in many countries for babies to be inoculated routinely against the disease. Primary tetanus inoculation involves a course of three injections administered over a period of 6 months and confers long-lasting immunity. Most people have received these initial injections at young ages, in schools and in the military service. An incomplete course means incomplete protection, and people should be encouraged to be aware of their inoculation status and to comply with instructions given by their doctor. It is usual for a booster dose of vaccine to be given at the time of any wound that needs medical attention and is potentially contaminated.

Blisters

Blisters on the feet are the scourge of athletes, and blisters on the hands can be a problem for crosscountry skiers, baseball players, basketball players, cricketers, rowers, tennis, badminton and squash players, and team handball players. Once a blister is broken it becomes a potentially painful open wound.

Athletes using wheelchairs are a special group who often have trouble with pressure sores and blisters. These can be difficult to treat because of impaired skin sensitivity and poor circulation (Figure 2.29).

Treatment

Blisters should be treated in the following way:
- When there is any tendency to a blister forming, a break from exercise should be taken in order to prevent further irritation. The problem area can then be protected with adhesive bandaging; avoid creases in the plaster which would encourage rather than prevent blister formation.
- Once a blister has formed, its surface should be retained intact as it acts as a barrier against bacteria. Never break a blister deliberately. Large blisters can be punctured at their edges with a sterile needle. The blister can be protected from pressure by means of a piece of plastic foam with its centre cut out.
- If a blister breaks naturally, it is important to clean it carefully with soap and water or antiseptic solution. A sterile nonadherent dressing or a bandage is used to cover the wound.

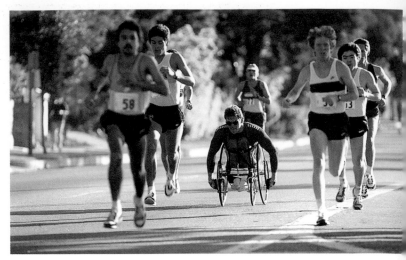

Figure 2.29 Athletes using wheelchairs or similar apparatus may be at risk of developing pressure sores or blisters (by courtesy of All Sport: photographer, Alvin Chung.)

Preventive measures

Blisters can be prevented by the following measures.

- All equipment should be designed for use in training as well as in competition. Footwear, in particular, should be well worn in.
- Socks should be free from holes, dry, clean, and of the correct size so that they do not crease. They should be changed frequently.
- Hygiene should be meticulous. The feet should be washed daily and can be rubbed with salicylic acid grease which softens calluses and keeps the skin supple.
- Sensitive skin areas can be protected with adhesive bandaging applied firmly and directly to the skin before exercise.

It cannot be stressed too strongly that blisters *can* be avoided if preventive measures are applied. They may seem trivial but they can necessitate long breaks from training, especially if they become infected.

Friction burns

An athlete who falls during training or competition on a synthetic surface or a synthetically treated floor runs the risk of sustaining friction burns (Figure 2.30). Usually the burn affects only the outer layer of skin and in its mildest form causes only superficial redness which needs no treatment, but if contact is hard it may result in an abrasion. If blisters appear in the skin, they should be covered with a clean dressing; if the skin is broken, the wound should be cleansed and dressed as soon as possible as described above, in order to prevent infection.

Treatment and prevention

The *athlete* or *trainer* should:

- prevent friction burns by making sure that the correct equipment and clothing for the protection of vulnerable areas is used;

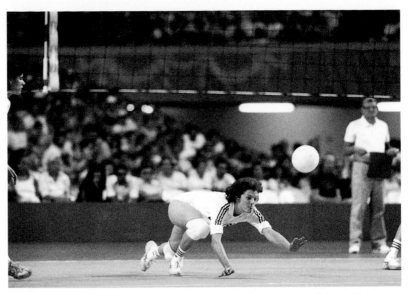

Figure 2.30 Falls onto a synthetically treated floor can result in a friction burn (by courtesy of All Sport: photographer, Alvin Chung.)

- reduce friction during falls by rubbing exposed parts with greasy ointment;
- treat frictional burns by cleaning the wound carefully with soap and water and dressing with medicated compresses held in place with a bandage.

Stitch

Runners who have not warmed up properly sometimes feel a sharp pain in the upper part of the abdomen a few minutes after they have started to run. It may be located on the right or the left and is more frequent when sporting activity is undertaken immediately after a meal. The pain may be made worse by deep expiration and relieved by deep inspiration.

The real causes of stitch are unknown, although some studies indicate that a purely mechanical effort may trigger it. The connective tissue that anchors the abdominal organs bears a much greater load just after a meal, and physical activity at this time could cause strain and minor internal bleeding. Other suggested causes are an insufficient supply of oxygen to the diaphragm, or pain arising from the internal abdominal organs, such as the spleen and the liver, as the blood flow is redistributed.

Treatment

The *athlete* should:
- avoid training and competition for a few hours after main meals;
- run bent forward, or stop so that the stitch has time to disappear before training is resumed;
- squeeze a hard object such as a stone, in the hands. Most athletes feel that this makes the stitch pains subside, but the mechanism of this phenomenon is unknown.

3 Mechanism and etiology of injuries

Running

Running is an effective way to exercise large muscle groups and has a documented effect in the preservation of health and in the prevention of cardiovascular problems. However, it is a potentially harmful activity, and running injuries are common—although 2–2.5 times less frequent than injuries from other sports. The overall yearly incidence rate for running injuries is about 37–56%. The incidence of all running injuries ranges from 3.6 to 5.5 injuries per 1000 hours of running. For competitive athletes, the range is 2.5–5.8 injuries per 1000 hours of running, depending on the specialization.

The examining physician must remember that most runners are dedicated to their running activity. Runners usually complain about problems associated with running, but they can often participate in sports activities, such as cycling, swimming, and crosscountry skiing, that involve lower levels of repetitive stress.

Running should be differentiated from sprinting, which is characterized by such factors as increased velocity, decreased shock absorption in early stance, and initial ground contact with the toe. Approximately 75–80% of runners have initial heel contact at distance running, and the remaining 20–25% have midfoot-forefoot contact.

Runners' problems occur because of the repetitive stress that running places on the lower extremities. The ground reaction force at the time of the midstance phase in running is equivalent to a vertical force ranging from 1.5 to 5 times body weight. A man running with stride length of 1.6 m (4.5 ft) will take approximately 1175 steps per mile. Considering an impact of 250% of the body weight (68 kg; 150 lb), the runner absorbs at ground contact a total of 220 tons, or 110 tons on each foot per mile. At a pace of 7 minutes per mile, stance time is approximately 0.2 second, which translates into approximately 5100 contacts during 1 hour of running. Considering those huge loads on the tissues, it is clear that even small biomechanical abnormalities can result in a significant concentration of stress and load.

Etiology of running injuries

The etiology of running injuries is multifactorial. Factors may be extrinsic or intrinsic.

Extrinsic factors

Extrinsic factors are present in 60–80% of reported injuries in runners. The most common of these are training errors.

Training errors

The most common errors are sudden changes in the running activity, such as increased distance or intensity. An example of this is a novice runner starting to run regularly, or an injured runner returning to running, who may attempt too much, too soon, resulting in an overuse reaction. Specific training errors include:
- persistent high–intensity training without taking easy days with lower intensity;
- sudden increases in distance and intensity without adequate rest;
- single severe training or competitive sessions, such as marathon or other long-distance events;
- repetitive hill training.

The injury rate is proportional both to the absolute level of training and to changes in the relative intensity and volume of training. The total weekly distance run is significantly associated with injury. The relationship between running speed and injury risk remains unclear. Running experience has not been proven to be significantly related to running injuries.

Running terrain

Too much downhill running can cause problems in the knee joints, because the body weight is mainly behind the knee's vertical axis, which requires high forces on the quadriceps muscles to protect the knee. In downhill running there are increases in knee flexion, net extensor moment, patellofemoral forces, power absorption of the knee extensors, and contraction of the knee extensors. Running up and down hills has been reported to produce injuries. There is no association between the rate of running injuries and terrain. Downhill running can produce pain symptoms from injury syndromes such as patellofemoral pain and iliotibial band friction syndromes. Too much uphill running can cause problems such as Achilles peritenonitis and plantar fasciitis.

Running surfaces

The running surface may be of importance. Certain surfaces may triple or quadruple the frequency of injuries in selected sports activities. Running on hard surfaces such as asphalt or concrete, which causes mechanical shock and thereby overloads joints and tendons, may be associated with a greater incidence of running injuries. Running on too soft a surface allows hypermobility of the joints, fatigues the muscles, and may cause overuse injuries. Wooden chips provide an excellent surface (Figure 3.1).

Running on uneven or artificial surfaces or on slippery roads can also cause overuse injuries. Running on a banked surface, or on the camber of a road in one direction, is apt to cause an abnormal stress on one side of the body. The result is a functional leg-length discrepancy, which may result in iliotibial band friction syndrome or trochanteric bursitis.

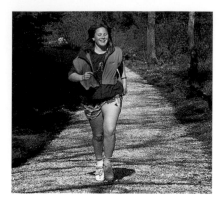

Figure 3.1 A trail with wooden chips.

Running shoes

A poor choice in sports shoes can be responsible for the development of sports injuries, because shoes can alter forces in specific anatomic structures by more than 100%. Sports shoes may also influence the site, type, and frequency of sports injuries. However, a study of three popular brands of well-constructed running shoes showed no difference in injury incidence.

Inadequate or worn-out shoes can cause increased stress and overuse. It is not acceptable to use tennis or basketball shoes during a regular running program. These shoes do not have the appropriate features to protect the runner from injuries. Improvements in footwear have led to a decrease in injuries of the foot and lower leg as a whole, but there have been increases in certain injuries, such as iliotibial band friction syndrome.

The shock-absorbing capacity of running shoes is considered important in injury prevention. Shock absorption can be increased by shoes fitting well. Shock-absorbing qualities are reduced in wet shoes, and also with wear, being reduced by 30–50% after only 400 km (250 miles) of running.

Technique

Running technique varies from one sport to another (Figure 3.2). Long-distance runners generally strike first with the heel, followed by the toe, while short-distance runners tend to be either midfoot strikers or run on their toes only. The most common technique faults are striking too hard with the heel, and running flat-footed. These can result in overuse

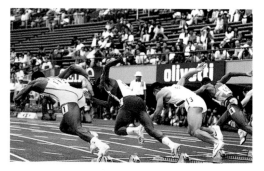 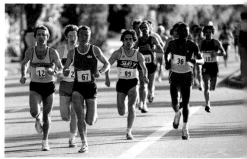

Figure 3.2 Running technique differs between (**left**) sprinters and (**right**) marathon runners (by courtesy of All Sport: photographers, Mike Powell and Alvin Chung).

injuries. Repeated incorrect running or jumping techniques nearly always result in overuse injuries.

Intrinsic factors

Intrinsic (body-related) factors can be divided into basic, primary, and secondary (acquired). Basic intrinsic factors include sex, age, growth, weight, and height. Important primary intrinsic factors are malalignments, leg-length discrepancy, muscle imbalance and inadequate strength, and poor flexibility and neuromuscular coordination. Secondary acquired factors, such as kinetic chain dysfunctions and previous injuries, are also important.

Running injuries—intrinsic etiological factors
Basic factors
    Gender
    Age
    Growth
    Weight
    Height
Primary factors
    Bone alignment
        Foot, tibia, knee, hip, pelvis, leg length
    Structural variations
    Muscular condition
        Strength
        Flexibility
        Neuromuscular coordination
        Ligamentous laxity
Secondary or acquired dysfunction
    Mechanical
        Foot, ankle, knee, hip, back, sacroiliac joints
    Muscular asymmetries
        Imbalance
        Localized weakness
        Localized inflexibility
    Previous and recurrent injuries

Basic intrinsic factors

Sex: sex and age are not important predictors of running injuries in general. Women have a weaker musculoskeletal system, 25% less muscle mass per body weight, less bone density, and a wider pelvis and more mobile joints than men. These factors can predispose women to specific injuries, such as pelvic stress fractures and patellofemoral pain syndrome. It is also known that menstrual irregularities constitute a risk factor for certain overuse injuries such as stress fractures. Overall, however, there is not an increased risk for running injuries in women.

Age: changes in the musculoskeletal system associated with aging include decreases in bone density, muscle strength, water content, metabolic activity, and collagen in tendons. Elderly people have greater degenerative changes in their tissues, with a decreased ability for shock absorption and, thereby, an increased risk for injuries. People with more than 30–40 years of extensive running experience did not have an increased incidence of osteoarthritis of the hip. There is no increased incidence of running injuries with age as a primary factor. This could be because the elderly run for enjoyment, at a slower pace and over shorter distances, and because they are more careful in general.

Growth: adolescents aged 12–15 years often have an imbalance between lever arm muscle strength, tightness, joint mobility, and coordination. Muscle–tendon units are relatively shortened at this age. Some diagnoses are age- and growth-dependent, such as Osgood–Schlatter disease, apophysitis injuries, and certain avulsion fractures. After the growth spurt, adolescents usually need a more flexible training program, including stretching.

Weight and *height*: although being overweight often is considered to be a potential problem for long-distance runners, no relationship has been found between body weight and running injuries. The development of knee and hip symptoms and osteoarthritis is, to some extent, associated with being overweight, as running may further accelerate the osteoarthritic process. Height is not related to running injury incidence.

Primary intrinsic factors

Malalignments in the foot can be simplistically divided into pes planus (flat foot) and pes cavus (claw foot), each of which occurs in approximately 20% of the population. Pes planus results in an excessive pronation through midstance. Pronation is discussed on p. 397. Excessive pronation can be physiologic, but it can also be secondary to tibial varum (leg directed inwards) of more than 10°, functional equinus (foot directed downwards), talar varus, and/or forefoot supination. Many good runners have a mild genu varum. There may be a low likelihood of injury if the total varus is less than 8°, and an increased incidence in running-related injuries if the varus is greater than 18°.

Different malalignments can be combined. The 'miserable malalignment' syndrome which can be seen in some runners, combines femoral neck anteversion (forward angling) with internal rotation of the hip and genu varum (with or without knee hyperextension), squinting patellae, excessive Q angle, tibial varum, functional equinus, and compensatory foot pronation. A miserable malalignment syndrome can cause such problems with regular running that it is reasonable to say that some people with this malalignment simply should not be running long distances.

Cavus feet (p. 398) are also associated with running injuries. Cavus feet were found to be present in about 20% of a group of injured runners. Athletes with cavus feet have decreased motion of the subtalar joints, with resulting decreased flexibility of the midfoot and excessively weighted rearfoot varus. At foot strike, the heel remains in varus, the longitudinal arch is maintained, and the foot does not unlock. The tibia remains in external rotation, and the net result is increased stress because the arch continues to be rigid through the midstance phase of running. With a reduction in internal tibia rotation, stress is passed through the lateral foot and knee, resulting in injuries such as iliotibial band friction syndrome, trochanteric bursitis, stress fractures, Achilles tendinitis, peroneal muscle strain, plantar fasciitis, and metatarsalgia, which are common in runners with cavus feet.

A functional *leg-length discrepancy* can be created by running on cambered roads; functional leg shortening can also be the result of sacroiliac joint dysfunction, unilateral excessive pronation, lumbar muscular pain, contractures, or imbalance of muscles. Leg-length discrepancy can result in pelvic tilt to the short side, functional lumbar scoliosis, increased abduction of the hip, excessive pronation, increased knee valgus, and outward rotation of the leg. During running, the legs are not on the ground at the same time, and an absolute leg-length discrepancy should not be a problem. A change in soft tissue biomechanics caused by a functional difference might result in overload, however. Leg-length discrepancy may be associated with such injuries as iliotibial band friction syndrome, trochanteric bursitis, low back pain, and stress fractures. Leg-length discrepancy unaccompanied by other orthopedic disorders usually does not require any compensation. If orthopedic disorders are present, leg-length discrepancy greater than 20 mm (0.8 in) usually does require correction. In runners with repetitive high loading and overuse problems, a leg-length discrepancy greater than 5–10 mm (0.2–0.4 in) usually requires compensation.

Structural variations can predispose to injury. A prominent posterior calcaneus can cause Achilles tendon and/or bursa problems. A large os trigonum or a prominent posterior talar beak can cause posterolateral ankle pain. Tarsal coalition of different kinds can cause abnormal painful motion. An accessory navicular can cause medial midfoot pain (see Chapter 14).

Good *flexibility* is stressed by many as important in the prevention of running injuries. Running itself causes tightness of hamstrings and calf muscles. These regional inflexibilities can contribute to injury. There seems to be no association between stretching habits and the incidence of injury.

Muscle strength: muscles stabilize the lower extremity and attenuate the forces and impact of running. Because of the important role of muscles in both stability and shock absorption, muscle weakness may predispose to stress fractures.

Neuromuscular coordination: a breakdown in balance and motor control can predispose a runner to injury. Any deficit in proprioceptive capacity may lead to functional instability that could make the athlete more prone to injury.

Ligamentous laxity: generalized laxity of the ligaments in excessive pronation can increase the risk of injury.

Secondary or acquired factors

With the kinetic chain the lower extremity is seen as a series of mobile segments and linkages that allow forward propulsion during gait. The kinetic chain is closed when the foot is in contact with the surface in stance phase and is open when the foot is off the ground in the swing phase. Anything that interferes with the normal progression and mechanics of force transfer can lead to alterations in gait and compensatory changes in the motion at other sites in the chain. In patients with recurrent and previous injuries, it is especially important to focus on the dysfunction of the kinetic chain. Because kinetic chain function is very complicated in nature, it is frequently overlooked as an etiology of running injuries.

The role of secondary or acquired dysfunction in causing injury remains controversial. These dysfunctions usually result from hyper- or hypomobility of a segment of the kinetic chain after an injury. Any dysfunction in the kinetic chain can lead to compensatory alterations in stance and gait that, in turn, can lead to tissue microtrauma, breakdown and overt injury.

Mechanical dysfunction: changes in the position and motion of the sacroiliac joint are fairly common. Although the sacroiliac joint is usually stable, with little motion, it has been claimed that motion can occur with anterior subluxation and rotation and can lead to asymmetry of the pelvic ring structure. This dysfunction is characterized by locking or hypomobility at the involved sacroiliac joint. The main symptom, pain, is usually localized to the sacroiliac joint but may also radiate to the buttocks and the groin region. In order to identify sacroiliac joint dysfunction, one must be aware of its existence and understand the biomechanics involved. A high index of suspicion should be present when treating patients with recurrent injury.

Previous injuries: most injuries heal sooner or later, but they can leave a residual scar in the tissue. This scar may have an elasticity different from that of normal tissue and can create a weak area with an increased risk of injury. Multiple and recurrent injuries may be indicative of kinetic chain dysfunction. Previous injuries can lead to fibrosis, with adhesion and limited joint motion and function. Long-standing joint injuries resulting in chronic instability, or even the slightest effusion, can result in a reflex inhibition of the muscles and secondary alteration of gait. Restricted motion of knee, ankle, or subtalar joints will increase stresses on other areas. Joint instability will result in muscle hypotrophy and increased compensatory stress on other structures.

Diagnosis of running injuries

The precise diagnosis of running injuries is often a challenge. An understanding of the injury mechanism and of different diagnostic options is important. Physicians often focus on the injury site when treating overuse running injuries. Any injury should, however, be regarded as a manifestation of dysfunction in the kinetic chain, and the entire chain must be examined to rule out any asymptomatic underlying injury or dysfunction. This approach is especially important in individuals with previous or recurrent injuries.

History

The history of running injuries is important, because it forms the basis on which a diagnosis is made. The physician should be aware of the demands and biomechanics of running. It is important to analyze the entire running program, including changes in distance and training conditions. The shoes the runner has been wearing and the use of orthotic devices should also be discussed.

Physical examination

An evaluation of the entire lower extremity and back can be carried out with the runner in standing, sitting, prone, and supine positions. The whole lower extremity should be carefully examined for asymmetries of both static and dynamic alignment and function. Any biomechanical imbalance in the foot or the lower extremity should be noted. The dynamic examination can be direct and should include gait, functional foot movements, patellar tracking, leg-length evaluation, and functional sacroiliac joint tests. The dynamic evaluation can also be indirect—for example, the runner's shoes can be examined for wear patterns. A full functional examination should include testing of the various linkages of the kinetic chain and running on a treadmill could be helpful.

Radiographs are sometimes of value. Indications for their use include suspicion of an arthritic joint or stress fractures. A bone scan is positive 2–8 days after the onset of stress fracture symptoms. Magnetic resonance imaging is a noninvasive imaging technique that provides excellent soft tissue contrast in multiple planes without exposing the patient to ionized radiation. It can provide a detailed assessment of the intrinsic abnormalities in tendons. Ultrasound evaluations have been shown to be valuable in the diagnosis of 'jumper's knee', meniscus lesions, and Achilles tendon lesions. The development of arthroscopy has also been of great importance in the diagnosis and treatment of injuries to the knee and ankle.

Running overuse injuries constitute a diagnostic problem because the symptoms of these injuries are often diffuse and uncharacteristic. The diagnosis of a runner's injury rests with the identification not only of the affected tissues but also the underlying predisposing conditions.

Principles of treatment

When treating running injuries, it is important to treat not only symptoms of the injury, but also the cause of the injury. It is, therefore, important to determine the primary problem and any secondary problems that may have resulted. Identification of kinetic chain dysfunctions is important. A correct diagnosis is the base for a successful treatment.

The cause of injury

Training routines must be checked, and training errors identified. An effective biomechanical strategy to reduce load and stress on the locomotive system can be:
- alter the movement (change the running style);
- alter the surface (run on a soft surface rather than a hard surface);
- change the shoe;
- diminish the frequency of repetition of movement (reduce the distance run).

Normal alignment and symmetry of the kinetic chain must be restored. Orthoses—rigid, semiflexible, or soft—may be the treatment of choice when malalignment or asymmetries are present. An orthotic device can significantly affect the amount of maximum pronation, time to maximum pronation, maximum pronation velocity, period of pronation, and movement of rear foot angle in the first $10°$ of foot contact. Undercorrection is common, and orthoses rarely provide the exact hindfoot and forefoot posting necessary to ensure a neutral subtalar joint. The common approach, to post the subtalar position to the maximum of $4°$ of varus, will provide adequate control. Despite their popularity, the use of orthotic devices is still controversial, and there are failures with this type of treatment. These failures may be caused by neglecting to adjust or change the orthotic devices as needed from time to time. No prospective scientific studies are available to show the effects of these devices. We have found that more than 80% of runners were satisfied with their orthotic treatment and experienced improvement after 1 year of wearing their orthosis regularly. Most runners adjusted to their orthosis after only 2–3 weeks, which is a much shorter time than had been anticipated.

It is important to use well-constructed running shoes, to provide cushioning support and friction. Running shoes give a maximum point of pronation, which occurs significantly later when barefoot than when wearing a running shoe. Shock absorption can be increased by well-fitting shoes. A runner's shoe should be a stable shoe with optimal shock absorption in the sole or insole and a well-fitted heel counter that is rigid around the heel pad.

With very few exceptions, stretching exercises should always be used by runners, who, in general, have very tight muscles and tendons. If the athlete is very flexible, strengthening exercises may be indicated. Adequate muscle strength, balance, flexibility, and coordination are essential, as are normal alignment, mobility, and symmetry of the kinetic chain.

Surgical correction may be indicated for some malalignments.

The symptoms

When treating running injuries, it is important to have an exact diagnosis before a specific treatment is initiated. The stage of healing should determine the mode of treatment to be used. Treatment should start as early as possible. Initially, pain and inflammation are treated with rest, avoidance of weightbearing, elevation, cryotherapy, compression, immobilization, and protection. Crutches are often indicated. Anti-inflammatory medication can be helpful. Heat, which increases the extensibility of collagen in connective tissue, decreases joint stiffness, and gives pain relief, should be used after 24–48 hours. Local heat can be generated by heat retainers.

Exercises should begin as early as possible. The initial program should be prescribed according to the slow progression principle, with a gradual increase of the load within the limits of pain. Because strength training alone has a negative effect on joint flexibility, it should be counteracted by flexibility training, including stretching. Crosscountry skiing, swimming, and cycling are valuable alternatives to maintain a good conditioning level if running is not possible. Pool running can also be effective.

Surgery should be avoided until conservative therapy has failed. Excision of scar and degenerative tissue secondary to delayed healing in tendons, such as chronic partial tears to the Achilles tendon and adductor longus injuries, has shown good results. Although the postoperative rehabilitation period may be long, the overall results are good.

Type and location of running injuries

Running injuries can involve most of the tissues in the body, including muscle, tendon, fascia, bone, bursae, nerves, and cartilage (Figure 3.3). The structures reported to be most commonly involved in overuse injuries were muscle and fascia, 27.2%; tendon and muscle insertion, 21.6%; joint surfaces, 15.9%; tendon and tendon sheath, 15.1%; bursae, bones, and nerves, 21.4%. The knee—the most common site of injury—was involved in 48% of all running injuries, followed by the lower leg, 20.4%; foot, 17.2%; hips, 6.0%; upper leg/thigh, 4.2%; and lower back, 4.1%. The most common running injuries are listed in Table 3.1.

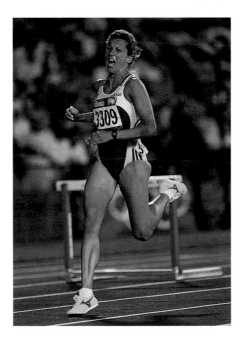

Figure 3.3 Running injury involving the Achilles tendon (by courtesy of All Sport: photographer, Gary M Prior).

In order to be successful, treatment must be based on the specific diagnosis. It is important to hear and understand the special wishes of each runner because patient compliance is the single largest factor determining the success or failure of treatment.

Bibliography

James J, Jones D (1990) Biomechanical aspects of distance running injuries. In: Cavanagh PR (ed.) *Biomechanics of Distance Running*, pp. 249–269. Champaign: Human Kinetics.

MacIntyre JG, Taunton JE, Clement DB, et al. (1991) Running injuries: a clinical study of 4173 cases. *Clinical Journal of Sports Medicine* 1: 81–87.

Table 3.1 Most common running injuries

	Men (%)	Women (%)
Patellofemoral pain	24.3	29.6
Tibial stress injury	7.2	11.4
Iliotibial band friction	7.2	7.9
Plantar fasciitis	5.2	4.0
Patellar tendinitis	5.1	3.1
Achilles tendinitis	4.7	2.7
Metatarsal stress syndrome	3.1	3.8
	n = 2359	n = 1814

Modified with permission from MacIntyre JG, Taunton JE, Clement DB, et al. (1991) Running injuries: a clinical survey of 4173 cases. *Clinical Journal of Sports Medicine* 1: 81–87.

Throwing

Throwing injuries are of increasing importance in both professional and amateur sports. They affect adults and children alike. Sports prone to throwing injuries include baseball, American football, tennis and other racket sports, javelin throwing, team handball, cricket, and sports with other overhead motions such as swimming and volleyball.

Throwing mechanism

The basic principle in throwing is the use of a kinetic chain to generate and transfer energy from the larger body parts (legs and trunk) to a smaller (more injury-prone) upper extremity. This kinetic chain in throwing includes the following sequence of motions: stride, pelvis rotation, upper torso rotation, elbow extension, shoulder internal rotation and wrist flexion. This biomechanical motion is a combination of true glenohumeral rotation, trunk hyperextension, and shoulder blade motion against the rib cage. For example, when a ball is released, there has been significant energy and momentum transferred to the throwing arm and ball. After the ball is released, the kinetic chain must decelerate the moving arm.

The throwing mechanism (here using baseball pitching as an example) can be divided into six phases: wind-up, stride, arm cocking, arm acceleration, arm deceleration with ball release, and follow-through (Figure 3.4).

Wind-up

During wind-up, the shoulder is hyperextended, externally rotated and abducted, and the elbow is flexed to an angle of about 45°. At this stage the anterior structures of the shoulder are under mild tension. The objective of this phase is to put the thrower in a good starting position.

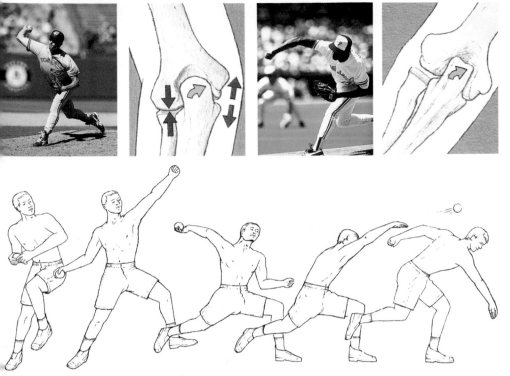

Figure 3.4 Wind-up; stride/arm cocking (with lateral compression and medial tension); arm acceleration; arm deceleration; follow-through (compression of posteromedial olecranon). **(Insets)** Arm cocking and follow-through in baseball (by courtesy of All Sport: photographers, Otto Greule and Jim Commentucct).

Stride

In this phase the thrower turns the lead side towards the target. The stance foot is planted, the arm abducts, and the athlete stretches the body. Forward movement is initiated by hip abduction of the stance leg, followed by knee and hip extension. During the stride, the throwing shoulder externally rotates and horizontally abducts. Wrist and finger extensors have very high activity during the stride phase. The stride phase ends when the lead foot contacts the ground.

Arm cocking

Arm cocking begins as the lead foot contacts the ground and ends at maximum shoulder external rotation. The shoulder girdle muscles stabilize the shoulder blade and position the shoulder socket (glenoid). The rotator cuff and other shoulder muscles are also active in stabilizing the glenohumeral joint. The shoulder remains abducted at approximately $90°$ throughout the cocking phase. At the end of the cocking phase, the shoulder is externally rotated $150–180°$. Competitive throwing can stretch out the shoulder capsule and increase shoulder flexibility. A competitive pitcher will often have $10–15°$ more external rotation in the throwing shoulder than the nonthrowing shoulder (Figure 3.5).

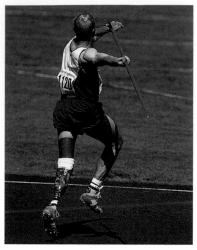

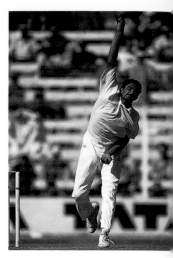

Figure 3.5 Arm cocking in javelin throw (by courtesy of All Sport: photographer, Stu Forster).

Figure 3.6 Arm acceleration in cricket (by courtesy of All Sport photographer, Chris Cole).

Arm acceleration

Arm acceleration is the explosive phase when the trunk flexes forward to a neutral position and the ball is released. The throwing shoulder remains abducted at approximately 90° during this phase. The shoulder internal rotator muscles contract to produce maximal internal rotation velocity. The rotator cuff muscles are highly active to stabilize the glenohumeral joint (Figure 3.6, 3.7).

Arm deceleration

Arm deceleration is a short phase that begins at ball release. During this phase the shoulder maximally rotates internally to approximately 0°. A shoulder posterior force is produced to resist anterior humeral translation. The teres minor muscle has the highest activity of all the glenohumeral muscles during this phase.

The acceleration and deceleration phases can cause injury to the internal rotator muscles of the shoulder. In adolescents, an injury to the proximal humeral growth zone (epiphysis) can occur. This causes widening and absorption of the epiphysis of the proximal humerus that is similar to a stress fracture (Figure 3.8).

Follow-through

Follow-through begins at maximal shoulder internal rotation and ends when the arm completes its movement across the body and the athlete

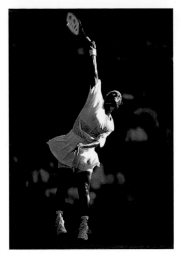

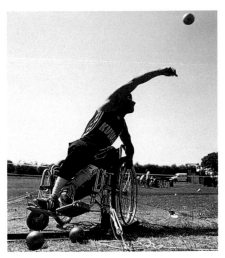

Figure 3.7 A tennis serve causes similar stresses to arm acceleration in a throw (by courtesy of All Sport: photographer, Clive Brunskill).

Figure 3.8 Arm deceleration in shot put throw (by courtesy of All Sport: photographer, Trevor Jones).

is in a balanced position. The kinetic chain during this motion helps to reduce the stress placed on the throwing arm by transferring the body weight and momentum to the lead leg. The posterior shoulder muscles continue to be active throughout the follow-through. The serratus anterior is the most active scapular stabilizer during this phase. In addition, during follow-through the forearm is rotated into pronation. This may cause rotational and shearing forces on the outside (lateral) side of the elbow, as well as compression on the back (posterior) of the elbow.

Treatment

Overuse injuries from excess throwing are common. An athlete who begins to develop signs of overuse from repeated overhead activities must limit the activity to avoid pain and possible further injury. Most of these problems will resolve with rest and a graduated return to activity: for details, see Chapters 6 and 7.

Skiing

Since the 1960s participation in downhill skiing has increased at least 40-fold in the USA. The number of skiers is estimated to be around 8 million on an annual basis. The number of ski injuries annually is probably more than 1 million per year worldwide.

Etiology of skiing injuries

Skier-related factors

Relative to the population at risk, men tend to have a higher incidence of collision injuries than women. Avoidance of reckless skiing habits and using care when skiing near fixed objects are probably important factors in preventing injuries.

Equipment

From the standpoint of skiing safety there can be no doubt that the ski bindings are the most important factor. The number of injuries caused by the ski acting as a lever to bend or twist the leg has diminished significantly, especially during the 1980s. However, the perfect ski binding has yet to be invented. Boots should be comfortable and fit correctly; they should distribute the load widely on the leg in both forward and backward lean. At the binding interface the boot should conform to internationally accepted standards.

Type of injury

The most common injuries in alpine skiing are knee sprains, representing around 23% of all injuries. Other common injuries are: ligament injuries to the thumb, 10%; lacerations, 8%; shoulder contusion, 5% and boot-top contusion, 4%. Tibia fractures constitute around 3.4% of all injuries, which is a dramatic decrease compared with the 1970s.

Since 1980 there has been an enormous increase in the number of anterior cruciate ligament (ACL) injuries, which in the early 1970s accounted for less than 1% of all skiing injuries. There are significant differences between skiers with predominantly severe medial collateral ligament (MCL) injuries and those with isolated ACL injuries. More ACL injuries result from backward falls. Individuals sustaining ACL injuries were more skilled and were more likely to be male than those who sustained MCL injuries. Those sustaining ACL tears wore higher and stiffer boots than a control group of skiers in one study.

Injury mechanism

During the 1970s excessive external rotation loading of the lower extremity was the most important factor in production of ski injuries. Other mechanisms have been described including internal rotation of the tibia relative to the femur (Figures 3.9, 3.10). In the 1990s new mechanism of injury have been responsible for severe injuries, especially ACL injuries.

In one common mechanism the skier falls backwards while the upper shell of the boot produces anterior drawer loading to the proximate tibi

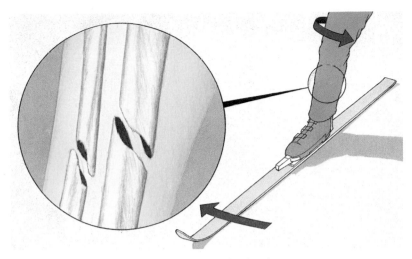

Figure 3.9 A fracture resulting from twisting load.

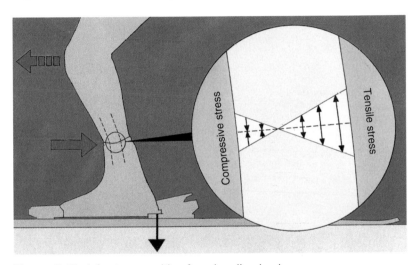

Figure 3.10 A fracture resulting from bending load.

(Figure 3.11). The mechanism involved in complete tears of the ACL has been the boot-induced ACL injury. After a jump the skier lands on one ski while slightly off balance, with the upper body leaning backwards. The tail of the ski hits the snow first, the ski is driven into the snow and the boot top drives the tibia shaft forward. At the moment of landing the skier's knee is in full extension and the opposite arm is thrown back in an attempt to regain balance. The actual injury to the ACL occurs at about the time the foot is driven flat on the snow. The fixed forward lean built into modern ski boots is instrumental in the production of this type of injury.

A second mechanism of injury of the ACL is when the skier is falling out of control. The only way this injury could be prevented would be for the toe of the boot to release or to allow the ankle to plantar flex. The injury mechanism here is unique to skiing accidents and is called

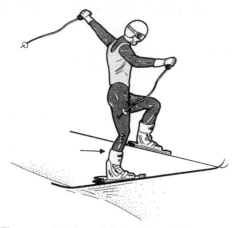

Figure 3.11 Skier falls backwards (by permission of Blackwell Scientific Publishers).

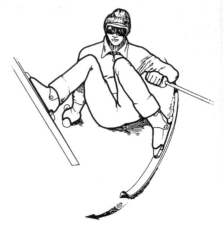

Figure 3.12 Skier falls out of control (by permission of Blackwell Scientific Publishers).

the 'phantom foot' mechanism (Figure 3.12). In this injury the skier falls backwards, and the ski leaves the surface of the snow so that only the inside edge of the portion of the ski behind the skier's foot is in contact with the snow. As soon as this set of circumstances occurs the ski carves a turn and produces an internal rotation of the tibia in relation to the femur. This occurs when the knee is flexed past 90°. This mechanism can produce isolated injuries to the ACL or injury resulting in some damage to the lateral and posterior lateral aspects of the knee. This mechanism is probably more common than the boot-induced anterior drawer mechanism.

The combination of high, stiff boots and bindings that are incapable of releasing upwards at the toe is at least partly responsible for the unfortunate increase in ACL sprains. It is now apparent that modern ski equipment is not very effective at protecting the ACL.

In skiing the high velocities to which the unprotected human body is exposed by the unnatural lengthening of the foot by the ski–binding–boot system generate a large number of devastating injuries. As many as 30% of all ski injuries are probably the result of failure of the ski binding to function properly.

Good binding design, along with correct adjustment and regular maintenance, is essential if the risk of injury is to be reduced.

Bibliography

Johnson RJ, Renström PA (1994) Injuries in alpine skiing. In: Renström PA (ed.) *Clinical Practice of Sports Injury: Prevention and Care*, pp 676–698. Oxford: Blackwell Scientific.

4 Sports and protective equipment

Footwear

Normal daily activities make considerable demands upon the feet, which are required constantly to support the entire body weight. These demands are far greater during sporting activities, and in most sports shoes are by far the most important item of clothing or equipment.

Use the correct shoe for the purpose. A number of factors have to be considered when choosing sports shoes, including the proposed training program, the surface involved, the anatomy of the foot, previous injuries, and the requirements of the particular sport. Soccer players who are improving their fitness by running on asphalt, for example, should not wear cleated boots or shoes.

Shoe construction

The sole of the shoe determines the amount of shock absorption that the shoe provides, and thus a sports shoe should be constructed of layers with different properties. The out sole should insulate from cold and be water-repellent and hardwearing, as it is this surface that determines the durability of the shoe, and reduces the amount of friction against the playing surface (Figure 4.1).

The heel counter of a sports shoe should be made of a firm material, cover the whole of the heel area, and fit well around the heel. A well-fitting heel counter should give improved lateral stability, with restriction of the movements of the joints below the ankle. The construction of the shoe varies with the different sports.

Shoes are the most important items of clothing in most sports, and the right shoes are a good investment.

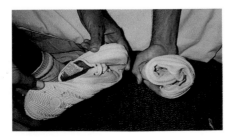

Figure 4.1 The quality of shoes varies considerably.

Equipment design and standards

Rapid technical developments in the field of sports equipment have meant both advantages and disadvantages for athletes. Performance is improving at the expense of an increase in the risk of injury. Modern alpine skis and boots, for example, have contributed both to improved performance and to a changed pattern of injuries. The design of the ski boot is such that most injuries now occur not in the area immediately above the ankle but mainly at mid-shin level and especially at the knee joint. Technical developments have also contributed to better results in athletics, for instance in pole-vaulting, where a change in design and material has resulted in a change in the technique of vaulting and the achievement of greater heights.

When new equipment is being designed, medical opinion concerning its requirements should be sought at an early stage. This enables the designer to avoid errors that could lead to an unforeseen increase in the number of injuries. If there are obvious elements of risk, then safeguards should be incorporated into the equipment from the outset. A change in one type of equipment can affect the functioning of another: for example, the shape of a ski-boot sole markedly affects the functioning of the ski binding, and the openings in the face guard used by both goalkeepers and players in ice hockey should be adjusted with the design of ice-hockey sticks in mind.

Safety standards
- Standard norms in protective equipment are a necessity.
- Equipment may cause serious injuries, especially if the rules governing its use are not followed. It is the duty of every athlete and coach to adhere to the rules of the game.
- If the rules of the game are thought to contribute to increased risks of injury, they should be changed.
- When new rules are being considered, due attention should be given, before they are finally approved, to the fact that they could lead to further risk of injury.

Protective equipment

Any protective device should prevent—or at least reduce—both long-term and short-term injuries to the part of the body for which it is designed. This is usually achieved by relieving the relevant part of the body of the full force of the impact and redistributing it over as large an area as possible. Protective equipment should not hamper the athlete's activity or technique, although the human ability to adapt is considerable. There may be restrictions in movement when, for example, a guard is first being used, but the athlete's adaptability will soon overcome any problems.

In many fields of sport there is no standard design or specification for protective equipment, so it is left to the individual athlete to evaluate its effectiveness. *Poorly designed guards give a false sense of security* which may have disastrous consequences.

Athletes and spectators alike often have preconceived ideas of what athletes should wear. If this attitude can be changed by enlightened and objective information, the use and range of protective clothing could be increased with a corresponding reduction in the number of injuries suffered.

All personal protective equipment should (and soon will) be regulated by standards, norms, and test procedures.

Helmets

Safety helmets are used by boxers, American football players, lacrosse and ice hockey players, cyclists, riders, alpine skiers, and racing drivers. Different sports have specific safety and design requirements relating to helmets, but the principles are generally similar for those used in ice hockey, cycling, riding, and American football. Considerably higher safety standards have to be met by the helmets used in alpine skiing and motor racing, because of the potentially much greater speeds of impact in these sports. Head injuries are discussed in Chapter 15.

The head must be protected from contact with other players, the ground and surrounding objects, and from blows from sticks, pucks, or balls. Safety helmets are usually made of a hard outer shell separated from the skull by a softer lining (Figure 4.2). When the helmet is subjected to a violent impact the energy is transferred to the softer lining. In some helmets, e.g. ice hockey helmets, the outer shell is semisoft, and can be partially deformed without coming into direct contact with the skull. The force of the impact is moderated by the change of shape and the remaining energy is both distributed over a larger area because of the soft lining of the helmet and further moderated when the lining is compressed.

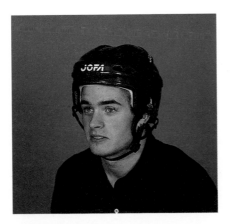

Figure 4.2 An ice hockey helmet.

For a protective helmet to fulfill its task properly, it must be fastened securely so that it does not fall off or fall down in front to block the player's vision.

Bicycle helmets

There are about a thousand fatal bicycle accidents in the USA each year half of these deaths occur in children and adolescents, and most of the victims do not wear helmets. Some studies have indicated that bicycle helmets can reduce the risk of head injuries by 85%.

In the sports in which the wearing of safety helmets is compulsory, serious head injuries have become rare, and the injuries that have occurred in spite of the helmets have been less severe. Safety standards are present for all sports helmets.

Face guards

Face guards are used by players of American football and youth hockey by goalkeepers in ice hockey, and by fencers, cricketers, and alpine skier (Figure 4.3). Facial injuries can occur as a result of a blow from a stick puck, or ball, or through collision with surrounding objects or other players. It is essential that face guards are designed with due regard for the shape and size of the equipment used in the sport concerned Standards have been laid down for the design of face guards for ice hockey and American football players.

Face guards prevent eye injuries which may cause permanent disability; cuts and gashes; and bone and dental injuries. Their success is borne out by the fact that virtually no such injuries have occurred in athletes wearing guards that completely cover the face. There is a strong case for their compulsory use in sports such as ice hockey.

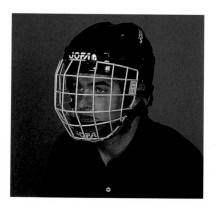

Figure 4.3 A ice hockey face guard.

A *visor*, made of Plexiglass (Perspex), covers the upper half of the face and serves mainly to protect against injuries to eyes, nose, and temple bones. A *mask* made of steel wire covers the whole or part of the face, and protects against eye injuries, fractures of facial bones, cuts and gashes to the face, and dental damage. Protective eye frames or glasses are essential for squash and other racket sports. Ski goggles are valuable protectors against snow, sun, and wind.

Gum shields

Dental injuries are serious and expensive and can present a great problem, particularly in contact sports such as rugby, boxing, ice hockey, and American football. As the loss of a tooth can influence the development of the jawbone and maxillary bone, a dental injury must be considered more serious in a young, growing athlete than in an adult. In boxing it is compulsory to use gum shields (mouth guards), which may be designed in one of two ways. An *intraoral* gum shield is made from a cast of the upper teeth and is worn inside the mouth, while an *external* shield is worn in front of the mouth. The surest protection against dental injuries is probably using both types of protection in combination.

Standards for extraoral gum shields have been established.

Neck protection

Serious injuries to the neck can be prevented by neck protection (Figure 4.4).

Shoulder padding

Shoulder padding is used by ice hockey, American football and lacrosse players, and in motor racing. Similar padding could probably also be used in other sports such as riding, cycling, alpine skiing, and ski-jumping, in which injuries to the shoulder area often occur. Shoulder injuries are discussed in Chapter 6.

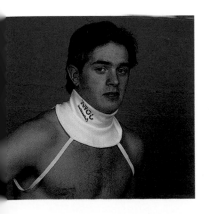

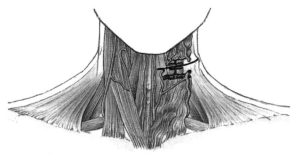

Figure 4.4 Neck protection against (e.g.) vascular traumatic injuries in skating and skiing sports.

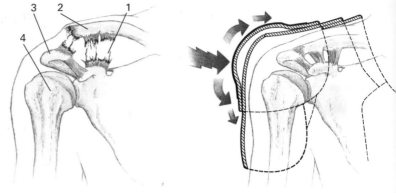

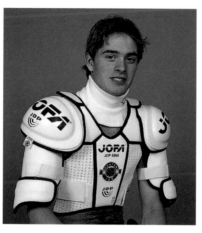

Figure 4.5 (**Left**) Shoulder acromioclavicular ligaments torn on impact; (**right**) protection afforded by padding; (**bottom**) shoulder padding. 1, Acromioclavicular ligaments; 2, clavicle; 3, acromion; 4, humerus.

Shoulder padding chiefly protects the front and outside aspect of the shoulder from impact (Figure 4.5). The padding should cushion the ball and socket joint and distribute the energy of the impact over the more robust surrounding tissues. The most common causes of shoulder injuries are falls on the outside of the shoulder, shoulder-to-shoulder tackles, or collision with the board in ice hockey. Such injuries can be prevented by shoulder padding. In American football, the tackle often hits the shoulders from above. These areas are especially protected with shoulder pads.

Shoulder padding can prevent many common injuries to the shoulder area. These are often difficult to treat and take a long time to heal.

Elbow guards

Elbow guards are used in sports such as basketball, team handball, volleyball, ice hockey, American football and lacrosse. The most common cause of elbow injuries is falling and landing on the tip of the elbow. The guard should completely cushion this area and prevent it from hitting the surface (Figure 4.6). Elbow injuries are discussed in Chapter 7.

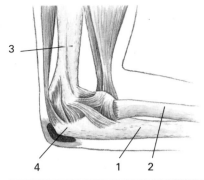
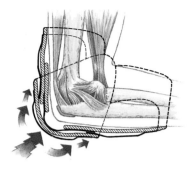
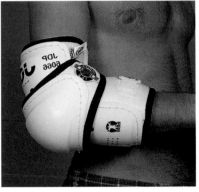

Figure 4.6 (**Left**) Elbow area vulnerable to impact; (**right**) protection afforded by padding; (**bottom**) elbow guard. 1, Ulna; 2, radius; 3, humerus; 4, olecranon.

In the short term, elbow guards prevent injuries to the bursa and the tip of the elbow, and in the long term, they prevent cartilage injuries in the elbow joints.

Wrist guard

Wrist guards should be used in sports such as inline skating, skateboarding, or snowboarding (see Figure 4.7).

Genital protectors

Boxes (cups) are used by ice hockey and soccer players, cricketers, and boxers, and sometimes by American footballers, team handball players and others. A box should enclose the penis as well as the testicles and protect them against direct impact.

In the short term, a box protects against the acute pain caused by a direct blow to the genitals. As these organs are invested with a good blood supply, they are very susceptible to bleeding after a blow to this area. The bleeding can be difficult to treat and may cause recurrent problems.

Hip or thigh guards

Hip or thigh guards are used by cricketers, ice hockey and American football players, and by goalkeepers in team handball and field hockey; they should be used more extensively. There are only a few hip guards on the market and they are generally badly designed. A hip or thigh guard should cushion the upper end of the femur and thus unload the hip joint itself. Groin and thigh injuries are discussed in Chapter 10.

> In the short term, hip or thigh guards prevent the pain and bleeding that may occur after falls and during tackles by an opponent. In the long term the guards prevent cartilage injuries in the hip joint by diverting direct impact.

Knee pads

Knee pads protect the knee joints only during falls, and not when they are subjected to blows from the side or to twisting, which may cause meniscus or ligament injuries (Figure 4.7). Combined knee and shin pads are used by ice and field hockey players, while separate knee pads are used by basketball, team handball and volleyball players, and by American footballers, cricketers, and soccer goalkeepers.

The pads should cushion the force of the impact from falls as well as from blows to the knees and shins. The patella is especially sensitive and should be completely cushioned from impact, so that a blow to the knee is redistributed over the surrounding tissues (Figure 4.8). Knee injuries are discussed in Chapter 11.

> It is important that the knee joint is cushioned to avoid cartilage injuries to joint surfaces, especially in the patellofemoral joint.

Shin pads

Shin pads are used to protect the shin from kicks and painful contact with the surroundings (Figure 4.9). Further development and research are needed to improve the shock absorption provided by shin pads and ultimately to reduce the risk of injury to bone and soft tissue. Lower leg injuries are discussed in Chapter 12.

> Shin pads should be capable of preventing the occurrence of bone and soft tissue injuries, or at least of reducing their severity, by distributing the force of the impact on the shin over a larger area.

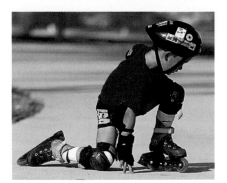

Figure 4.7 Knee pads protect the knee against a fall (by courtesy of All Sport: photographer, Simon Bruty).

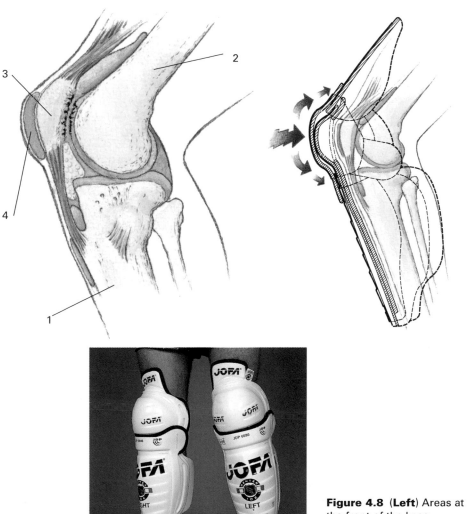

Figure 4.8 (**Left**) Areas at the front of the knee vulnerable to impact or twisting; (**right**) protection afforded by padding; (**bottom**) knee pads. 1, Tibia; 2, femur; 3, patella; 4, bursa.

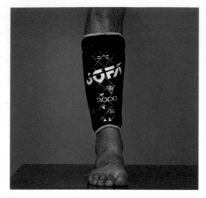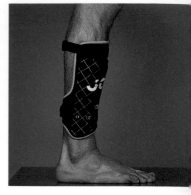

Figure 4.9 Shin pads.

Ankle and foot protection

For many athletes, shoes or boots are of prime importance since the protect against overuse injuries and sprains. The development of th protective properties of shoes, however, has been neglected, and we hav for example, only a limited knowledge of the relationship between th playing surface, the shoe and the foot, and of the importance of th design of the sole with regard to studs, profile, resilience, and so on.

The skating boot offers ice hockey players a built-in protection again: injuries to the ankle and foot; alpine skiers have a similar protection i the ski boot. Skating and ski boots protect the ligaments and bon in the foot and ankle. Ankle and foot injuries are discussed in Chapte 13 and 14.

Ski safety bindings

Ski injuries continue to be common in spite of improved equipment an better facilities. The safeguard of importance in preventing injuries i skiing is the safety-release binding of the ski, providing it has bee correctly designed and set. The type of ski binding has a direct effect c the overall injury rate in skiers. Some injuries occur because the relea: bindings are poorly designed and adjusted, and the binding fails to relea properly, or releases at the wrong time. During the past few years the has been a significant reduction in binding-related injuries. There evidence that a better-functioning ski binding is the single most impo tant factor contributing to this trend, but approximately 30% of a injuries still remain related to improper binding performance.

The binding can be a multidirectional release, which releases in a direction the skier might fall. Bindings today still most commonly ha a limited release function such as a side-to-side or twist release capabi ity at the toe, and a forward lean mechanism on the heel. Few bindin; incorporate several of these modes. The choice of ski binding for beginner, who tends to fall frequently, should be a multimode relea system.

Binding function should be checked regularly and well maintained. Mechanical checks should be carried out at least once before each season. The boots, bindings, and skis should be kept clean. The bindings should be tested each time someone uses the skis. The bindings should be tested in each and every direction before going on the slopes.

Ski poles and gloves

Injury to the ulnar collateral ligament at the base of the thumb is the most common upper extremity injury to the skier, and is to some extent related to the design of the poles. A ski pole should be designed so that it can readily be discarded (Figure 4.10). Another technique is to avoid placing the hand through the strap, so that the ski pole can be dropped during the fall.

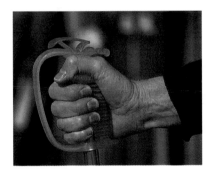

Figure 4.10 This ski pole can easily be discarded.

Gloves protect against fractures of the bones of the hand and painful bruising. They are used mainly by ice hockey and American football players, cricketers, and boxers. Injuries to the ligaments of the thumb and wrist may also be prevented. Wrist and hand injuries are discussed in Chapter 9.

General advice

It is in the interests of every athlete to obtain the best possible protection in order to prevent injury.

Athletes should form their own opinions about the risks of injury in their particular sport, and should then test the protective clothing available. If this advice were followed more widely it would be possible to reduce the injury rate in many sports, especially in sports such as rugby in which traditionally little or no protection is employed.

5 Principles of treatment

Acute phase

Soft tissue injuries include:
- muscle and tendon damage (hematoma and/or rupture);
- joint and ligament damage (dislocation and/or rupture);
- soft tissue injuries associated with fractures.

When muscles, tendons, or ligaments are damaged, blood vessels in the area are also torn, and bleeding spreads rapidly into adjacent tissues. The bleeding causes swelling, placing increased pressure on surrounding tissues, which become tense and tender. The increased pressure causes pain in sensitive tissues, and the combination of bleeding, swelling, and increased pressure can adversely affect and delay the healing process (Figure 5.1).

In cases of soft tissue injury, it is important to inhibit and control bleeding as soon as possible. Treatment should be started immediately. Correct initial treatment of a soft tissue injury can be the most important factor influencing recovery.

Once bleeding has been controlled, some blood remains in the tissues and has to be resorbed. This function is performed mainly by the lymphatic system. A variable amount of scar tissue forms in the area and constitutes a weak spot in the injured muscle, tendon, or ligament. If too

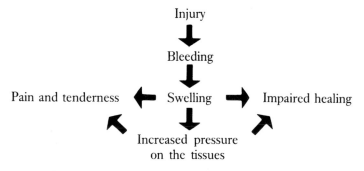

Figure 5.1 The soft tissue injury process.

early or too heavy a load is applied to this scar tissue, injury is liable to recur.

Sports injuries may take so many different forms that it is impossible to create a standard protocol for their management. Certain guidelines for immediate treatment can, however, be drawn up.

Immediate management

- An on-the-spot assessment of the extent of injury should be made by the injured athlete or by the trainer (Figure 5.2). A more careful examination can follow in a quiet place such as the changing room.
- The injured athlete should be undressed to the extent necessary for a full examination of the injured area. Tapes, strapping, and protective pads are removed.
- The course of events should be analyzed. Listen to the injured athlete's description of how the injury occurred and what symptoms are present.
- The injury should be examined in the light of the history. Is there any effusion of blood, swelling, an open wound, or any other abnormal sign?
- A simple functional assessment of the injured part should be made. Can the injured athlete carry out normal movements of the part (with or without a load) without pain?
- The area around the injury should be examined. Is there tenderness in soft tissues or bone? Can a defect be felt in any soft tissue?

If there is swelling and tenderness together with pain when movements are made or a load is applied, treatment should be started as follows.

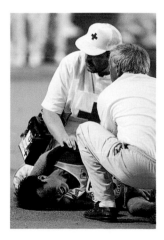

Figure 5.2 On-the-spot assessment (by courtesy of All Sport: photographer, Mike Powell).

Compression

A compression bandage is intended to provide counterpressure to the bleeding developing within the injured area, so that the body's own

91

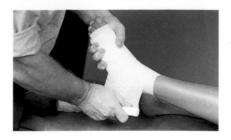

Figure 5.3 Immediate compression is most effective in acute injuries.

hemostatic functions can take effect more easily. A compression bandage is an elastic bandage applied with careful tension. It should be applied as soon as possible (Figure 5.3). It is convenient to position an ice pack with the aid of an elastic bandage so that cooling and compression effects are achieved simultaneously. The compression bandage should be kept in position usually for another 2 days after cooling has ceased, provided the location and extent of the injury allow it. Later it may be replaced by a supportive bandage or strapping.

> A compression bandage is the most effective way to limit a hematoma and swelling and should be applied as soon as possible. Be careful not to apply too much tension to the bandage.

Cryotherapy (cooling)

When soft tissue injuries occur, the first priority is to attempt to stop the bleeding, since this results in swelling, pain, and tenderness. The general rule is that the lighter the bleeding, the faster the effusion of blood disappears, and the less scar tissue forms in the injured tissue. Therefore, in soft tissue injuries, reduce the extent of the bleeding by compression bandaging, rapid cooling, an elevated position of the injured limb, and rest. This enables the hemostatic functions of the body itself to take effect more easily. Cooling of body tissues brings about:

– *a local pain-relieving effect* which makes the injured athlete feel better and may encourage a return to sporting activity. Here trainers and coaches have a great responsibility: if an injury needs cooling it is probably of such severity that further exertion will only delay healing. Common sense should prevail;

– *contraction of the blood vessels* so that the blood flow is reduced in the injured area. The effect of the treatment is limited and does not really start for 15 minutes. Less swelling may occur and healing proceed more rapidly.

> In the presence of signs of extensive soft tissue injury with bleeding or injury to the skeleton, the injured person must not resume sporting activity until the injury has healed. Nothing is gained by endangering future health.

Cryotherapy is usually applied for 15–20 minutes per treatment and may be applied hourly for the first 24–72 hours after the injury. During each application of cold therapy, four progressive sensations will be experienced: cold, burning, aching, and numbness.

Cryotherapy is beneficial for sports injuries because:
- the patient quickly feels an improvement in symptoms;
- the treatment is easy to carry out and is well tolerated;
- there are few risks;
- it is inexpensive.

Cryotherapy cooling is mainly a treatment for pain and can be applied in several ways.

Ice massage

Ice massage is most commonly used prior to range-of-motion exercises, for friction massage, and for its localized analgesic effect. Ice is rubbed over the area in small circular movements for 5–10 minutes until numbness is reached.

Ice packs and contoured cryo-cuffs

Ice packs made with ice cubes or ice chips are by far the most popular, effective, and easiest method of application. The ice pack is applied to the area for 15–20 minutes, often wrapped on with an elastic bandage for compression and perhaps a light layer of material between the skin and ice for skin protection (Figure 5.4). Ice packs may be molded to the body contour and elevated above the heart to minimize swelling.

Contoured cryo-cuffs use ice water flowing into a contoured insulated pack, while a moderate amount of compression is maintained at the same time, thus combining cold and compression. However, they are more expensive.

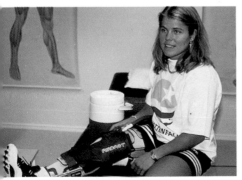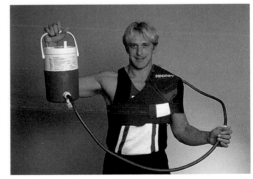

igure 5.4 (Left) Cryo-cuff on knee; **(right)** cryo-cuff on shoulder.

Ice immersion, cold whirlpools

Ice immersion and cold whirlpools are often used to combine the analgesic effect of the cold and the buoyancy of water to treat the inflammatory phase and allow early range-of-motion exercises. The water should be maintained at a temperature of 10–15 °C (50–60 °F). Treatment lasts 5–1. minutes. As pain is relieved, the body part is removed from the water and functional movements are performed.

Commercial cold gel and chemical packs

Commercially available cold packs are generally made up of a chemica or gelatinous substance enclosed in a strong vinyl case. The packs are activated by squeezing or hitting the pack against a hard area, thereby setting off a chemical reaction to produce the cold. These packs are convenient to carry, and many are single-use disposable packs. They can be expensive and are usually do not maintain their coldness as well a real ice. The packs can be molded to the body area and used with eleva tion just as with ice for treatments.

Cold water

Cold water can be used for cooling injuries when ice packs are not a hand, and also when the injuries involve larger areas which cannot easil be covered with packs of the usual size.

Neither cold water nor ice packs should be used directly on open wounds.

Cooling sprays

A cooling spray may be used when local pain relief is the only objective This applies to areas where the skin is in close contact with the skeletor such as the shins, knuckles, and ankles. The cold from such a spra penetrates only 3–4 mm (0.12–0.25 in) into the skin and therefore doe not affect underlying injured tissue. There may be some contraction o deeper blood vessels triggered by reflex action, but this effect is probabl only slight and transitory. Cooling ceases after spraying has stopped, and the blood flow subsequently increases, *causing an effect entirely opposite t that desired*. Apart from this disadvantage, there is also a risk of inducing cold injuries to the skin when a cooling spray is used.

Cooling has mainly a pain-inhibiting effect. Cooling will therefore mask the real extent of the injury. There is a great risk that an injury will get worse if the athlete resumes activity after cooling.

Rest

It is generally true to say that an injured athlete should rest the injure part for 24–48 hours and that it should not be subjected to loading. I follows, therefore, that the athlete should be assisted from the scene of th injury and taken home or to a doctor, as soon as possible. Crutches are usually very helpful in the acute phase.

Elevation

When an injured part is elevated, its blood flow is reduced, and expelled blood is transported away from the site of injury more easily, thus reducing swelling. An injured leg that is elevated should be supported at an angle of more than 45° when the patient is lying supine. Four or five cushions or a stool placed under the leg will achieve this effect. In cases of extensive bleeding and swelling the injured part should be kept elevated for 24–48 hours if possible. Subsequently, it should be elevated whenever the opportunity arises.

Pain relief

Cooling, compression, and rest usually provide relief from pain in soft tissue injuries. Pain-relieving medication may be given if the examination is complete but should be avoided in the early stages as it can complicate further treatment if continued analysis and medical examination are required.

Preparation

At sporting venues available equipment should include (as well as the trainers' and physicians' kits) crutches, stretchers, and immobilization splints. An emergency plan should be in place to provide adequate acute treatment and transportation. Staff should be well educated and trained.

Treatment within 24–48 hours

When a soft tissue injury does not require further medical treatment, but effusion, pain, and impaired functioning of the injured part are present, treatment should continue along the following lines:

compression bandaging replaced after a few hours by a support bandage;
- *further cooling* if pain relief is the objective;
- *rest* the injured area if there is persistent pain;
- *elevation* of the injured part. If walking is necessary, use crutches to unload the injured area if the lower limbs are involved.

A limb that has suffered a soft tissue injury should not be loaded or used until a definitive diagnosis has been made. In cases of extensive bleeding, persistent pain, and impaired functioning, or when there is uncertainty about the correct treatment method, a doctor should be consulted.

Injured athletes should seek a medical opinion within 24–48 hours in cases of:
- persistent symptoms arising from injuries to muscle, tendon, joint, or ligament;
- severe pain.

It is generally true to say that a doctor should be consulted if there is any uncertainty about the diagnosis, and thus the treatment, of any sports injury.

Urgent conditions

For lifethreatening injuries, see p. 428. A medical opinion should be sought *urgently* in any of the following circumstances:
- unconsciousness or persistent headache, nausea, vomiting, or dizziness after a head injury;
- breathing difficulties after blows to the head, neck or chest;
- pains in the neck after impact, whether or not they extend to the arms;
- abdominal pain;
- blood in the urine;
- fracture or suspected fracture;
- severe joint or ligament injury;
- severe muscle or tendon injury;
- dislocation;
- severe eye injury;
- deep wound with bleeding;
- injuries with intense pain;
- any injury in which there is doubt about its severity, diagnosis or treatment.

Remember that if free breathing is secured and any bleeding stopped the seriously injured can be saved.

Treatment after 48 hours

As well as the treatment options described in this section, exercises are an important part of long-term treatment and are described in Chapter 21.

Rest

After any injury it is usually necessary to avoid painful activities and to rest the affected part, and occasionally confinement to bed is justified. In cases of overuse injuries and in certain ligamentous injuries accompanied by swelling, adhesive strapping or tape may provide relief. Rest is also recommended after an operation. It is usually continued until pain and swelling are negligible before loading the injured part.

Even if an injured athlete is obliged to wear a cast or a brace, other parts of the body can still be trained and muscle exercises and conditioning carried out. A lower leg in a cast or brace does not prevent physical fitness being maintained by activities such as cycling. The immobilized part should be held in an elevated position and exercised by repeated isometric contractions.

Although rest and immobilization are beneficial in the acute stage they have deleterious effects on all tissues in the long term. Early motion is essential.

Heat treatment (thermotherapy)

Heat has been used for thousands of years in the treatment of different types of pain. Experience shows that it has a beneficial effect on pain arising from inflammation, which is the body's defense mechanism in cases of injury due either to accident or to overuse. Injuries caused by trauma or overuse, such as ligament injuries and muscle ruptures, are often treated during the acute stage by cooling and bandaging so that the bleeding in the injured area is limited. After the initial 48 hours, heat treatment can be introduced to help the healing process. Heat may be started once the risk of hemorrhage is over, and aids healing by increasing the blood flow to the injured area.

If an injury is treated by heat applications in its acute stage the blood vessels expand, and the blood clotting procedure may be disrupted. The amount of fluid in the tissue increases. This leads to increased bleeding in the injured area, increased swelling and higher pressure in the surrounding tissues. The result may be more pain and slower healing than would otherwise be the case.

Heat treatment should not be started until at least 48 hours after the injury has occurred. The same applies to massage.

Perhaps the most important effect of heat treatment is its influence on collagen fibers. A tendon is composed of 90% collagen fibers and 10% elastic fibers. Collagen has viscous and elastic properties, which means that the more rapidly a tendon is loaded, the stiffer (less elastic) and less extensible it becomes. Heat increases elasticity and plasticity, so after its application the collagen fibers become more extensible and more capable of rehabilitation exercises. Heat also decreases joint stiffness and relieves muscle spasm. This reduces the risk of injury.

Heat can be used in both the prevention and rehabilitation of overuse injuries and to combat the after-effects of torn muscles and tendons. It can be valuable during warm-up before training sessions and competitions and in cold weather, increasing the mobility of joints.

Heat treatment provides pain relief, makes collagen fibers more extensible, and is of great importance as a means of both preventing and rehabilitating injuries.

Heat therapy is used after the acute inflammatory stage to increase blood flow and promote healing to the injured area. It increases circulation and cellular metabolism, decreases muscle spasm, and has an analgesic effect on surrounding tissues. Heat is typically used before activity to increase the extensibility of connective tissues, leading to an increased range of motion. The depth of heat penetration depends on the method of application.

Superficial heat treatment

Superficial modalities transfer heat by conduction, convection, and radiation. The heat penetrates to a depth of less than 1 cm (0.4 in).

Whirlpools

Whirlpools combine warmth with a hydromassaging effect to increase superficial skin temperature, decrease muscle spasm and pain, and facilitate range-of-motion exercises. Treatment times are from 20–30 minutes with the body part to be treated immersed in water at temperatures of 37–40 °C (100–105 °F).

Hydrocollator packs

Hydrocollator packs provide superficial moist heat to a slightly greater tissue depth than whirlpool treatment. The packs consist of a silicone gel encased in canvas fabric compartments, and are stored in a hot water unit. The pack is wrapped in terry toweling or a commercially available hot-pack cover and placed over the injured area for 20 minutes.

Contrast baths

Contrast baths combine cryotherapy and thermotherapy to reduce edema and restore range of motion in subacute or chronic injuries. One whirlpool or container is filled with cold water and ice at 10–15 °C (50–60 °F) and the other is filled with hot water at 37–43 °C (98–108 °F). The injured body part is alternated between the two containers at a 3:1, 3:2 or 4:1 ratio of hot to cold for approximately 20 minutes, or 4 or 5 cycles. The treatment should end in the cold water.

Heat retainer

A heat retainer is a support made of synthetic material which generates and retains heat in the parts of the body which it encloses. It can be effective at rest as well as in training and competition. Heat retainers are made of a fine, porous material with low fluid absorption and good heat retention. They have an elasticity which keeps them in place without hampering movement in the bandaged part of the body. In addition, they give some support and exert counterpressure which may be of value when there is swelling. They are available in versions suitable for most joints and most types of injuries (Figure 5.5).

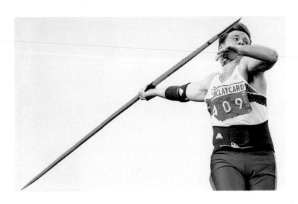

Figure 5.5 A heat retainer is often effective.

Heat retainers have been tested clinically to assess their effect on prevention as well as treatment of sports injuries, and results have been good. By relieving pain, improving tissue elasticity, and maintaining and extending the range of mobility, they assist not only the rehabilitation of ligament injuries in the knees and ankles but also the treatment of pain arising from muscle injuries and osteoarthritis.

Heat retainers are a simple form of thermotherapy and are a valuable addition to the range of treatments available. They can be useful at rest as well as in training for the prevention and treatment of injuries due to overuse and trauma, both in sporting and other activities.

Deep heat treatment

Ultrasound

Ultrasound waves are of a higher frequency than those detectable by the human ear. The penetration of ultrasonic waves is inversely related to their frequency. As the ultrasonic beam travels through tissue, the energy is absorbed, producing heat. Ultrasound energy can produce temperature increases in tissue as deep as 10 cm (4 in). The technique is especially suitable for the treatment of pain in tendon attachments.

The indications for ultrasound treatment are pain and inflammatory conditions that are deeply located. Ultrasound can reduce the pain as well as increase the extensibility of the collagen fibers. It has been shown to be effective in combination with stretching. It may have some effect on calcium deposits in various tissues, but this is debatable.

Phonophoresis

Phonophoresis uses the mechanical energy of ultrasound to introduce medications such as cortisone through the skin to deeper tissues. In one study, 68% of those receiving phonophoresis with hydrocortisone cream obtained relief from pain and improved range of motion, compared with 28% of patients receiving ultrasound alone. This medication has been found 10 cm (4 in) deep within the tissue after 5 minutes of treatment, but it is not known how long it remains. This procedure is used in the postacute stage of inflammatory conditions such as tendinitis, bursitis, contusion, or arthritis. The advantage of this treatment is that the medication is delivere directly to the injury site but it is less invasive than an anti-inflammato injection, and may be used where an injection is contraindicated.

Electrical stimulation

Electrical stimulation is increasingly widely used (Figure 5.6). It has thr recognized applications for the treatment of soft tissue injuries:
- pain reduction by transcutaneous stimulation of sensory nerves; this known as transcutaneous electrical nerve stimulation (TENS);
- muscle strengthening; electrotherapy is sometimes used after surge when hypotrophy is serious;
- enhancement of healing

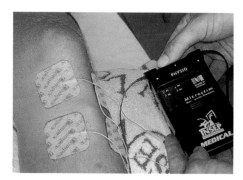

Figure 5.6 Electrical stimulation device.

More research concerning the effects of electrical stimulation is neede Although electrical stimulation may control pain and be beneficial muscle strengthening, it should not be used in routine rehabilitatio Treatment should be given by knowledgeable physical therapists only.

Iontophoresis

Iontophoresis uses a direct current to drive charged molecules of medic tion into damaged tissue. The medication is placed under the electro with the same polarity and the molecules are pushed away from t electrode into the skin toward the injured site. Anti-inflammator analgesic or anesthetic drugs may be used.

TENS

Transcutaneous electrical nerve stimulation enhances the body's abili to control pain. A weak electric current is applied to the skin in t painful area by means of superficial electrodes. The response to TEN varies, and some, but not all, patients find it very effective in relievi pain. It probably exerts its effect by activating a 'gate' mechanism in t spinal cord which prevents painful sensations from reaching the brain

Acupuncture

Acupuncture is widely used in China where the method was developed and is used increasingly all over the world. Traditional acupuncture is based on the assumption that each half of the body has 12 meridians, representing certain organ systems. Along these meridians are a number of points that are connected with particular organs, and these points can be stimulated by needles of varying shape and length, effecting changes in the organs concerned. The connection between the meridians and anatomical nervous pathways has not yet been explained. The effect of the acupuncture needles is intensified by rotating them or connecting them to a low-voltage power source (electroacupuncture).

Scientific evaluation of acupuncture is as yet incomplete and inconclusive, but it does seem to benefit a significant number of people.

Massage

Massage has been used in the world of sport from time immemorial. It was once thought that it increased the blood flow in muscles and thus relieved pain, stiffness, and tenderness. However, studies have not been able to prove that blood flow is increased, although massage does bring about symptomatic improvement.

Massage should not be too vigorous, and should work inwards from the extremities towards the heart. Carried out by a trained and capable masseur, massage can produce a feeling of general well-being and relaxation (Figure 5.7).

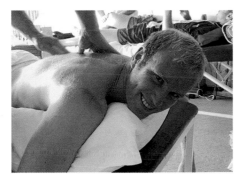

Figure 5.7 Massage is a popular therapy.

Water massage

Water massage is usually carried out in hot water. The injured part is immersed for about 20 minutes during which time air is injected under high pressure into the water, providing an effect similar to that of manual massage. Use of a whirlpool or jacuzzi enables the whole body or individual part to be immersed alternately in hot and cold water, which is supposed to stimulate circulation and facilitate healing and rehabilitation.

Support bandages

Different types of support bandage are used depending on the degree of stability required.

An *elastic bandage* is made of cotton woven together with strands of rubber. It can be used for securing dressings or ice packs over injured areas and also provides compression in acute injuries, such as ankle sprains. The elastic bandage is flexible and stretches after use, which makes it unsuitable for long-term support. It has the advantage of being washable, and can be reused.

An adhesive elastic bandage is firm and flexible and its adhesive properties provide a strong hold. It is particularly useful for injuries of the knee, ankle, and wrist. Adhesive elastic bandages can also be used for taping as a preventive measure. Disadvantages of this type of bandage are that it is bulky and cannot be reused.

Self-adhesive elastic bandages consist of closely packed, unwoven polyester fibers. This type of bandage adheres to itself but not to the skin. It does not interfere with the normal functions of the skin, and is nonallergenic. It remains in place during bathing and dries quickly after getting wet. Self-adhesive elastic bandaging can be used as a preventive measure as well as during rehabilitation after an injury. It provides a stable but flexible dressing which is not bulky and even fits inside a shoe when applied to the foot. If the correct technique is used when applying the dressing and its elasticity is not overstretched, self-adhesive elastic bandage can be used as a semi-permanent support in ligament and other soft tissue injuries.

Braces

Braces are increasingly used in sports. They are mostly used for the ankle and knee, but are increasingly used for the shoulder, elbow, hand, and wrist.

Knee braces

Knee injuries are often serious. The risk of knee injuries is 6–22% each year for a college American football player. Many of these injured players use knee braces of some kind during the treatment phase. Knee braces can be divided into three types: prophylactic, rehabilitative, and functional.

Prophylactic knee braces

Prophylactic knee braces are designed to distribute applied loads away from the knee joint and, thereby, reduce the load on the medial collateral ligament (MCL) and perhaps also on the anterior cruciate ligament (ACL). Biomechanical studies indicate that there may be a limited protection to the MCL and ACL when they are subjected to valgus loads. Research indicates increased stiffness to valgus loads, with highest efficiency around 20°. The benefits have, however, been documented only for low nonphysiologic loading. The few clinical studies available indicated a trend in the reduction of serious MCL injuries. There has been only one report of a prospective randomized study controlling playing surface, shoe wear and type of brace, that also included a control group: this study indicated that a prophylactic knee brace can reduce the amount of knee and MCL injuries in defensive players in American football.

Rehabilitative knee braces

Rehabilitative knee braces are at least as effective as a plaster cast in treatment of complete MCL injuries, since they allow controlled early motion. They are valuable during the first weeks of conservative treatment of knee ligament injuries and after knee ligament surgery.

Functional knee braces

Functional braces (Figure 5.8) are valuable in supporting the knee so that the joint can function without 'giving way'. The brace operates by interacting with ligament, meniscus, and muscle function. The functional knee brace supports the following:
- varus/valgus (side-to-side) instability with medial and lateral side posts;
- anterior tibial translation (tibia moves forward in relation to femur) by preventing hyperextension ;
- rotational control—this is extremely difficult to achieve and at present no brace can really control rotation;
- suspension is the most difficult part to control in these braces as the thigh muscles are very giving and their motions are difficult to control.

Biomechanical studies show that functional knee braces can reduce anterior translation at low physiological loads and during weightbearing. Clinical studies show that the athlete experiences positive effects from the brace, although many may continue to have some instability episodes

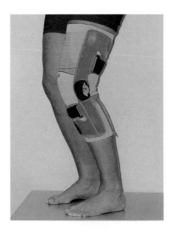

Figure 5.8 Functional knee brace.

despite brace wear. The braces have a verified effect on activities of daily living, but during physical activities benefits are not well documented and vary from individual to individual.

Braces for patellofemoral pain syndrome

Braces for use in patellofemoral pain syndrome (p. 310) have unloading areas designed to fit against the patella. They usually incorporate horseshoe-shaped lateral supports to stabilize the patella and prevent lateral subluxation. Medial straps may give extra stability. Some studies indicate that these braces improve the performance of these patients. Bracing seems to make it possible to include isotonic and isokinetic exercises in the rehabilitation program and to allow early return to recreational and athletic activities.

Ankle braces

Ankle injuries account for 15% of all athletic injuries. To reduce the incidence, athletic tape and bracing are extensively used to support the ankle joint (Figure 5.9). Ankle braces do not, as a rule, significantly affect performance. There may be a slightly decreased performance in vertical jumping.

Biomechanical studies indicate that some support is provided by these braces, especially in the loading situation. Clinical studies show that braces decrease the severity of ankle sprains and also decrease the recurrence of ankle sprains. Other studies show that the combination of low top shoes and ankle stabilizers are the most effective means of preventing ankle injuries in college American football players.

Taping and bracing are both effective in rehabilitation after ankle injuries. Taping will, however, lose its biomechanical support over time and ankle braces seem to be more effective in reducing ankle injuries. Taping is, however, still popular with athletes who perceive it not to affect performance. The use of ankle braces will increase as the designs become lighter and more effective.

In the treatment of acute first-time ankle sprains research shows that the combination of an ankle brace and an ace wrap seems to be the most effective (Figure 5.10).

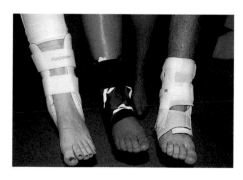

Figure 5.9 Ankle braces.

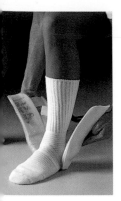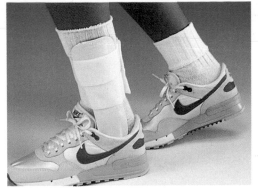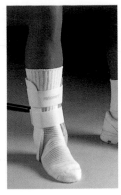

Figure 5.10 (Left) An ankle brace in combination with an ace wrap is a very effective treatment in acute and subacute ankle sprains, whether with (**middle**) or without (**right**) a shoe.

Shoulder braces

Surgery for anterior shoulder instability can be successful, but the use of bracing is controversial. A few shoulder braces are commercially available. The aim of these braces is to limit abduction and external rotation, and prevent the shoulder from being placed in unstable positions. These braces are large and affect the performance of highly skilled athletes. They can be used by ice hockey players, for example, who do not perform overhead shoulder movements. No clinical or biomechanical studies have evaluated these braces.

Elbow braces

Elbow braces are available for tennis elbow (p. 166) or elbow hyperextension injuries.

Braces for tennis elbow are based on the counterforce principle. An elastic strap placed on the proximal portion of the forearm provides a counterforce to muscle contractions either by constraining full muscular expansion and thereby decreasing the potential force the muscle can generate, or by dispersing pressure from the area of injury, which lessens the stress at the lateral epicondyle. The counterforce brace thereby controls the muscle forces and directs the tension overload to healthy tissue. Studies indicate that the counterforce brace decreases the electromyographic activity in the proximal lower arm muscles. In athletes with tennis elbow, the counterforce brace may produce significant increases in wrist extension and grip strength, although no significant effect on perceived pain has been reported. Although scientific evidence is limited, these braces seem valuable in the management of tennis elbow.

Traumatic hyperextension injuries may occur in contact sports such as American football and wrestling. Braces are available that can prevent elbow hyperextension.

Hand and wrist braces

Functional wrist orthoses for ligament injuries of the wrist can be fabricated to protect the injury and allow return to sports. Even distal radius and scaphoid fractures can be protected this way.

Stener's lesion (p. 198), which is an injury to the ulnar collateral ligament, can be treated by protective devices. These often have to be properly padded as the hard and nonyielding materials used are not allowed in many sports. Less severe cases can be well treated by taping.

Bibliography

Ough JV, Clancy WG (1993) Functional knee braces: review *Orthopaedics* 16: 171–176.

Rovere GD, Clark TJ, Yeats CS et al. (1988) Retrospective comparison of taping and ankle stabilizers in preventing ankle injuries. *American Journal of Sports Medicine* 16(2): 228–233.

Taping

Tape was known to be in use in Egypt around 300 BC. Tape is still extensively used, especially for ankle ligament injuries. Taping is mainly used for the protection of uninjured ankle ligaments, but it is also used after injury to prevent recurrence or worsening of the injury. After a recently healed ankle ligament injury, the ankle needs long-term rehabilitation to regain strength and nerve muscle function. During this time it is valuable for the ankle to be protected in order to prevent recurrence.

The object of taping is to *support a weakened part of the body without limiting its function, by preventing movements that would stress the weakened area*. However, this goal is difficult to achieve, even when taping is correctly applied.

Indications for taping

The primary purpose of taping is to provide a semirigid or rigid splint around a joint and/or surrounding tissue. Taping has stabilizing effects mainly on structures and joints where there is little soft tissue, and where the skin can not move too freely around the joint, such as the ankle and wrist joints. Taping soft tissue injuries such as a ruptured thigh muscle may be questioned since it is doubtful whether tape has a stabilizing influence in this case. There may, however, be a compression effect which can be beneficial.

Taping and performance

Taping an injured ankle will decrease its range of motion for 2–3 hours of physical activity. Correctly applied tape probably does not affect performance in sports very much. Biomechanically the support of tape is limited, but clinically it does seem to have an effect. Studies on tiltboards indicate that taping has a proprioceptive effect on unstable ankles.

Applications

Acute injury

It can be risky to use tape on acute injuries, and overtight taping of an area in which swelling and bleeding are occurring may cause serious impairment of circulation.

If an acute injury is to be taped, this should only be done by a doctor experienced in these injuries, using elastic tape.

Before taping an acute injury a detailed medical examination should be carried out, including a careful stability test. If there are any indications of a total rupture, taping should not be used. The taping of an acute injury may unfortunately lull the athlete into a false sense of security, encouraging the resumption of sporting activity which will make the injury considerably worse.

Preventive taping

There has been some suggestion that taping healthy ankles as a preventive measure could, by changing mechanical conditions, increase the occurrence of knee injuries. Research has shown that this is not the case, and has confirmed that preventive taping can decrease the number of ligament injuries to the ankle. It is of particular value in sports in which the ankles are vulnerable to violent impact, e.g. soccer, team handball, and volleyball.

Ligaments such as those around the ankle joint can be subjected to repeated impact and injuries with a result that they become weak and stretched. *In such cases taping plays an important part in contributing to the stability of the joint.* If, despite precautions, progressive instability of the joint is seen, surgery should be considered.

Taping during rehabilitation

Taping is most useful in rehabilitation after an injury has been treated surgically or has healed spontaneously. It is becoming common for athletes to use taping when they resume sporting activity after an injury, though the value of this practice has not been proven. Studies have shown that taping the knee joint does not provide stability to any significant degree. In cases of medial instability of the knee, taping gives virtually no support after 5 minutes' hard physical activity.

Used correctly, taping can be of value after an injury, but it should not be considered to be a miracle cure for all cases.

Types of tape

The tape in general use is inelastic and is available in a range of widths; 38 mm (1.5 in) and 50 mm (2 in) widths are often used. The tape is perforated so that strips can be torn off easily. By stretching the tape before application it is possible to achieve a firm restriction early in the range of movement.

Risks of taping

- In certain situations, for example in acute injuries, taping may restrict circulation.
- The long-term effect of taping is limited. It can never provide a permanent solution, and there are few justifications for using it continuously for as long as a week.
- Skin irritations may occur if tape is in contact with the skin for a long period. This problem is unlikely to occur in less than a week, but as a rule tape should not be used directly on the skin for more than a few hours at a time. If it is necessary to exceed this limit, a protective material should be worn under the tape.

Tape may cause irritation by mechanical or chemical means or because of allergy, and the effects may be exaggerated by sweating, itching, and bacterial infection. In order to reduce the risk of skin irritation some tapes are backed with zinc oxide.

Applying the tape

Knowledge of taping is gained first by instruction and thereafter by experience. It is only possible to learn how to tape quickly and safely by constant practice. Figure 5.11 demonstrates the technique, but the following points should also be noted:

- Any body hair in the area to be taped should be shaved. If the skin is damaged or infected it is advisable to wait until it has healed before tape is applied.
- The skin in the area to be taped must be cleaned, as grease or sweat will stop the tape adhering. An adhesive spray may also be used.
- Various types of tape underlay in the form of thin plastic foam, adhesive cream, or plastic dressing can be applied to the skin. One of these underlays should be used if the tape is to be worn for a long time or if skin allergy occurs.
- A tape bandage must never be applied around a swollen joint as it may impede circulation.
- In principle, application of a tape bandage should begin distal to the injured part, be built up over the injury, and be fastened below it.
- Tape adheres better to itself than to skin, so an 'anchor' of tape should be applied on each side of the injured joint. The injured ligament which is to be supported should be held in a shortened position during taping. If, for example, the ligament on the lateral (outer) aspect of the ankle is injured, the lateral (outer) edge of the foot should be directed upwards and the tape stretched over the outer side of the joint.

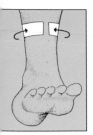 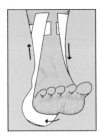 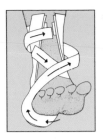 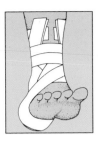 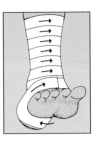

Figure 5.11 How to tape an injury to the lateral ligaments of the ankle.

– Folds and creases in the dressing should be smoothed out, as they may cause blisters and skin irritation. The effect of the bandage is also reduced if the tape is 'concertinaed'.
– The tape should be removed with care. It is better to try to 'push' the skin away from the tape rather than to tear or pull the tape away from the skin. The edges of the wound are often difficult to free, but it can sometimes be effective to hold the skin tight and pull it from the tape. Alternatively, tape bandages can be removed with the help of tape cutters or tape scissors; solvents are also available.
– The athlete should always be listened to, and if the tape is causing any discomfort, it should be adjusted.

Walking boots

Walking boots are particularly useful because they limit motion of the ankle during weightbearing and walking, but can be removed to allow non-weightbearing early motion exercises.

Casts and splint

When there is a need for rigid support (e.g. in fractures and ligament injuries) or complete immobility (e.g. in acute peritendinitis), a plaster cast or splint is the best solution. Depending on the nature of the injury, some activity, such as isometric exercises, can be allowed on the muscles encased in the cast. In principle, a plaster cast or splint should include the injured area and the joints above it, not those below it.

Waterproof cast

Casts can be made of many synthetic materials; some are composed of fiberglass impregnated with a plastic compound which hardens in cold water. The plastic cast becomes pliable 5–7 minutes after it has been dipped into cold water and can then be wrapped around the injured part of the body or applied as a splint. After 30 minutes it can withstand a certain amount of load. These casts are suitable as a temporary or permanent support for various parts of the body without the need for any restrictions on bathing, showering, or swimming.

During the last few years there has been a rapid development of bandages made from plastic material. Various types with different properties (and colors) are available.

Medication

Medication may be used for soft tissue injuries.

Pain relieving and anti-inflammatory medication

Acetylsalicylic acid (*aspirin*) is effective on mild and moderate pain, particularly that caused by headache and muscle and joint problems, but is inadequate in controlling serious pain such as is caused by a fracture. Side-effects include gastric irritation. Paracetamol is as effective as aspirin against some forms of pain although its inflammatory activity is not great. It may reduce raised temperature. There are no real side-effects.

Medications with combined pain-relieving and anti-inflammatory effects are widespread in sports medicine. The most commonly used are diclofenac sodium, which is effective against inflammation and has some pain-relieving effect (there can be gastric irritation) and ketoprofen, naproxen and ibobrufen, which have relatively good pain-relieving and anti-inflammatory effects, which last for a relatively long time (there is some gastric irritation). The COX-2 (cyclooxygenase 2) inhibitors celecoxib and rofecoxib are also useful: they seem to be effective and give possibly less gastric irritation.

Cortisone preparations (corticosteroids) for local injections

These injections can be of great value for overuse injuries but should not be given directly into muscles or tendons or into young joints, since they may cause weakening and consequent tendon injury. They can be given around the muscle or tendon attachment or into the surrounding sheath. Refraining from exercises with loading activities is recommended for 1– weeks after injection.

Local injection with pain-relieving drugs can sometimes be valuable to secure a diagnosis.

Ointments and liniments

Ointments may be used for muscle pain, stiffness and medial tibial stress syndrome. These products may increase skin circulation and produce a feeling of local heat without really affecting muscular blood flow. The psychological effects on athletes from the act of rubbing in the ointments and liniments cannot be denied.

Shoulder and upper arm

Impingement
syndrome
(p. 131);
subacromial
bursitis (135);
calcific tendinitis
(136)

Rotator cuff
injury (137)

Subscapularis
endon injury
142)

Pectoralis major
rupture (152)

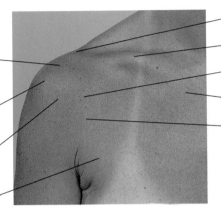

Acromioclavicular separation
(p. 118)

Clavicle fracture (117)

Coracoid impingement syndrome
(143)

Sternoclavicular separation (121)

Shoulder dislocation (123) and
instability (125); glenoid labrum
tears (128)

Figure 6.1 Anterior aspect of the
shoulder and location of
associated injuries.

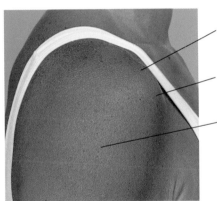

Rotator cuff injury (p. 137);
coracoid impingement syndrome
(143)

Biceps long tendon overuse (147);
dislocation (149); tear (150)

Deltoid tear and inflammation
(152)

Figure 6.2 Lateral aspect of the
shoulder and location of
associated injuries.

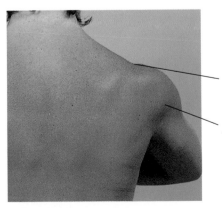

Acromioclavicular separation
(p. 118)

Triceps tendon tear (150)

Figure 6.3 Posterior aspect of
the shoulder and location of
associated injuries.

Shoulder motion

Shoulder motion is guided by the integrated motion of several joints such as the sternoclavicular, acromioclavicular, scapulothoracic, and gleno humeral joints (Figure 6.4).

– The glenohumeral joint is the main shoulder joint, comprising the head (ball) of the humerus and the glenoid (socket) of the scapula (shoulder blade). The surrounding capsule is loosely applied and allows a wide range of movements. The articular surface of the socket is enhanced by the glenoid labrum, which is an extension of the joint that increases its stability.

– The sternoclavicular joint is the joint between the clavicle (collar bone) and the sternum (breast bone). The joint is surrounded by the joint capsule and strong ligaments.

– The acromioclavicular joint is the joint between the clavicle and the scapula. The clavicle is a rather flattened and elongated S-shaped bone and is connected by strong ligaments to the scapula.

– The scapulothoracic joint is a pseudojoint (it acts like a joint) where the scapula moves against the rib cage.

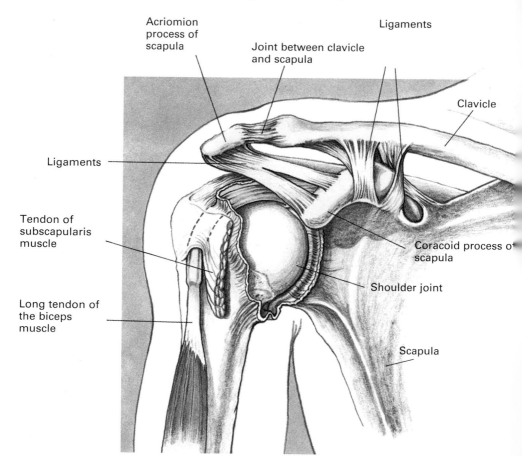

Figure 6.4 Anatomic representation of the shoulder region.

The total range of motion of the shoulder is extensive because the shoulder joint itself has a shallow socket and a loose capsule. The arm is allowed to move from 0° to 180° of elevation and for approximately 150° of internal and external rotation. Anterior and posterior rotation in the horizontal plane is about 170°. Twenty-six muscles are required to control the various joints for optimal shoulder function.

Shoulder stability

The shoulder is a lax joint with great mobility; it is mainly the muscles and tendons of the rotator cuff that are responsible for stability.

Static stability

The shoulder does have some *static stability* from capsular ligaments, the articular components, negative intra-articular pressure, and the glenoid labrum.

The *capsular ligamentous complex* consists of the superior, middle, and anterior and posterior inferior glenohumeral ligaments, as well as the coracohumeral ligaments.

1. The *superior glenohumeral ligament* is present in approximately 90% of shoulders. It originates on the glenoid (shoulder socket) anterior to the tendon of the long head of the biceps and courses inferior and lateral to insert on to the lesser tuberosity, which is located on the lateral aspect of the humerus. This ligament resists inferior translation of the humeral head with the humerus at the side of the body.

2. The *middle glenohumeral ligament* is present in 70% of shoulders and courses from the labrum to insert medially to the lesser tuberosity under the subscapularis tendon. This ligament protects against instability by acting as a secondary restraint to anterior translation.

3. The *inferior glenohumeral ligament* is present in 90% of shoulders, and consists of an anterior and a posterior band. The origin is on the inferior half of the glenoid labrum and the insertion is on the humerus. This ligament provides most of the stability, especially when the shoulder is abducted (moved out from the body) and externally rotated.

4. The *coracohumeral ligament* originates from the coracoid process, blends into the capsule and attaches onto the humerus. This ligament is put in tension in external rotation and resists inferior subluxation to the joint.

The effects of *articular geometry* are limited. The concavity of the glenoid, however, when combined with a compressive force, does provide significant stability of the humeral head.

The *negative intra-articular pressure* at rest is −4 mmHg (−0.5 kPa). A 52% increase in the humeral head translation (anterior–posterior motion) after incision of the capsule has been documented.

The stability of the glenohumeral joint is enhanced by the *glenoid labrum*, which is a fibrous structure that forms a ring around the periphery of the glenoid and provides an anchor point on the glenoid for the

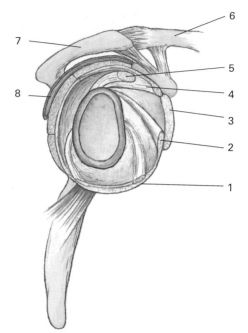

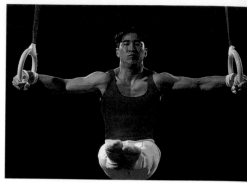

Figure 6.5 (Left) Capsular ligaments around the shoulder. 1, Inferior glenohumeral ligament; 2, middle glenohumeral ligament; 3, subscapularis; 4, superior glenohumeral ligament; 5, biceps tendon; 6, clavicle; 7, acromion; 8, bursa. **(Right)** The shoulder muscles in action (by courtesy of All Sport: photographer, Mike Powell).

capsular ligaments (Figure 6.5). The labrum attaches to the glenoid artic ular surface. It contributes to glenohumeral stability by increasing th depth of the glenoid socket. Loss of the glenoid labrum decreases the dept of the socket by 50% in either direction. The labrum also contributes t stability by increasing the surface area of the glenoid and acting as loadbearing structure for the humeral head. The labrum is consistentl attached tightly to the glenoid articular cartilage below the equator, anc therefore, detachment in this area is more likely to represent instability.

The *rotator interval* is the triangular region between the anterior borde of the supraspinatus tendon and the upper border of the subscapulari tendon. An injury to the capsular structures in the rotator interval are of shoulder may result in instability.

Dynamic stability

Dynamic stability is provided by the muscles around the shoulders. Th rotator cuff is the key to dynamic glenohumeral stability. The *supraspina tus* muscle tendon plays a major stabilizing role, as exemplified by th throwing movement (p. 72); peak supraspinatus activity occurs durin late cocking when the arm is already abducted and is most susceptible t subluxation. The supraspinatus contributes to stability by drawing th humeral head toward the glenoid.

The *infraspinatus* and *teres minor* muscles are activated after th supraspinatus and they externally rotate the humerus in addition to stabi lizing the shoulder by joint compression. The peak activity is shown t be in late cocking and follow-through phases of the throwing motion.

The *subscapularis* muscle is active during the late cocking phase c throwing to protect the anterior shoulder structures. Thereafter, functions as an internal rotator during acceleration and follow-through

The long head of the *biceps tendon* is activated during shoulder flexion and abduction. It acts as a humeral head depressor. The *pectoralis major* and *latissimus dorsi* muscles are internal rotators of the glenohumeral joint. The *trapezius* muscles act as an important scapular stabilizer and also decelerate scapular protraction during follow-through.

The *deltoid* muscle functions in three sections. The middle deltoid participates in all arm activities. The anterior deltoid acts in flexion and is assisted by the pectoralis major and biceps. The posterior deltoid provides extension of the arm.

Investigation of shoulder and upper arm injuries

History

Thorough history-taking is the key to correct diagnosis. This involves asking the correct questions—and more importantly—giving the athlete adequate time to answer. The physician must listen carefully to the answers and also watch the patient during the interview to obtain clues through body language. The primary questions should focus on the following areas.

- *What happened?* This is particularly important in acute traumatic injuries. If the athlete can recreate the mechanism of injury, a general biomechanical analysis can indicate which tissues were abnormally stressed. The more detail that the athlete can recall, the better the cause and mechanism of the injury can be recreated to point to the injured structure.
- *Where does it hurt?* The best way to approach this is to have the injured athlete place one finger on the most painful area. Sometimes this can be difficult because the pain may be deep and/or diffuse.
- *What is the nature of the pain?* Burning pain that radiates down the extremity can indicate nerve pain. Throbbing pain can indicate pain of vascular origin. Pain of brief duration that disappears quickly can indicate possible mechanical problems from tissues rubbing or locking together. Dull, aching pain is more likely to be caused by chronic overuse problems.
- *What makes it better or worse?* Activities that can change the course of the pain can give clues to the diagnosis. For example, stress fractures will become worse with prolonged activity, and injuries that respond well to anti-inflammatory medications are probably due to inflammatory processes.
- *Has the athlete been injured before?* Often injuries are recurrences of previous problems, or can be related to changes in training habits from previous injury.
- *What treatments have been used, and did they help?* Perhaps the treatment has exacerbated the injury rather than relieved it.
- *What other health problems are present, and what medications are used?* Many musculoskeletal problems are due to disease and not injury. Many times these diseases will have other associated problems that the

patient believes are unrelated to the musculoskeletal injury. Finally, a
medicines have side-effects, which can sometimes affect the muscu
loskeletal system.

The history should direct the doctor towards tests that may confirm
the diagnosis. A good, accurate history-taking will secure the correct
diagnosis in at least 80% of cases.

Physical examination

Both shoulders should be exposed for comparison. Lost range of motio
muscle hypotrophy, bone deformity, and shoulder asymmetry should b
looked for. A prominent scapular spine suggests rotator cuff hypotrophy
which may indicate a rotator cuff tear or a suprascapular nerve lesion. Deltoi
hypotrophy can be noted in association with axillary nerve lesions or fracture

Range-of-motion testing

Range of motion should be examined in both the upright and the supin
positions. The examination includes assessment of total range an
rhythm of motion, as well as pain at the limits of motion. To determir
total active elevation, the arm is observed from the side, and the angl
between the arm and the chest is measured. Evaluation of external an
internal rotation is important. Abduction (moving the arm from th
body) can give useful information relating to impingement and strength
Pain between 80° and 120° of abduction is a reliable indicator of tendin
tis due to impingement. This is called the 'painful arc' (see Figure 6.28

Strength testing

The strength of forward flexion, abduction, adduction, and external an
internal rotation should be documented (Figure 6.6). The strength
decreased in abduction and external rotation when there is rotator cu
disease. Specific testing of the supraspinatus is performed by abductin
the athlete's arm to 90°, then forward flexing 20°, and maximal rotatio
of the arm internally into the thumb-down position. Muscle strength i
this position is a test of the *supraspinatus* and a small portion of th
central deltoid. This is an important test, since rotator cuff tears usuall
involve the supraspinatus.

The muscles providing external rotation are the infraspinatus and ter
minor. External rotation (strength) is assessed with the arms at the sic
in a neutral position; resistance is applied and compared with th
opposite side. Internal strength is a test of subscapular strength.

Stability testing

The apprehension test, relocation test and drawer stability test are essenti
procedures, described under the injury concerned (p. 127).

Figure 6.6
Strength testing
of the shoulder.
(**A**) Adduction
and neutral; (**B**)
abduction and
neutral; (**C**)
external rotation;
(**D**) internal
rotation.

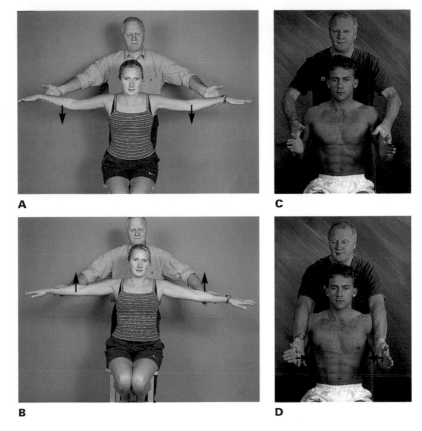

A

C

B

D

Clavicular injuries

Fractures of the clavicle

Fractures of the clavicle occur as a result of a tackle or falling on the shoulder or the outstretched hand (Figure 6.7). Clavicle fractures commonly occur during skiing, cycling, riding, and contact sports. The fracture is often located in the middle third or towards the outer third of the bone.

Symptoms The area over the fracture is extremely tender and swollen. Pain is felt when moving the shoulder. A crackling sensation (crepitus) can be felt between the bone ends when movement is attempted.

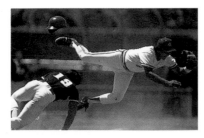

Figure 6.7 Falling on the shoulder or an outstretched hand carries a risk of a clavicle fracture (by courtesy of All Sport.)

117

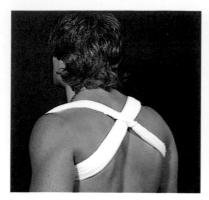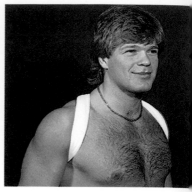

Figure 6.8 A figure-of-eight bandage seen from the back and the front.

Treatment

A fracture of the clavicle is treated with a sling or figure-of-eight bandage to immobilize both shoulders (Figure 6.8). With the bandage in place, the arms can still be moved freely below the horizontal plane. This treatment is usually sufficient, but surgery may be necessary in certain cases, for example, if the fracture is situated at the lateral end of the bone and the fracture ends threaten to penetrate the skin.

Healing

Fractures of the clavicle generally heal well. Conditioning exercises such as running should not be resumed until the fracture has healed or does not cause pain (about 3–8 weeks after the injury). Cycling and nonpounding activities can often be continued during the recovery period.

Separation of the acromioclavicular joint

Separation of the acromioclavicular joint is a relatively common injury in contact sports, riding, cycling, skiing, and wrestling. The joint is surrounded by ligaments running between the clavicle and the acromion process of the scapula (the acromioclavicular ligament), and is further stabilized by other ligaments running between the clavicle and the coracoid process of the scapula (the coracoclavicular ligaments). The joint sometimes contains a cartilaginous meniscus or disk.

The vast majority of acromioclavicular injuries are due to direct force produced by the athlete falling on the point of the shoulder with the arm in the adducted position (close to the body) or when an ice-hockey player is tackled against the board. Force is transferred up the arm through the humeral head and the acromion process. Acromioclavicular joint injuries occur less commonly as a result of indirect force, for instance when the athlete falls on an outstretched arm.

Classification

These injuries may be classified according to the extent of ligamentous disruption to the acromioclavicular joint and coracoclavicular ligaments

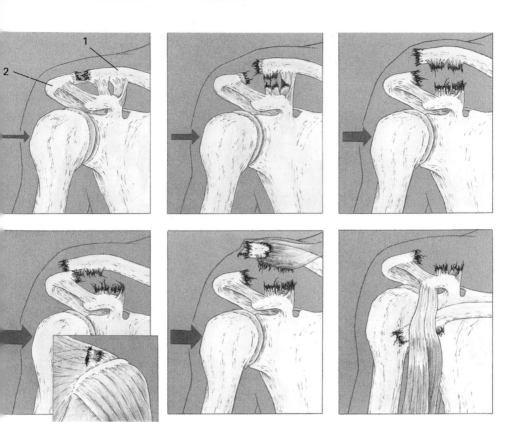

Figure 6.9 Grades I–VI of acromioclavicular joint separation: 1, clavicle; 2, acromion.

The most common injury types in athletes are grades I–III; grades IV–VI are very rare (Figure 6.9). They can be characterized as follows:

– *Grade I*: a sprain of the acromioclavicular ligament, causing pain over the acromioclavicular joint and minimal pain with shoulder motion. There is mild tenderness.

– *Grade II*: disruption and widening of the acromioclavicular joint with some elevation of the distal end of the clavicle. There is moderate to severe pain near the acromioclavicular joint and shoulder motion is restricted. The athlete will usually withdraw from competition.

– *Grade III*: disruption and dislocation of the acromioclavicular joint with superior displacement of the clavicle. The coracoclavicular ligaments are disrupted and the coracoclavicular space is greater than in the normal shoulder. The upper extremity is seen to be depressed and the clavicle can be free-floating, possibly lifting the skin. Moderate to severe pain is present. There is tenderness over the joint. The athlete is usually unable to continue sports. The lateral end of the clavicle is reducible.

– *Grade IV*: the acromioclavicular joint is dislocated, with the clavicle displacing posteriorly into or through the trapezius muscle. The coracoclavicular ligaments are completely disrupted. The clinical findings are similar to type III injury, except that more pain is usually present and the clavicle is dislocated posteriorly and not reducible.

– *Grade V*: disruption of the acromioclavicular ligament as well as the coracoclavicular ligaments. The acromioclavicular joint is displaced with gross disparity between the clavicle and the scapula. The clinical finding are similar to type III, but there is more pain and displacement betwee the distal clavicle and acromion. The skin may be tented so much tha there is a threat it will be penetrated. This injury is rarely seen in athletes

- *Grade VI*: The acromioclavicular and coracoclavicular ligaments ar disrupted and the joint is dislocated with the clavicle being displace inferior to the acromion or the coracoid. The shoulder has a flatte appearance superiorly. This injury is rare in athletes owing to the grea trauma necessary to produce the subcoracoid dislocation. There is high incidence of associated fractures.

Symptoms and diagnosis

A complete history will often secure the diagnosis.

- Pain is localized to the anterior superior aspect of the shoulder (Figur 6.10). The pain does not radiate and the severity is often proportior ate to the degree of injury.
- Physical examination shows swelling, abrasion, skin color change (ecchymoses), and sometimes deformity of the joint. The involved arr is usually held at the side and all shoulder motions are restricte because of pain.
- There is localized tenderness over the joint.
- Passive adduction at shoulder level (Figure 6.11) is often painful.
- Injection of local anesthetic solution may relieve pain.
- Depending on the degree of separation, the lateral end of the dist clavicle may be displaced upward. A partial separation (grade I and I involves tearing of the acromioclavicular capsule and ligaments, and complete separation (grade III) will also have a complete tear of th coracoclavicular ligament.
- The diagnosis is confirmed by X-ray, which is more likely to reve the abnormality if it is carried out with the joint loaded. In grade I separation, there is no contact between the articular surfaces.

Treatment

The *doctor* may

- prescribe early mobility exercises, especially in grade I–III injuries;
- use a bandage to reduce the clavicle back into position. The results this technique are limited;

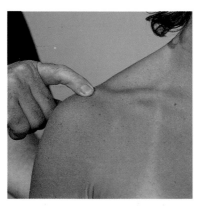

Figure 6.10 Location of pain in acromioclavicular joint separation.

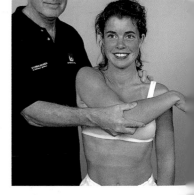

Figure 6.11 Passive adduction at shoulder level.

– recommend surgery in grade IV–VI lesions. The treatment of grade III injuries remains controversial, but there is a definite trend toward nonoperative management with early mobilization. A surgical approach should be considered in young athletes (15–25 years) in sports with overhead activities. With nonoperative management the athlete may have a residual displacement but the end result and function are largely the same. In most cases, therefore, early symptomatic treatment is recommended with progression to resistance exercises as soon as tolerated. The athlete can return to sports when there is pain-free range of motion, which usually occurs in 4-8 weeks.

Healing and complications

In grade I and II injuries degenerative changes and arthritis occur in the joint in 8–9% of cases. If this injury continues to cause pain, an excision of 1 cm (0.4 in) of the distal end of the clavicle is indicated. This usually results in early pain-free return to sports. If there is residual pain or disability interfering with performance after a grade III injury, an excision of the distal clavicle may be indicated, with restoration of the coracoclavicular ligaments. Return to sports is usually possible within 2–3 months.

Chronic acromioclavicular joint injury

Persistent pain after acromioclavicular joint injury may necessitate surgery, which includes removal of the lateral end of the clavicular bone.

Separation of the sternoclavicular joint

The sternoclavicular joint is seldom separated, but it is an important injury to recognize. The medial end of the clavicle, and hence the shoulder, is anchored to the sternum by the sternoclavicular ligaments (Figure 6.12). The joint cavity lies obliquely and contains a meniscus (disk). If the shoulder is subjected to a violent impact, the sternoclavicular joint can slip and the ligaments can tear, causing the medial end of the clavicle to move either in an anterior direction making it more prominent, or posterior.

Symptoms and diagnosis

– Pain may be located towards the shoulder region rather than in the sternoclavicular joint itself.
– Tenderness occurs when pressure is applied to the joint.
– The clavicle is usually only partially separated, but its medial end can be completely detached from the sternum.
– An X-ray and CT scan should be obtained.
– If the clavicle is displaced backwards (posteriorly) towards the major blood vessels, life-threatening injury can occur.

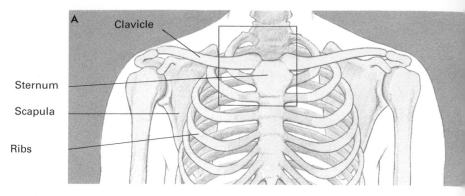

A

Clavicle

Sternum

Scapula

Ribs

Ligament and capsule
over the joint between
sternum and clavicle

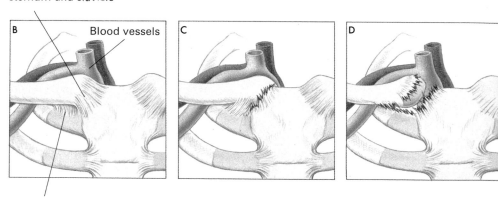

B Blood vessels C D

Ligament between
clavicle and first
rib

Figure 6.12 (A) Diagram of the shoulder region. The lined area shows a
normal joint between clavicle and sternum. (**B**) A normal joint between
clavicle and sternum. Note the position of the large blood vessels that go up
to the head and down the arm. (**C**) Partial dislocation (subluxation) of the
joint between clavicle and sternum. The ligaments and the capsule around
the joint are torn. (**D**) Total posterior dislocation (backwards) of the joint
between clavicle and sternum. The ligament between the clavicle and first
rib is also torn. In some cases, the end of the clavicle may pierce blood
vessels.

Treatment   The *doctor* may:
– in cases of partial separation, suggest that the injured person rest fo
  1–2 weeks with mobilization of the shoulder as tolerated;
– in cases of posterior separation, make sure that there is no pressure o
  damage to the underlying vessels. Surgery is indicated in cases c
  complete posterior dislocation;
– operate in cases with chronic pain or major discomfort. The surger
  usually involves excision of the medial end of the clavicle bone.

Healing   In cases of partial separation of the sternoclavicular joint, the injure
                 athlete can generally resume sporting activity early; however, pain an
                 other symptoms may remain for several months.

Shoulder injuries

Dislocation of the shoulder joint

Dislocation of the shoulder joint is a relatively common injury in sports such as ice hockey, team handball, American football, rugby, riding, alpine skiing, skating, and wrestling. Shoulder dislocations are 3 times more common in men 20–30 years old, than in persons aged over 30 years. The male to female ratio for primary dislocation is 9 : 1.

Injury mechanism

When falling, it is instinctive to lift the arm and turn it outwards to protect the body. Dislocation can occur when the arm, held in this position, receives the impact of the fall. The joint can also be dislocated by falling directly on the lateral aspect of the shoulder or by a violent collision with another player. This injury can also occur when the arm is caught by another player and pulled vigorously outwards and backwards.

Types of dislocation

- *Anterior dislocation (diverted forward and downward)* is most common and has a tendency to recur in young, active people.
- *Posterior dislocation (backward)* is unusual; the injury is commonly missed, and needs special attention. It can be difficult to diagnose and treat.

Pathology

Complete dislocations of the shoulder are characterized by lesions of the labrum, capsule, muscles, and/or bone. The labrum can be avulsed from the rim; this is called the *Bankart lesion* and is the most common cause of recurrent dislocation (Figure 6.13).

A dislocation of the shoulder may include varying degrees of rupture or stretching of the capsule off the glenoid. Fracture of the rim of the glenoid or rupture of the capsule off the humeral head occurs occasionally. Excessive laxity of the capsule can follow repeated injury. There are no major muscular lesions associated with dislocations.

A bony lesion is produced by the impaction or compression of the posterior humeral head against the anterior rim of the glenoid at the time of the dislocation. This is called the *Hill–Sachs (Hermodson) lesion* of the humeral head, and this is most commonly associated with recurrent dislocation (Figure 6.14).

Symptoms and diagnosis

- Excruciating pain is felt at the time of injury and as long as the joint is dislocated.
- Lack of mobility; the arm hangs loosely beside the body.
- The upper part of the humerus can be felt as a lump in the armpit, and, where it is normally located, an empty joint socket can be felt.

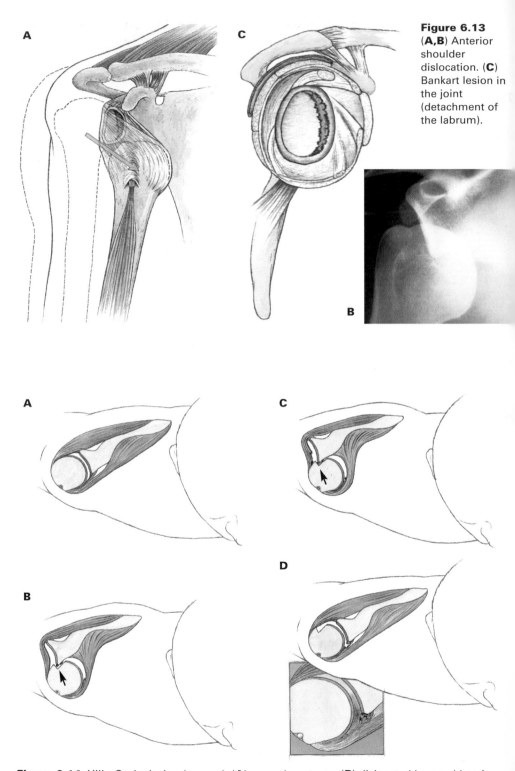

Figure 6.13 (**A,B**) Anterior shoulder dislocation. (**C**) Bankart lesion in the joint (detachment of the labrum).

Figure 6.14 Hills–Sachs lesion (arrows): (**A**) normal anatomy; (**B**) dislocated humeral head (posterior aspect) in contact with the anterior glenoid (socket) rim; (**C**) additional overstretching of the posterior capsule; (**D**) reduced shoulder, showing the bony and labral lesions.

- The outline (contour) of the injured shoulder looks uneven in comparison with the rounded outline of the undamaged shoulder.
- The diagnosis can be verified by X-ray. A posterior dislocation often requires an X-ray examination using special techniques.

Treatment

The injured athlete should be taken to a doctor for immediate treatment. As a rule, the earlier the joint is reduced, the fewer the complications and the shorter the healing period. It is more considerate to manipulate the joint back into position after the patient is anesthetized. An X-ray should be taken before the reduction to exclude a concurrent fracture and again after the reduction to check alignment.

After manipulation, the arm is immobilized against the body in order to reduce pain and to allow the joint capsule and ligaments to heal. The time of immobilization is controversial. The older athlete may use a sling for 1-2 weeks, but should intermittently remove the sling to perform range-of-motion exercises. The period in a sling may be extended for the young athlete in whom the danger of redislocation is high, especially if this is a first dislocation. In recurrent dislocations, an early, thorough muscle-strength training program can be initiated. Range-of-motion exercises (pp. 495, 502) should under all circumstances start early.

In very active athletes with a first-time dislocation, acute arthroscopy can be of value with lavage and/or debridement, and stabilization of the labral lesion. This acute treatment is becoming more and more common, as it seems to decrease the recurrence rate in athletes aged 16–25 years which is currently more than 85%.

Healing and complications

- If there are no complications, a dislocated shoulder heals well. Light conditioning and gentle exercise can be resumed after 2–4 weeks.
- Return to sporting activity involving the injured arm should not take place until full mobility and strength are regained, usually 2–3 months after injury.
- Sometimes a dislocation of the shoulder joint is complicated by a fracture of the upper part of the humerus or the scapula.
- In rare cases, nerve and blood vessel injuries and muscle ruptures may occur.

Patients who sustain their first dislocation before the age of 25 years are at great risk of recurrent dislocations. If dislocations occur more than three or four times, surgery to stabilize the joint should be considered. The results are good to excellent. With open stabilization, such as the Bankart procedure, the results are excellent in 90–95% of the cases; arthroscopic reconstructions have excellent results in about 80–85% but are continuously improving. In young athletes, the open procedure is therefore still the treatment of choice. However, in older athletes, arthroscopic treatment can be attempted, provided the athlete is aware of the lower success rate. Return to sports involving the affected arm is usually possible after 4–6 months.

Shoulder instability

It is important to make a distinction between *laxity* and *instability*. Shoulder laxity is a translation of the humeral head on the glenoid (socket) in the absence of clinical symptoms or pathologic changes. This means that normal shoulders may be lax without being unstable. When the laxity results in clinical symptoms and is associated with pathologic changes, instability results. Shoulder instability is mostly a chronic, recurrent condition. The direction of the shoulder instability can be anterior and inferior, posterior and inferior, posterior, or multidirectional. The degree can also vary from dislocation to subluxation.

Shoulder instability and impingement are a continuum of shoulder disease. Too many classification systems exist but a practical one in sport could be:
- type I is pure impingement;
- type II is secondary impingement and primary instability caused by capsular trauma;
- type III is secondary impingement with primary instability from associated hyperelasticity;
- type IV is pure instability.

Chronic shoulder instability is most common in athletes participating in sports involving throwing or other overhead activities. Chronic fatigue of the dynamic anterior shoulder stabilizers seems to initiate most problems. As these dynamic stabilizers fatigue, increased and repetitive stress is placed on the static anterior, glenohumeral (shoulder joint) stabilizers which result in gradual stretching of these stabilizers. A relative imbalance between the anterior and posterior capsule may be the result. This fatigue may result in changes in the throwing or hitting mechanism, which may include scapular lag and/or a dropped elbow. In the early phases there is mostly fatigue or loss of consistency, but no major decrease in performance. At this stage training program may have good effects with time. Gradual stretching of the anterior structures will occur with anterior subluxation. This will allow the rotator cuff to impinge on the posterior superior surface of the glenoid in the abducted and externally rotated position of the arm, which may eventually progress to fraying of the undersurface of the rotator cuff. This pattern can be seen in throwing athletes, and in baseball, volleyball, and tennis players. Swimmers have similar shoulder problems. Stress combined with laxity predisposes to internal impingement. Exercises at this stage are very important. The gliding of the joint within the socket may cause pain during and after sporting activity. The athlete often feels as if the shoulder has almost slipped out of the socket in sports such as pole-vault, ice hockey, team handball, volleyball, basketball, American football, and in throwing and racket sports. In order to treat these injuries successfully, it is important to determine the direction and the magnitude of the instability.

Symptoms and diagnosis
- Pain in the shoulder joint occurs during and after exercise and competition.
- 'Dead arm' sign is present. This sudden onset of weakness, numbness and tingling in the arm is provoked by certain actions and can be due to a sudden transient subluxation of the shoulder.
- A feeling of dislocation is experienced when the arm is lifted above the horizontal plane and externally (outwards) rotated.
- The diagnosis can be made with the aid of the apprehension and stability tests.

The **anterior apprehension test** is a test for anterior shoulder instability. The arm is forced in abduction and external rotation. The test can be performed in the upright or the supine position. The examiner raises the arm to 90° of abduction (with the elbow flexed 90°). The right hand of the examiner is placed over the humeral head with the thumb pushing from the posterior aspect of the humeral head for extra leverage (Figure 6.15). With increasing external rotation and gentle forward pressure against the humeral head, an impending feeling of anterior instability may be produced—the 'apprehension sign'.

The **relocation test** is performed in patients with a positive apprehension sign and suggests the finding of instability. The examiner places the arm in 90° of abduction and external rotation to cause apprehension. Pressure is then placed on the anterior humeral head to push it posteriorly and 'relocate' the glenoid. Immediate relief of pain is considered a positive result.

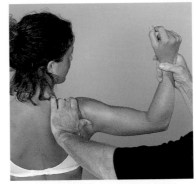
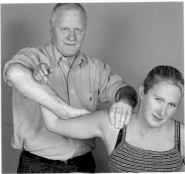

Figure 6.15 Anterior apprehension test: two different methods.

Stability assessments can be carried out with the athlete in the supine or seated position. The shoulder is positioned in the scapular plane with neutral rotation maintained. Anterior and posterior forces are applied to the proximal humerus and the amount of translation is graded (the drawer test) (Figure 6.16):
- grade 1: the examiner can translate the humeral head further in an anteroposterior direction, compared with the contralateral shoulder;
- grade 2: the examiner can subluxate the humeral head over the glenoid rim, but the humeral head spontaneously returns to a neutral position when the applied force is withdrawn;
- grade 3: the examiner can lock the humeral head over the glenoid rim.

For anterior stability, grade 1 or greater is pathological. For posterior instability, only a grade 3 examination is pathological, as many normal shoulders can be subluxated up to 50% out of the joint posteriorly.

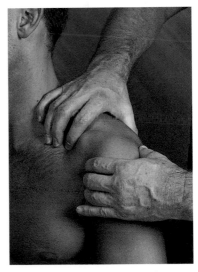

Figure 6.16 Anterior drawer test.

Inferior laxity is measured by the sulcus test (Figure 6.17). The shoulder is held in 0° abduction, neutral rotation and neutral flexion/extension. The examiner applies traction downward on the arm. If a sulcus appears between the humeral head and lateral acromion the sulcus sign is positive. The sulcus sign is graded as 1 if the acromial humeral interval increases up to 1 cm (0.4 in); a grade 2 indicates an increase of 1–2 cm (0.4–0.8 in); and a grade 3 indicates an increase greater than 2 cm (0.8 in). The sulcus sign is pathological for examination grades 2 or greater. Normal shoulders can translate 1 cm (0.4 in) inferiorly by pulling on the arm. The measurement is often clinically difficult to assess.

- An X-ray examination reveals skeletal changes along the anterior edge of the joint socket.
- An MRI (Figure 6.18) or preferably an MR arthrogram may show a labral tear, intra-articular changes, and the redundant capsule. This test is excellent but expensive.
- Arthroscopy and examination under anesthesia will confirm the diagnosis.

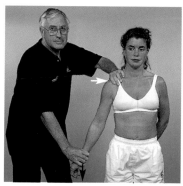

Figure 6.17 Sulcus test. The white arrow indicates where the sulcus will appear.

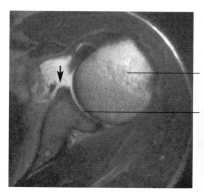

Figure 6.18 MRI showing labrum with separation from anterior glenoid (arrowed). 1, Head of humerus; 2, glenoid.

Treatment

The *athlete* should improve the function of the joint with active strengt exercises.

The *doctor* may operate in cases of prolonged problems. It is ofte enough to stabilize a tear of the labrum, but if there is multidirectional inst bility, open surgery with a capsular shift procedure may still be needed.

Glenoid labrum tears

The glenoid labrum is a fibrocartilage rim surrounding the articul surface of the glenoid cavity (the socket of the shoulder joint) (Figu

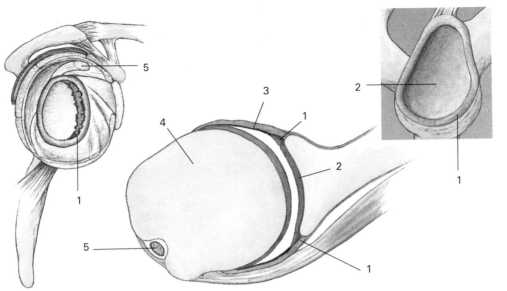

Figure 6.19 (**Left**) Labrum injury. (**Middle**) Glenoid labrum in cross-section. 1, Labrum; 2, glenoid socket; 3, joint capsule; 4, head of humerus; 5, biceps tendon. (**Right**) Glenoid area with labrum.

6.19). The labrum contributes to stability by increasing the depth of the glenoid socket. The loss of the glenoid labrum decreases the depth of the socket by 50% in either direction. A glenoid labral tear is commonly associated with anterior dislocation or subluxation of the shoulder or with a degenerative lesion. An isolated glenoid labral tear, without instability, can occur in younger throwing athletes, in wrestlers and boxers, and in racket players.

Symptoms and diagnosis
- Pain in the shoulder occurs during activity, especially during overhead movements such as throwing. The pain is often deep and located anteriorly. If an athlete localizes the pain to the anterior aspect of the shoulder joint, labral tears should be suspected.
- There is a popping, catching or locking sensation.
- Sometimes there can be a feeling of instability and a slight limitation of motion.
- During examination the doctor can detect a clicking or locking. This is felt during overhead abduction and rotation.
- There is tenderness to palpation over the joint line.
- The anterior slide test (Kibler test: Figure 6.20), where the arm is pressed upwards from behind, may cause pain.
- The diagnosis is confirmed by an MRI (with accuracy of around 76–90%) or an MR arthrogram (accuracy: 90–93%) or shoulder arthroscopy.

Treatment
The *athlete* should:
- rest from painful activities;
- carry out open and closed kinetic chain exercises for strength training.
The *doctor* may perform arthroscopic surgery to reattach the labrum using sutures or absorbable tacks (Figure 6.21). The healing time is about 3–4 months and return to throwing takes 3–6 months.

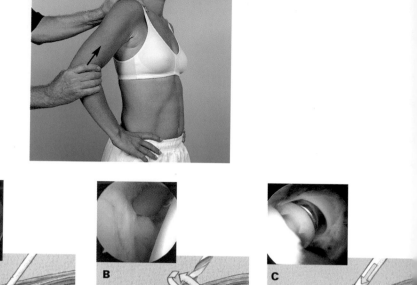

Figure 6.20 Kibler test.

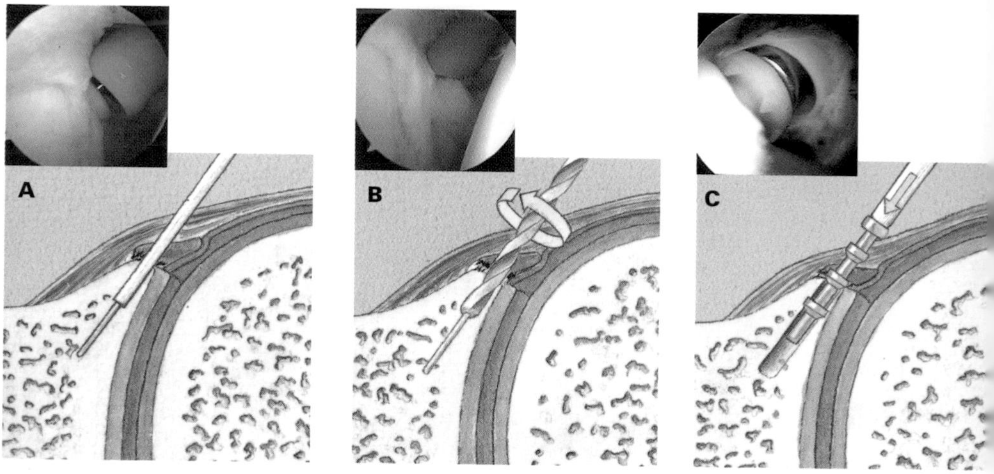

Figure 6.21 Arthroscopic fixation of an unstable labrum with a resorbable tac or screw. (**A**) Pin is inserted in labrum to the bone through a sheath; (**B**) resorbable tac or screw is inserted over the pin; (**C**) tac or screw goes into the bone.

SLAP lesions

Labral injuries are usually located at the anterior aspect of the glenoid. However, some glenoid labral lesions are located in the superior labrum from anterior to posterior, at the biceps tendon insertion. These are known as Superior Labrum from Anterior to Posterior (SLAP) lesions. They are treated with the help of arthroscopy if they cause symptoms. There are four types:

- Type I is characterized by fraying in the superior labrum, but the labrum remains firmly attached to the glenoid. Treatment is by arthroscopic debridement if the injury is causing problems.
- Type II includes an injury where the superior labrum and biceps tendon are stripped off the underlying glenoid. The frayed labral tissue may be debrided or reattached, after which the arm should be immobilized to allow the biceps labral complex to heal. The optimal treatment of this injury is controversial.
- Type III includes fragmentation of the superior labrum with an intact biceps tendon. The treatment is by excision of the labral fragments.

- Type IV is a labral tear across the superior labrum into the biceps tendon. Treatment usually consists of excision of the labral and biceps fragments.

Impingement syndrome

Impingement can be defined as a trapping of the soft tissues in the subacromial space, between the acromion and the humeral head. The entrapment of the soft tissues when moving the shoulder may lead to a painful reaction. Athletes, including tennis players, swimmers, throwers, and weightlifters, who make repetitive movements of the arms above the horizontal plane, are at risk of developing this painful condition.

The soft tissues can become too large and may be pinched between the head of the humerus, the acromion process of the scapula, and the coracoacromial ligament. The soft tissues in the limited subacromial space include the tendons of the long head of the biceps, the supraspinatus, infraspinatus, teres minor, and subscapularis muscles, and the bursa overlying the supraspinatus tendon. The subacromial space can also be inadequate. If the ligament is thickened or calcified, or becomes inelastic, or if the anterior–inferior edge of the acromion process over the acromioclavicular joint becomes irregular with bony outgrowths or spurs, the space can be further compromised. This occurs most often in elderly people.

The contour of the anterior–inferior acromial bone is important since it may affect the size of the space below the acromion. The shape of the anterior acromion is studied by plain radiographs (supraspinatus outlet or arch view). The contour of the anterior–inferior acromion is classified according to Bigliani (Figure 6.22) as follows:
- Type 1: the acromion is flat on the undersurface with the anterior edge extending away from the humeral head.
- Type 2: the acromion is gently curved on the undersurface with the anterior edge extending parallel to the humeral head.
- Type 3: an inferiorly pointing, or hooked, anterior bone spur (osteophyte) narrows the outlet of the supraspinatus muscle and tendon.

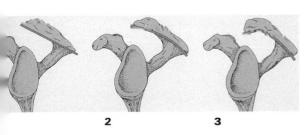

2   3

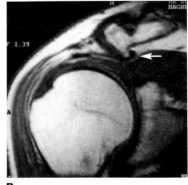

Figure 6.22 (A) Classification of contours of the anterior–superior acromion. (B) MRI showing bone spur under the acromion causing impingement.

B

131

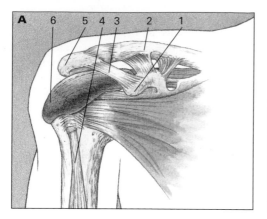
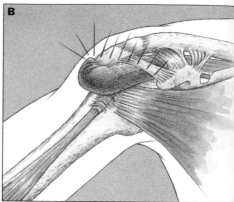
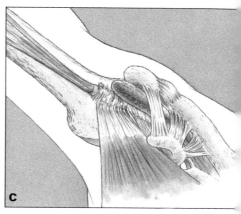

Figure 6.23 (**A**) Arm at rest: 1, coracoid process; 2, clavicle; 3, coraco-acromial ligament; 4, biceps tendon; 5, acromion; 6, bursa. (**B**) Arm is abducted (lifted outwards) 60–120°. The bursa is compressed between the acromion and the rotator cuff tendons. (**C**) Arm is abducted above 120° and the pressure on the bursa decreases.

When the upper arm is moved forwards and upwards (its usu functional position) to an angle of 90° to the body and the arm is th further internally rotated (inward), the soft tissues are compressed agai the sharp edge of the coracoacromial ligament. During movement t tendons and the bursa rub against the ligament, causing mechani irritation that gives rise to painful inflammation (Figure 6.23). As infla mation is accompanied by swelling, the space is even further reduced a the condition may become progressively worse. Repeated loading caus thickening of the soft tissues and leads to a chronic inflammato reaction. The subacromial bursa and the vulnerable areas of t supraspinatus and biceps tendons are most affected by this process.

Etiology

Impingement syndrome may be caused by extrinsic or intrinsic factor

Extrinsic factors

– Primary extrinsic factors arise from mechanical attrition of the tend against the undersurface of the anterior acromion. The majority cases have this etiology.

– Secondary extrinsic factors arise from a relative decrease in the size of the supraspinatus outlet due to instability of the glenohumeral joint. This is more commonly seen in young throwing athletes and swimmers, many of whom have some generalized ligamentous laxity.

Intrinsic factors

Intrinsic factors, such as degenerative changes (p. 43) within the rotator cuff tendons, are likely to cause problems because of subsequent weakness causing superior migration of the humerus, thus producing a secondary mechanical impingement.

Classification

– Grade 1: pretear condition with subacromial bursitis and/or tendinitis.
– Grade 2: impingement with partial rotator cuff tears.
– Grade 3: impingement with complete rotator cuff tears.

Symptoms and diagnosis

– When the arm is used for overhead activities and is lifted above the horizontal plane, pain is located at the lateral and upper part of the shoulder.
– When the arm is above 90° of abduction (elevated to the side), the athlete will often substitute scapulothoracic motion for glenohumeral motion—i.e. will use the shoulder blade more than normally. This can be seen to hunch the affected shoulder up during abduction of the arm. The pain is often worse after the arm is lowered than when it is raised.
– Pain occurs at night, especially if there is involvement of the rotator cuff.
– Tenderness can be felt in the upper aspect of the head of the humerus, and also over the biceps tendon.
– Active range of motion can be limited in abduction and forward flexion secondary to pain, especially above shoulder level. There may be a subtle loss of internal rotation.
– Crepitus can be palpable in the subacromial region.
– Hypotrophy of the deltoid and the spine muscles may be present.
– Impingement tests will, if positive, verify the diagnosis.

Neer impingement test
The Neer impingement test consists of full forward passive elevation of the humerus in the scapula plane (Figure 6.24). This causes the critical area of the supraspinatus tendon to impinge against the anterior inferior acromion. If this produces pain, it is a positive impingement sign.

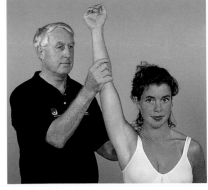

Figure 6.24 Neer impingement test.

133

Hawkins's impingement test

Hawkins's test can be performed by forward flexing the shoulder to 90° and then forcibly internally rotating the shoulder (Figure 6.25). This maneuver drives the greater tuberosity further under the lateral acromion and coracoacromial ligament, thereby reproducing the pain.

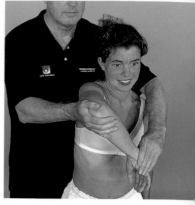

Figure 6.25 Hawkins's impingement test.

Impingement injection tests

The impingement test compares the athlete's response to impingement testing before and after the injection of an anesthetic agent into the subacromial bursa. Significant reduction of the athlete's pain is a positive sign of impingement.

Plain X-rays, including an anteroposterior view of the glenohumeral joint (that is, an internal rotation view of the humerus with 20° upward angulation to show the acromioclavicular joint), an axillary lateral view and the supraspinatus outlet or arch view, will show the subacromial morphology well.

Preventive measures
- Perform warm-up exercises and flexibility training.
- Exercise the whole kinetic chain, including strength training.
- Avoid abuse (pain-causing situations).

Treatment

The *athlete* should:
- carry out active movements of the shoulder and maintain range of motion (p. 501);
- keep up conditioning exercises;
- apply local heat and use a heat retainer after the acute phase;
- resume sports training gradually when the pain has resolved.

The *doctor* may:
- give instructions for specific strengthening and stretching programs. A maintenance program to prevent loss of motion and stiffness is important;
- prescribe anti-inflammatory medication;
- use steroid injections selectively (when local steroids are justified, the injection should be followed by a few days of rest);
- operate if conservative therapy fails.

As long as the patient is making progress and other significant lesions do not exist, conservative treatment should be continued. If a plateau is reached, surgery may be indicated. A subacromial decompression includes removal of the bursa and the undersurface of the acromion which can create more space for the soft tissues. The surgery can be performed with the aid of an arthroscope. In the elderly, more extensive measures may be necessary. After surgery, early mobilization with active strength training is recommended. A return to overhead sports is often possible 2–3 months after surgery.

Subacromial bursitis

One large bursa in the shoulder is located between the supraspinatus muscle and the deltoid muscle and acromion process of the scapula. In its inflamed state the bursa is about the size of a golf ball. Inflammation of the bursa (subacromial bursitis) commonly occurs.

Causes
- A fall or blow to the shoulder or a supraspinatus tendon rupture can cause bleeding into the bursa resulting in inflammation.
- Repetitive movements can cause bursitis which, in turn, causes accumulation of fluid in the bursa. The effusion causes tension in the tissues and pain in the anterior (front) and upper part of the shoulder and a thickening of the bursa.
- Inflammation in an adjacent tendon can easily spread to include the bursa.

Symptoms and diagnosis
- Pain occurs in the anterior, upper part of the shoulder.
- Impingement testing is positive (p. 133).
- Tenderness is found on palpation.
- Sometimes the bursa feels 'spongy' on palpation.
- Examination using an arthroscope and/or bursography can confirm the diagnosis.
- Aspiration of the bursa can also be diagnostic.

Treatment

The *athlete* should:
- rest until the pain has resolved, and avoid pain-causing situations;
- apply local heat and use a heat retainer after the acute phase.

The *doctor* may:
- aspirate the bursa when bleeding or effusion is accompanied by pain;
- prescribe analgesic and anti-inflammatory medication;
- advise mobility exercises (p. 495);
- administer a steroid injection and advise short-term rest in cases of chronic inflammation;
- use arthroscopic surgery to remove the bursa in chronic cases.

Healing

When bursitis is treated promptly, symptoms usually resolve in 2–3 weeks, after which sporting activities can be resumed.

Thickened subacromial bursa

A previously unrecognized form of rotator cuff injury can occur contact sports. After an acute traumatic injury to the shoulder, the athle may develop weakness on elevation and external rotation. The clinic symptoms are the same as for a torn rotator cuff (p. 137). An MRI revea only hypertrophic changes (enlargement and thickening) on the burs side of the cuff. Symptoms may persist despite rehabilitation.

These patients can be treated arthroscopically. Diffuse proliferation the subacromial bursa may be noted. After resection of the hypertroph bursa the athlete tends to rapidly improve. This syndrome should l considered in an athlete with persistent cuff pain and weakness wl participates in contact sports.

Calcific tendinitis

The degenerative changes that occur in the supraspinatus tendons as pa of the aging process can, in combination with exertion, cause chron inflammation with deposits of calcium (Figure 6.26). This can occur athletes as young as 30–35 years. The calcium deposits can rupture in the bursa overlying the supraspinatus tendon; this brings about a temp rary improvement of the condition but may then cause bursitis. Alte natively, the deposits can disappear spontaneously 2–3 weeks aft formation, or simply remain without causing any symptoms.

Symptoms and diagnosis
– Intense pain can begin suddenly in the anterior upper part of t shoulder. It can be so severe that it prevents sleep. It can at le partially be relieved by holding the arm still against the body.

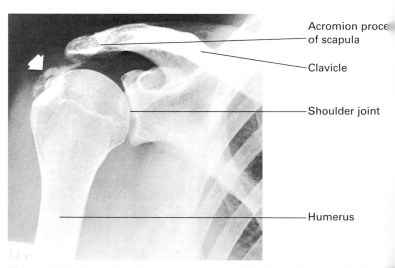

Acromion proce of scapula

Clavicle

Shoulder joint

Humerus

Figure 6.26 X-ray of a shoulder showing calcification. The arrow indicate a calcium deposit just above the joint head at the bursa.

– Because of the intense pain, a doctor is often consulted early. The doctor will detect a distinct tenderness over the anterior upper part of the shoulder, and X-rays will confirm the diagnosis.

The *athlete* should:
– maintain range of motion after the acute phase to avoid stiffness;
– take a pain-relieving preparation.

The *doctor* may:
– puncture and aspirate the calcium deposit;
– administer a local anesthetic and steroid injection;
– prescribe an analgesic preparation;
– advise flexibility exercises (p. 496);
– if the pain is persistent, operate in order to remove the calcium deposit.

Rotator cuff injury

In 75% of cases of shoulder pain, the main source is the supraspinatus tendon of the rotator cuff. The supraspinatus muscle, together with the deltoid, raises the arm to initiate abduction. If there is a complete tear, the athlete cannot hold the arm elevated in the scapular plane between 60° and 120° and has to drop the shoulder. The arm may swing laterally, at which point the deltoid takes over. The weakest point of the supraspinatus tendon is the part which forms the cuff over the joint in the area that is 1 cm (0.4 in) from the attachment of the tendon to the humerus. It is at this point that ruptures most often occur. They may be either partial or total. In the vulnerable area there is a network of capillaries. With increasing age or overuse there is decreased blood flow; this causes typical degenerative changes (p. 43), including reduced elasticity and increasing weakness. These changes are often apparent in elderly athletes, but may start at the age of 30–35 years. When the arm is abducted to an angle of 60–120° to the body, and during static work in this position, the blood vessels are compressed; this further impairs the blood flow and reduces the tissue oxygen supply to increase the risk of injury.

Etiology

Impingement syndrome (which can be primary or secondary to instability), traction overload tendinitis, and trauma can all cause rotator cuff problems.

Impingement syndrome
Primary impingement occurs mostly in persons aged 40 years or more, while secondary impingement is more common in younger athletes.

Traction overload tendinitis
Traction overload tendinitis is more common in younger athletes. These patients are less likely to have partial tears of the rotator cuff and are

more likely to have asymmetry in shoulder range of motion, as well as asymmetry in strength of the periscapular muscles. Posterior capsular tightness and periscapular weakness are common problems, which force the rotator cuff tendons to work harder, thus creating an overload or overuse condition. Symptoms similar to traction overload tendinitis can also be due to subtle shoulder instability.

Trauma

Trauma can cause rotator cuff injury by the following mechanisms:
- any force that rotates the arm internally against a resistance or that prevents the arm from turning externally, as may occur during team handball, American football, or wrestling;
- falling directly on the shoulder or on an outstretched arm;
- lifting or throwing heavy objects.

Classification

Rotator cuff tears can be of different degrees and distinct types. The location of the tear is important: rotator cuff tears can be located on the bursa surface of the tendon (the bursal side) or on the undersurface of the tendon (the articular side). The tear can also be partial or complete, connecting the articular and bursal sides.
- Primary compressive cuff disease is associated with a type III hooked acromion, degenerative spurs, or a thick coracoacromial ligament. A cuff tear originating on the bursal side of the tendon can be the result.
- Secondary compressive cuff disease is usually due to associated gleno-humeral (shoulder joint) instability.
- Tensile lesions occur on the articular side and are believed to occur secondary to cuff resistance to the high deceleration forces that occur during activities such as the later stages of throwing. There is a higher incidence of articular side tears in throwing athletes.

Partial tears

In a cuff with smooth coverings of synovial and bursal tissue, the severity of a partial tear can be classified as follows:
1. Minimal superficial bursal or synovial irritation, or slight capsular fraying with a partial tear less than 1 cm (0.4 in) in size.
2. Actual fraying and failure of some rotator cuff fibers in addition to synovial, bursal, or capsular injury. The tear is usually less than 2 cm (0.8 in) in size.
3. More severe rotator cuff injury, including the fraying and fragmentation of tendon fibers often involving the whole surface of the cuff tendon. The tear is usually less than 3 cm (1.2 in) in size.
4. Very severe partial rotator cuff tear that usually contains, in addition to fraying and fragmentation of the tissue, a tear that often encompasses more than a single tendon.

Complete tears

Complete rotator cuff tears are classified as follows:
1. A small complete tear such as a puncture wound.

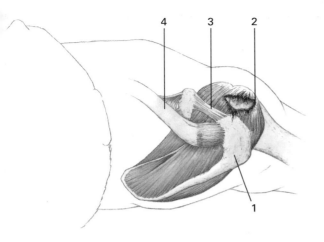

Figure 6.27 Moderate–large rotator cuff tear viewed from above. 1, Acromion; 2, rotator cuff tear; 3, coraco-acromial ligament; 4, clavicle.

2. A moderate tear that still encompasses only one of the rotator cuff tendons; the tear is usually less than 2 cm (0.8 in) in size, with no retraction of the torn ends (Figure 6.27).

3. Large complete tear involving an entire tendon with minimum retraction of the torn edges. The tear is usually 3–4 cm (1.2–1.6 in) in size.

4. A massive rotator cuff tear involving two or more rotator cuff tendons. This is frequently associated with retraction of the remaining tendon ends.

Symptoms and diagnosis

– Intense pain is felt when the injury occurs. The pain returns on exertion, may increase during the next 24 hours and may extend down the upper arm. A diagnosis of a tear of the supraspinatus tendon is suspected if the athlete has fallen on the shoulder, or has lifted or thrown a heavy object.

– Pain is often intense, or increased, at night. The patient often complains of problems with sleeping or lying on the injured side.

– Pain occurs when the arm is externally rotated or is raised upwards and outwards. When the tendon is only partially torn, the arm can be abducted to an angle of 60–80° to the body with little or no pain. The pain increases as the arm is lifted to an angle of 70–120°; it may increase once more when the arm is lowered (Figure 6.28). Between these angles the arm is also weak. When the tendon has sustained total rupture the arm can be held at an angle of more than 120° to the body, but when it is lowered further it suddenly drops. This is an important diagnostic sign (the 'dropping arm' sign).

– The rotator cuff test is positive. The arms are held in 90° of elevation in the scapular plane and the thumbs are rotated down towards the ground (Figure 6.29). When pressure is placed on the arm, the patient complains of pain and weakness.

– Injection of anesthetic solution into the subacromial space can give relief in 75% of athletes with a partial tear on the bursa side; the relief supports the diagnosis.

– X-ray views, including a supraspinatus outlet view, are helpful in demonstrating acromial morphology and bony spurs that originate from the acromioclavicular joint.

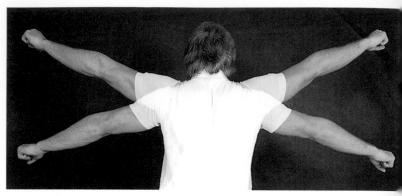

Figure 6.28 A rupture of the supraspinatus muscle causes muscle weakness in the range of movement of the injured arm. Pain will increase when the arm is lifted above an angle of 60–120° to the body.

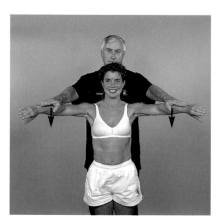

Figure 6.29 Rotator cuff test. With the patient's arms abducted (lifted up) at 90° and internally rotated (thumbs down), the examiner presses the arms down gently. If there is discomfort and weakness the test is positive.

- Ultrasonography can be sensitive and specific in identifying full-thickness rotator cuff tears.
- MRI (Figure 6.30) is highly sensitive in the diagnosis of rotator cuff tears. It can demonstrate not only the size of the tear, but also the exact location. It can be made more accurate when combined with an arthrogram.
- Arthroscopy can verify the diagnosis of a tear that can be seen on the bursal or the articular side.

Treatment

The *athlete* should:
- treat the shoulder with ice at the scene of the injury;
- rest;
- avoid abuse of the arm;
- consult a doctor if the symptoms persist.

The *doctor* may:
- prescribe an exercise program designed to promote dynamic stability of the humeral head (p. 498). Often a physical therapist or trainer needed to monitor the program. The program should consist

140

stretching the posterior capsule and maintaining good range of motion, as well as shoulder girdle strengthening. The goal of the rehabilitation should be to restore symmetry between the two arms with respect to (1) range of motion, especially internal rotation which is commonly decreased on the affected side; (2) quality of motion, with decreased compensatory shoulder blade motion; (3) strength, with an emphasis on strengthening the rotator cuff muscles to hold the humeral head centered within the glenoid; and (4) strengthening the periscapular muscles to provide a stable base for shoulder motion;

– if pain continues despite physical therapy, give a subacromial injection or operate in certain circumstances as described below.

Healing and complications

– Spontaneous healing of a *partial tear* appears to be clinically unlikely because of the poor circulation at the site of the tear, the physical separation of the stump ends, and the subacromial impingement. Bursal-side tears have a poor prognosis, so a more aggressive surgical approach is required.

– If there is a partial thickness tear of the rotator cuff, arthroscopic (or, if necessary, open) debridement of the lesion may be performed in the hope that this will reactivate the healing process. This procedure is often combined with an anterior acromioplasty where a part of the acromion is removed. If subtle instability is present, the surgery is focused on this problem. Postoperatively, a gradual progressive strengthening program is begun after full range of motion is achieved.

– If there is a *complete rotator cuff tear* (one with full thickness tear), surgery is usually recommended. Symptoms generally improve, but functional recovery is less predictable: 75% of patients usually have significant pain relief, but only about 40% of top-level throwers return to their preinjury level of function. A gradually increased rehabilitation program under supervision is important for this injury.

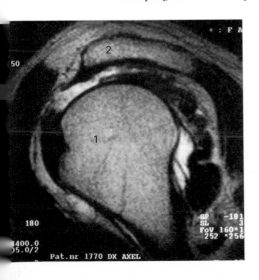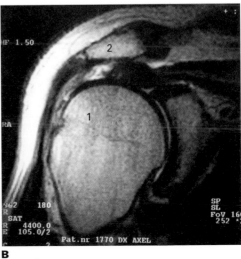

Figure 6.30 MRI showing rotator cuff tears: (**A**) lateral view of complete tear; (**B**) anterior view of full thickness tear. 1, Humerus; 2, acromion.

Athletes with conservatively treated traction overload tendinitis may
often be able to return to sports 3–4 months after the onset of symptoms.
Athletes with partial rotator cuff tears may need 4–6 months before the
return to sports after surgical treatment; athletes with complete rotator
cuff tears may need even longer. A tennis player can often start playing
again 4–6 months after the injury, but has to be careful with the serve
for up to 1 year after the injury. Range-of-motion and condition exercises
should start as soon as possible. Lifting and throwing exercises are
prescribed individually and should usually be avoided for the first 3–
months after surgery.

A neglected rotator cuff tendon tear can cause permanent disability
due to impaired function. This injury can sometimes be surgically
repaired at a later date, but the longer the wait, the lower is the chance
of a successful outcome.

Injury of the subscapularis tendon

The subscapularis muscle (which originates on the inner surface of the
scapula, runs anterior to the shoulder joint, and is inserted high into the
anterior aspect of the head of the humerus) is the most important internal rotator of the upper arm. Its tendon can be affected by partial or total
ruptures. A partial rupture, which is most common, may heal with thickening of the tendon as a result. A complete rupture is uncommon but
can occur in conjunction with dislocation of the shoulder joint.

Throwers and athletes whose sports require repetitive overhead activity
most commonly suffer from injury and degeneration of the subscapularis
tendon. Such sports include baseball, American football (quarterbacks),
racket sports, javelin, team handball, wrestling, weightlifting, and goalkeep-
ing. Tennis players and volleyball players make a similar movement when
serving or smashing, but they keep the elbow joint bent until it is extended
at the moment of impact. About 25% of top-level tennis players examined
had symptoms of overuse of the subscapularis tendon in one study.

– Internal rotation is limited (Figure 6.31).
– Pain is felt on moving the shoulder joint, particularly when the arm
  is held above the horizontal plane and is turned inwards.
– Pain is initiated by rotating the arm inwards against resistance.
  Another application is the 'lift-off' test (Figure 6.32).
– Tenderness is found when direct pressure is applied against the tendon
  and the tendon attachment anterior to the shoulder.
– The power of the arm is impaired during movements involving inward
  rotation.

Lift-off test
The arm is internally rotated so that the dorsal aspect of the hand
rests on the lower back. The hand is actively pressed away from the
back against resistance. This tests subscapular integrity.

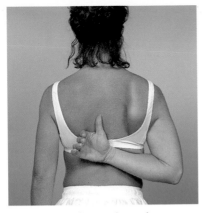
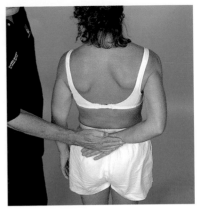

Figure 6.31 Internal rotation.   **Figure 6.32** The 'lift-off' test.

Treatment

The *athlete* should:
- start active mobility training;
- avoid pain-causing situations;
- apply local heat and use a heat retainer after the acute phase;
- see a doctor if pain is severe.

The *doctor* may:
- advise active flexibility training (p. 495);
- prescribe anti-inflammatory medication;
- arrange physiotherapy with flexibility training and heat treatment;
- when symptoms are chronic, administer a steroid injection around but not in the tendon, followed by a few days of rest;
- recommend surgery in chronic cases. If focal pathological changes can be verified, surgery (often arthroscopic) may be indicated.

Healing and complications

With appropriate treatment, the injured athlete can, in most cases, resume training after 1–3 weeks. If signs of injury in the subscapularis tendon reappear, the athlete should rest from sporting activity until symptoms resolve and consult a doctor. Otherwise, the injury may become chronic and force the athlete to interrupt training for several months or even give up the sport completely.

Coracoid impingement syndrome

Coracoid impingement syndrome is an unusual syndrome that causes anterior shoulder pain. The space between the coracoid process and the anterior part of the humerus can be reduced by changes in the structures around the process. This can be seen as a result of fractures of the arm, calcification within the subscapularis tendon, abnormal orientation of the shoulder joint, or simple prominence of the coracoid process itself. It is also seen as a complication of previous surgery for impingement, biceps tendon lesions, or instability.

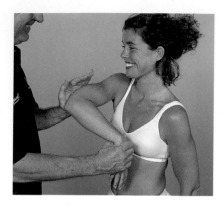

Figure 6.33 Coracoid impingement syndrome. Pain is experienced when the humeral head is pressed against the coracoid process.

Symptoms and diagnosis

- The patient has anterior shoulder pain localized to the coracoid process.
- The patient has tenderness over the anteromedial shoulder at the location of the coracoid process.
- The pain is made worse by forward flexion and medial rotation combined with adduction (the arm is moved forward against the chest). This maneuver can produce a painful click. This is called the coracoid impingement sign (Figure 6.33).
- An injection of local anesthetic solution between the humeral head and coracoid process can give relief.
- A CT scan can assist with the diagnosis, showing a lengthening of the coracoid process and/or a decrease in the distance between the coracoid process and the humeral head.

Treatment

The treatment in chronic cases is the surgical removal or shortening of the outermost anterior part of the tip of the coracoid process. Active exercises are started 2–3 weeks after surgery, but heavy loading is avoided for 6 weeks to allow the tendons to heal back to the coracoid process. Return to sports is possible after 3–6 months.

Bibliography

Jobe FW, Bradley JP (1988) Rotator cuff injuries in baseball: prevention and rehabilitation. *Sports Medicine* 6: 378–387.

Warner JP, Ding XH, Warren RF et al. (1992) Static capsular ligamentous restraints to superior inferior translation of the glenohumeral joint. *American Journal of Sports Medicine* 20: 675–685.

Bigliani LU, Kimmel J, McCann PD et al. (1992) Repair rotator cuff tear in tennis players. *American Journal of Sports Medicine* 20: 112–117.

Nerve injuries in the shoulder region

Nerve damage in the shoulder region is uncommon but should nevertheless be considered. It occurs mainly after injuries caused by impact and external pressure but it can also occur as a result of overuse.

Injuries to the suprascapular nerve

The suprascapular nerve supplies the supraspinatus and infraspinatus muscles. It runs in a groove on the upper edge of the scapula, and is held in the groove by a ligament. The suprascapular nerve can be damaged at the time of forward or backward dislocation of the shoulder joint, with the dislocation stretching the nerve over the edge of the scapula (Figure 6.34). In addition, the nerve can be damaged by a direct blow to the scapula, by external pressure (e.g. from a backpack) or by repetitive, one-sided overhead motions of the shoulder which cause tension in the nerve. Damage can also be caused by a local cyst.

Symptoms and diagnosis
- Pain radiates out toward the upper posterior part of the shoulder.
- Weakness in the supraspinatus and infraspinatus muscles is manifested by impaired abduction of the shoulder joint to an angle of 80–120°.
- Decreased volume (hypotrophy) of the supraspinatus and (especially) infraspinatus muscles can be pronounced and readily noticeable.
- Electromyographic examination will confirm the diagnosis.
- If only the infraspinatus is involved, compression of the nerve passing the spina scapulae should be suspected.

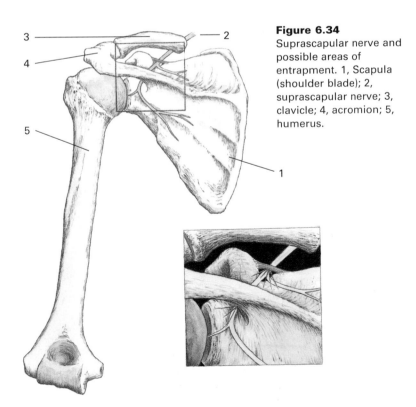

Figure 6.34
Suprascapular nerve and possible areas of entrapment. 1, Scapula (shoulder blade); 2, suprascapular nerve; 3, clavicle; 4, acromion; 5, humerus.

Treatment includes:
- avoiding abuse if there is pain;
- flexibility training and, if there is no pain, strength training;
- local steroid injection;
- if the complaints persist, surgery to free the nerve by cutting th overlying ligament;
- neurolysis (release of the nerve), which should be performed distal the spine.

Injuries to the axillary nerve

The axillary nerve supplies the deltoid and teres minor muscles and run close to the shoulder joint. Damage to this nerve usually occurs as complication of dislocation or fracture of the upper part of the humeru The symptoms include radiating pain and impaired sensation over th lateral aspect of the upper arm, along with weakness (due to paralysis the deltoid muscle) when the arm is abducted.

Since the course of the axillary nerve wraps around the upper part the humerus close to the bone, a hard blow to this area can sometim injure it. However, the symptoms are usually transitory.

Injuries to the long thoracic nerve

The long thoracic nerve supplies the serratus anterior muscle whic holds the scapula in position. An isolated injury to this nerve can occu during violent shoulder movements, e.g. during weightliftin Backstroke swimmers may also sustain similar damage as their arm moved through a combination of external rotation and forwards an upwards lifting.

When the long thoracic nerve is damaged, there is usually a dull acl which disappears spontaneously. The ability to lift the arm is impaire and, at the same time, *'winging' of the scapula* is seen—the medial side the scapula protrudes backwards on the damaged side. One way of revea ing the injury is to ask the athlete to perform press-ups (push-up against a wall; the medial side of the scapula will protrude posteriorl The treatment consists of anti-inflammatory medication and gradual increasing strength training.

Brachial plexus injuries (Burner syndrome)

Burner syndrome is not uncommon in contact sports such as America football. Following trauma to the head and shoulders, the athle complains of a burning pain and numbness extending down the upper extremity. The cause of this pain may be a traction injury to the brachial plexus (nerve bundle between the shoulder and the neck) and/or cervical nerve roots (typically the C5 and C6 roots). The extremity can feel weak and heavy for a short time, but these problems usually resolve within several minutes.

If there are prolonged motor and sensory deficits, these may represent a more severe injury. The athlete should not return to contact sports until a clinical examination, including an EMG and strength evaluation, has been carried out, and strength has returned to normal. It is important to differentiate a brachial plexus injury from a serious neck or spine injury. If there is any neck pain or tenderness, the athlete's neck should be immobilized and an emergency evaluation performed.

Injury to the brachial plexus can also occur without an inciting traumatic event and is characterized by acute onset of persistent severe pain. There may be a motor loss, but sensory loss is usually minimal. Treatment includes rest followed by rehabilitation. Weakness may persist for long periods or may be permanent.

Injuries affecting the upper arm

Overuse injury of the long tendon of the biceps

Overuse injury of the long tendon of the biceps is usually secondary to another shoulder injury such as impingement or instability. The biceps injury is usually of a degenerative nature. Midsubstance degenerative changes in a tendon are referred to as tendinosis (p. 43). This biceps tendon glides over the articular head of the humerus and leaves the joint through a special groove. When degeneration of the tendon occurs, tenderness at the uppermost part of the extremity is very noticeable. This injury occurs most commonly in canoeists, rowers, weightlifters, swimmers, javelin throwers, fencers, wrestlers, golfers, tennis players, table tennis players, badminton players, and squash players.

Symptoms and diagnosis
- Tenderness is felt over the anterior aspect of the upper arm and shoulder, especially when the elbow joint is flexed.
- Yergason's and Speed's tests are positive (see Figures 6.35, 6.36).
- In the acute stage tendon crepitus (creaking) can be felt over the anterior aspect of the shoulder during flexion and extension of the elbow.

Treatment
The *athlete* should:
- gradually progress through a carefully planned exercise program;
- apply local heat and use a heat retainer after the acute phase and before activities.

147

Yergason's test

The elbow is flexed to 90° and the forearm pronated. The examiner holds the athlete's wrist to resist active supination by the patient (Figure 6.35). Pain localized to the bicipital groove area suggests the presence of a lesion in the long head of the biceps.

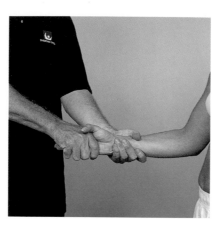

Figure 6.35 Yergason's test.

Speed's test

With the elbow extended and the forearm supinated, the arm is forward elevated against resistance to approximately 60° (Figure 6.36). The test is positive when there is pain localized to the biceps groove area.

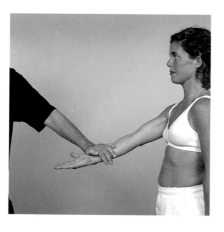

Figure 6.36 Speed's test.

The *doctor* may prescribe anti-inflammatory medication.

Healing

The injured person can resume sporting activity when symptoms ha disappeared.

Dislocation of the long tendon of the biceps

On the anterior aspect of the humerus, between the attachments of the tendons of the supraspinatus (greater tuberosity) and the subscapularis muscles (lesser tuberosity), is a ligament that holds the long biceps tendon in the groove in which it glides (Figure 6.37). If this ligament stretches or tears or if the groove is shallow, the biceps tendon may become partially or totally dislocated. Dislocation most commonly takes place medially, giving the tendon a straighter course during contraction. It can also dislocate laterally with abduction and external rotation.

Symptoms and diagnosis

– Bending of the elbow and abduction of the shoulder may cause pain extending up to the shoulder.
– Abduction of the humerus can cause pain over the anterior aspect of the shoulder.
– The examiner may feel the biceps tendon slipping in and out of its groove when the arm is externally and internally rotated.
– An MRI scan can assist with the diagnosis.

Treatment

The *athlete* should:
– rest;
– apply local heat and use a heat retainer after the acute phase.

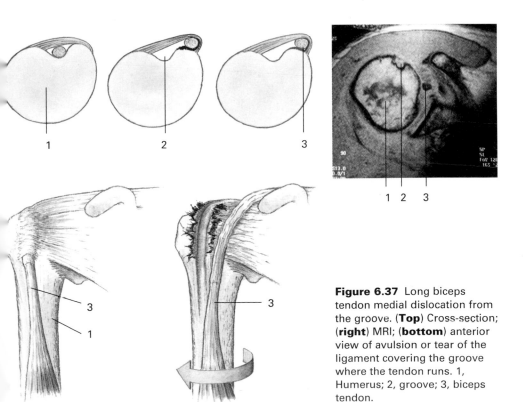

Figure 6.37 Long biceps tendon medial dislocation from the groove. (**Top**) Cross-section; (**right**) MRI; (**bottom**) anterior view of avulsion or tear of the ligament covering the groove where the tendon runs. 1, Humerus; 2, groove; 3, biceps tendon.

149

The *doctor* may:
- prescribe anti-inflammatory medication;
- immobilize the arm in acute cases;
- perform an MR arthrogram (with contrast medium in the joint) of th shoulder;
- operate if the tendon is completely dislocated or causes persistent problem.

Tear of the long tendon of the biceps

Tears of the long tendon of the biceps muscle are seen in gymnast tennis players and badminton players, wrestlers, rowers, weightlifter and javelin throwers.

The long biceps tendon is susceptible to degenerative changes, whic predispose it to rupture (Figure 6.38). The tears occur most often in athlet over the age of 40–50 years; in younger athletes this injury is relative unusual. The injury mechanism is a sudden eccentric (opposite-directe resistance during flexion and/or external rotation of the elbow or shoulde

Symptoms and diagnosis
- Moderate pain occurs over the anterior aspect of the shoulder joint.
- Swelling is visible over the anterior aspect of the upper arm.
- There is inability to contract the muscle against resistance in the acu stage.
- Strength is moderately impaired when the elbow joint is flexed ar the forearm is supinated.
- Slow contraction of the biceps produces a more prominent swellir than that produced by the normal biceps of the healthy arm. Th muscle fails to make its full contribution to flexing of the elbow join

Treatment
The *athlete* should consult a doctor for advice.
The *doctor* may:
- prescribe physiotherapy and mobility exercises (p. 495);
- operate when a complete rupture has affected a young athlete acti in overhead sports.

Healing
If surgery is not considered necessary, mobility and strength exercis can be started as soon as the pain begins to subside. After conservati treatment there may be some residual weakness.

If surgery is carried out, range-of-motion exercises start within 1 weeks. Conditioning exercises not involving the upper extremity can sta early. Gradually increased strength training should not be resumed un a few weeks later. Contact sports should be avoided for 2–3 months.

Tear of the tendon of the triceps

Falling on the hand when the arm is flexed or forceful throwing c; cause a rupture in the tendon of the triceps. Weightlifting with ve

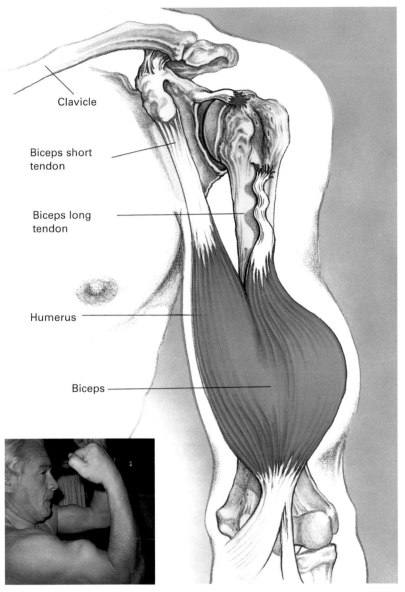

Clavicle

Biceps short
tendon

Biceps long
tendon

Humerus

Biceps

Figure 6.38 Rupture in the long tendon of the biceps of the upper arm.

heavy weights can also cause this injury. Most tricep tears are partial and are most commonly located at the insertion of the olecranon (the tip of the elbow); occasionally, however, the tendon attachment will be completely torn away from the olecranon.

mptoms
d diagnosis
– Pain occurs at the tip of the posterior aspect of the elbow.
– A gap can be felt in the tendon.
– Weakness and impaired ability to straighten the arm at the elbow are present.

– An X-ray should be carried out to exclude bony injury. An MRI scan can show the extent of the injury.

<table>
<tr><td>Treatment</td><td>– In cases of minor or partial tears, gradually increasing exercise is the main treatment.
– Surgery should be carried out when active athletes have suffered complete tear of the tendon or its attachment.</td></tr>
</table>

Tear and inflammation of the deltoid muscle

Tears of the deltoid muscle, though infrequent, do occur in team handball and volleyball players, American footballers, weightlifters, wrestlers, and other athletes. The muscle is damaged in most cases by direct impact, but it can also be injured by overuse. The tear affects only a small part of the muscle, making it difficult to raise the arm upwards and in abduction. Local tenderness is felt over the region of the tear. The treatment is rest.

Overuse injuries can affect the deltoid attachment to the humerus, particularly in young athletes who repeatedly elevate and abduct the arm under a heavy load. Overuse of the posterior part of the deltoid muscle occurs, for example, in butterfly-stroke swimmers because of their vigorous backward arm movements. Overuse of the anterior part of the muscle is not uncommon in certain contact sports when players use their outstretched arms to push or tackle. The treatment for these overuse injuries is, as a rule, rest and heat.

Rupture of the major pectoral muscle

The pectoral muscle has its origin on the anterior chest wall and its insertion on the anterior surface of the upper part of the humerus. Its function is to draw the upper arm towards the chest and to rotate the arm inward. When it is subjected to a heavy load, the pectoral muscle can tear. A complete tear can be induced by strength training (especially bench-press training), heavy weightlifting, and other strength sports such as wrestling, shot-putting, and discus and javelin throwing. It is usually the tendon close to the insertion of the muscle onto the humerus that is damaged.

<table>
<tr><td>Symptoms
and diagnosis</td><td>– Pain occurs at the insertion of the major pectoral muscle onto the humerus.
– Swelling and bruising (secondary to bleeding) appear over the anterior aspect of the upper arm.
– Tenderness is found over the anterior aspect of the upper arm.
– Impaired strength is noted when the upper arm is adducted (drawn inwards towards the chest) or is internally rotated against resistance.</td></tr>
</table>

- The major pectoral muscle fails to contract when the upper arm is pressed inwards against resistance. This can be felt by placing a hand over the muscle so that it covers both the damaged and healthy portions.
- There is visible deformity or loss of definition of the muscle.

Treatment

The *athlete* should:
- apply acute treatment (Chapter 5);
- carry out a gradually increasing strength training program when the tear is partial;
- consult a doctor.

The *doctor* may operate in cases of complete muscle rupture, especially in weightlifters, since this muscle has no agonist (muscle with same function) (Figure 6.39).

Healing

Following surgery, early range-of-motion exercises are recommended. A supportive sling should be worn for about 2–4 weeks. Strength training should not be resumed until at least 4–6 weeks after the injury and then only with gradually increasing light loads. Increasing the number of repetitions is preferable to increasing the loads.

Return to sport

In a partial tear, early strength training is initiated and sport is resumed when normal strength and pain-free normal range of movement are achieved. After a complete tear, return to sport is possible after 3–5 months.

Overuse injury at the insertion of the pectoral muscle

The insertion of the major pectoral muscle can be the site of local traction injury with inflammation. The injury occurs particularly in gymnasts, tennis players, badminton players, squash players, golfers, rowers, weightlifters, swimmers, and throwers. The usual cause is intensive strength training and overuse.

Symptoms and diagnosis

- Pain occurs in the region of the insertion of the major pectoral muscle tendon onto the humerus.
- Tenderness is observed at the tendon attachment.
- Pain, and sometimes weakness, are felt when the upper arm is adducted against resistance.

Treatment

The *athlete* should:
- rest the damaged area;
- apply local heat and use a heat retainer before activity and ice after activity.

The *doctor* may:
- prescribe anti-inflammatory medication;
- initiate strength and flexibility training (p. 495);
- give a local steroid injection and prescribe a few days of rest.

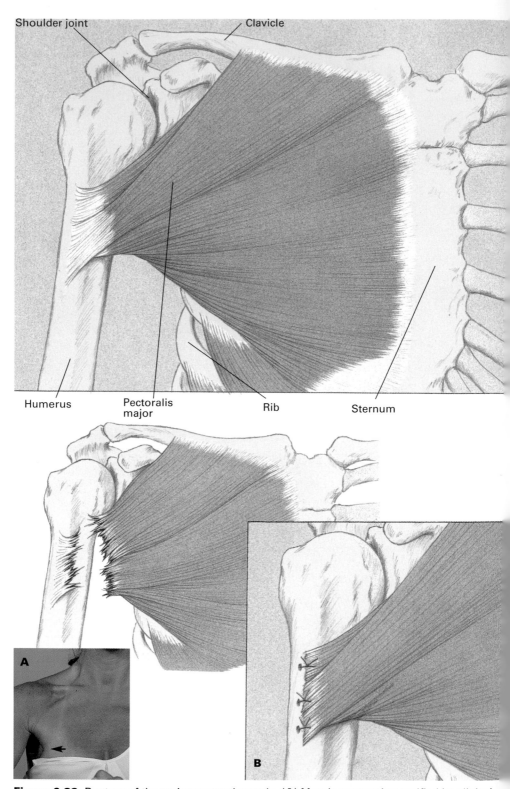

Figure 6.39 Rupture of the major pectoral muscle. (**A**) Muscle contraction verified by clinical testing. (**B**) Surgical reattachment.

Fractures of the humerus

Fractures of the *upper part* of the humerus occur most frequently as a result of falling on an outstretched arm, but they may also follow a direct fall on the shoulder during contact sports, such as rugby and American football, alpine skiing, and riding. Fractures of the upper part of the humerus occur most frequently through the surgical neck of the humerus. Sometimes they are avulsion fractures of the greater tubercle (supraspinatus tendon insertion) or the lesser tubercle (subscapularis tendon insertion).

Symptoms and diagnosis

Tenderness and swelling occur over the area of the injury, and pain is experienced on attempted movement.

Treatment

- The injured person should be taken to a doctor or a hospital for examination and an X-ray.
- A support bandage is applied and kept in position for a few days, after which mobility training is begun. Mobility training starts with pendulum movements and progresses to the exercises described on p. 495.
- Physiotherapy aids the process of rehabilitation. If the displacement of the avulsed tubercle is great or interferes with the range of motion, surgery should be considered.

Healing

As a rule, fractures of the upper part of the humerus heal well, and conditioning can be resumed after 4–8 weeks.

Fractures of the *midshaft* of the humerus can occur in riders, wrestlers, and other athletes. They are usually treated by cast bracing or occasionally by strapping the arm to the body for 3–6 weeks. Surgery may occasionally be necessary. A rehabilitation period of 3–6 months is advisable before resumption of any sporting activity involving the use of the injured arm.

Stress fractures of the humerus can occasionally occur, e.g. in javelin throwers. Management is suggested on p. 8.

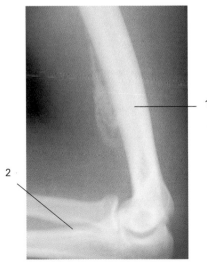

Figure 6.40 X-ray of myositis ossificans of upper arm. 1, Humerus; 2, radius and ulna.

Myositis ossificans

After a blow to the arm, an intramuscular hematoma can occur. Pain swelling, and impaired muscle function are common. In spite of early treatment with ice, compression, and rest, the injury may be complicated by bone formation within the muscle (Figure 6.40) secondary to the hematoma (p. 35).

Bibliography

Allen AA, Warner JJP (1995) Shoulder instability in the athlete. *Orthopedic Clinics of North America* 26: 487.

Arciero RA, Wheeler JH, Ryan JB, et al (1994) Arthroscopic Bankart repair versus nonoperative treatment for acute, initial anterior shoulder dislocation. *American Journal of Sports Medicine* 22: 589–594.

Snyder SJ, Karzel RP, Del Pizzo W et al (1990) SLAP lesions of the shoulder. *Arthroscopy* 6: 274–279.

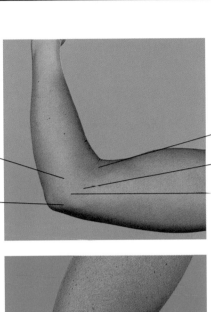

Figure 7.1 Medial aspect of elbow and location of associated injuries.

Elbow instability (p. 170)

Ulnar nerve entrapment (171)

Distal biceps tendon rupture (p. 176)

Median nerve entrapment (177)

Thrower's elbow (169); Little Leaguer's elbow (173)

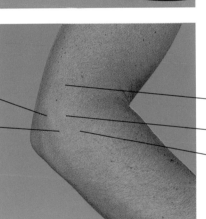

Figure 7.2 Lateral aspect of elbow and location of associated injuries.

Tennis elbow (p. 162)

Radial head fracture (168)

Humerus lower end fracture (p. 179)

Osteochondritis dissecans (167)

Radial nerve entrapment (177)

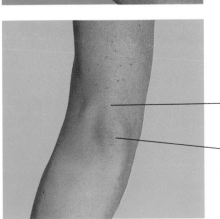

Figure 7.3 Posterior aspect of elbow and location of associated injuries.

Posterior tennis elbow (p. 173); triceps tendon strain (174)

Bursitis (174); olecranon fracture (176)

The elbow joint not only allows the arm to flex but also permits the forearm to rotate inwards and outwards (pronation and supination). Good elbow function is essential for everyday activities. Elbow injuries often occur during throwing or falling, and may result in serious complications owing to the proximity to the joint of major blood vessels and nerves (Figures 7.1–7.3).

Functional anatomy

The stability of the elbow is provided by the collateral ligaments and the fibrous capsules, as well as by the bones and their articulations, and the muscles and tendons (Figure 7.4). The medial ulnar ligament is well developed and forms three distinct bands: the anterior oblique ligament; a small, transverse, nonfunctional ligament; and the posterior oblique ligament. The anterior oblique ligament is very strong: it is taut through the entire arc of elbow flexion and is the primary constraint of valgus stress of the elbow. The posterior oblique ligament is taut in flexion and lax in extension and does not have a primary role in elbow stability. The lateral collateral ligament stabilizes for varus stress.

The anconeus muscle appears to provide lateral support, as do the forearm extensor muscles. The extensors carpi radialis brevis and longus, digitorum communis, digiti minimi and carporadialis originate at the lateral epicondyle and are mainly wrist and finger extensors. The three primary flexor muscles of the elbow are the biceps brachii, the brachioradialis, and the brachialis. The most important pronator muscles of the elbow are the pronator teres and the pronator quadratus. The triceps is the only effective extensor of the elbow.

The radial nerve runs anterior lateral of the elbow and divides into the posterior interosseous nerve and the lateral cutaneous nerve of the forearm; the former especially can be entrapped. The median nerve remains anterior of the elbow in its course and passes between the two heads of the pronator muscle and can also become entrapped. The ulnar

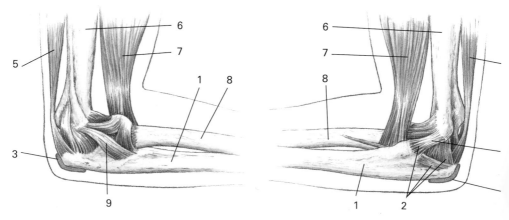

Figure 7.4 Elbow anatomy. 1, Ulna; 2, ulnar collateral ligaments; 3, bursa; 4, anterior oblique ligament; 5, triceps; 6, humerus; 7, biceps; 8, radius; 9, lateral collateral ligament. (**Left**) Lateral aspect; (**right**) medial aspect.

nerve passes through the triceps fascia as it approaches the cubital tunnel on the medial posterior aspect of the elbow, where it can be compressed and cause distal problems.

The elbow joint can be moved about a longitudinal and transverse axis. Flexion–extension is provided by the humeroulnar joint. The rotational motion is provided by the unique articulation of the radius with the capitellum portion of the humerus and the ulna so that forearm pronation and supination can be carried out.

The normal range of motion of the elbow is flexion and extension 0–145° with a functional arc of 0–130°. Pronation and supination can be carried out with 70–90° of pronation to 90° of supination. The axial rotation is around the center of the radial head.

Types of elbow injury

Elbow injuries in adults

Elbow injuries can be grouped into those occurring in medial, lateral, posterior or anterior areas.

Medial injuries

Medial injuries include medial epicondylitis, injury to the common flexors (myositis or acute rupture), compression of the hypertrophied pronator teres by the overlying fascia, chronic elongation and/or rupture of the medial collateral ligament with or without spur formation, and development of traction osteophytes medially. Ulnar nerve problems are also frequent.

Lateral injuries

Lateral epicondylitis is very common. As this area is subjected to compression rather than traction, other soft tissue injuries are less common. Osteochondritis dissecans can occur, resulting in loose bodies and post-traumatic arthritis.

Posterior injuries

Loose bodies may again result from traction injuries, such as overpull of the triceps or compression of the tip of the olecranon in the olecranon fossa. Posterior elbow injuries occur with sudden extension and hyperextension of the elbow, resulting in compression of the olecranon against the humerus. Older baseball pitchers may develop flexion deformities that limit full extension. In these cases, an injury thought to be due to compression of the olecranon into the olecranon fossa may actually be an avulsion injury.

Anterior injuries

The distal biceps tendon may tear.

Elbow injuries in children

Unique bony problems of the elbow are seen in children and adolescents. The pathology of these problems corresponds to each stage in the development of the elbow—that is, prior to the appearance of all the secondary centers of ossification in children; prior to fusion of the ossification centers in adolescents; and prior to the completion of bony growth in young adults. The majority of injuries are due to overuse resulting from an increase in frequency, rapidity, and duration of throwing.

Medial injuries

The medial side of the elbow is subjected to distraction forces which may cause injury to the medial epicondyle and the medial soft tissues, including the capsular structures and the ulnar nerve. In children, ossification of the medial epicondyle may be disturbed by enlargement of the epicondyle or by osteochondrotic (bone-cartilage) changes. In adolescent avulsion fractures of the medial epicondyle may occur. The epicondyle may occasionally displace in the joint causing mechanical derangement. After fusion of the medial epicondyle, muscular injuries are more frequent and may cause the development of osteophytes (bone spurs).

Lateral injuries

On the lateral side of the elbow, bony disturbance from repetitive compression and shearing forces may occur during childhood at both the head of the radius and the capitellum. Injury to the lateral aspect may affect the entire epiphysis with enlargements and fragmentation throughout. During adolescence, the periphery of the ossification center affected more with avulsion fractures damaging the articular cartilage and forming loose bodies. The capitellum and sometimes the head of the radius are affected by lesions.

Posterior injuries

In children, stress fractures and nonunion of the olecranon epiphysis (growth zone) may occur, as well as ectopic bone formation around the olecranon tip and loose body formation at a later date.

The various throwing injuries can be related to the various stages the throwing mechanism (see p. 72). An understanding of this mechanism, as well as of the stages of the skeletal maturation in the youthful athlete, is important in diagnosing and treating throwing injuries.

Clinical examination

Examination starts with inspection followed by palpation, evaluation of motion, strength testing, and instability testing.

Any gross swelling or muscle hypotrophy should be noted. Holding the forearm and hand supinated and the elbow extended, the angle formed by the humerus and forearm is determined (the carrying angle). The average is 10° for men and 13° for women. An inflamed olecranon bursa with swelling on the posterior aspect is a sign of olecranon bursitis.

The bony landmark needs to be palpated. Any tenderness is noticed as this usually indicates the area of injury.

Motion is important in assessment of elbow function. The motion occurs around two axes: flexion and extension and forearm rotation with pronation and supination. Flexion and extension ranges from 0° to 140° ± 10°. Pronation is often 70° and supination is 85-90°.

Flexion and extension strength testing is performed against resistance with the forearm in neutral rotation and the elbow at 90° of flexion (Figure 7.5). Elbow extension strength is normally 70% of flexion strength and is best measured with the elbow at 90° of flexion with the forearm in neutral rotation. Pronation and supination strength are also best studied with the elbow at 90° of flexion. Supination strength is normally about 15% greater than pronation strength.

The collateral ligament instability is evaluated with the elbow flexed and in 30° extension. Varus stress is applied with the humerus in full internal rotation and the lower arm pressed inwards. Valgus instability is best measured with the arm in full external rotation and the lower arm pressed outwards.

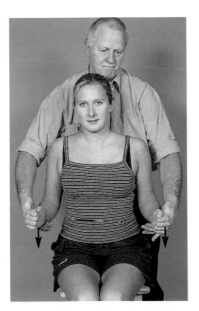 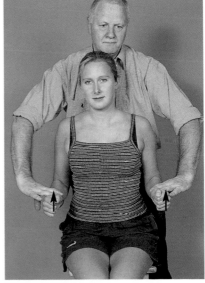

Figure 7.5 Elbow strength testing. (**Left**) Extension. (**Right**) Flexion.

Lateral elbow injuries

Tennis elbow (lateral epicondylitis, lateral elbow tendinosis)

Tennis is played by people of all ages, as it is a sport which in general does not produce severe medical problems. Problems do occur, however, in the elbow region. It should be remembered that only 5% of people suffering from tennis elbow relate the injury to tennis. This injury occurs in other racket sports such as squash, badminton, and table tennis. Golfers and others can also be affected, as well as those who carry out repetitive, one-sided movements in their jobs (e.g. electricians, carpenters) or leisure activities (e.g. needlework, knitting, gardening).

Etiology

Lateral elbow tendinosis is most common in tennis players 35–50 years of age. This group is characterized by a high activity level and they often play tennis three times a week or more, for at least 30 minutes per session. It has been shown that 45% of the athletes who play tennis daily, or 20% of those who play twice a week, may at certain stages suffer from lateral elbow tendinosis. Frequency of play has a direct relationship with pain. The more frequently a person plays, the greater is the incidence of pain. Players of higher ability, who play longer and practice more, more commonly have a history of elbow pain.

Tennis players most likely to sustain lateral elbow tendinosis are those who have demanding techniques and inadequate fitness levels. Faulty technique is one of the most common causes for lateral elbow tendinosis, especially a faulty backhand (Figure 7.6). The serve may also be associated with elbow pain.

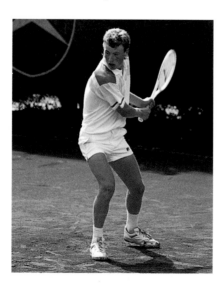

Figure 7.6 Tennis players with a double-handed backhand do not develop lateral elbow tendinosis.

Pathology

The pathoanatomy of lateral elbow tendinosis related to tennis involves primarily the extensor carpi radialis brevis and secondarily the extensor digitorum communis muscle tendons. The bellies of the relevant muscles are all located in the forearm, while the long tendons bridge the elbow and wrist joints, and insert on the metacarpals or phalanges (fingerbones). The lateral epicondyle of the humerus forms a common origin for at least parts of all the extensors of the wrist and fingers (Figure 7.7).

The disorder represents a degenerative process (see p. 43) that is secondary to tensile overuse fatigue, weakness, and possibly avascular changes (poor circulation). There are usually no inflammatory cells present. The term 'tendinosis' is therefore replacing the term 'tendinitis'.

Symptoms and diagnosis

- There is a history of repetitive activity or overuse, such as playing tennis intensively at a training camp, or resuming playing after a period of little activity.
- Pain mainly affects the lateral aspect of the elbow, but can also radiate upwards along the upper arm and downwards along the outside of the forearm.
- Weakness in the wrist can cause difficulty in carrying out such simple movements as lifting a plate or a coffee cup, opening a car door, wringing out a wet dishcloth, and shaking hands.
- A distinct tender point is elicited by pressure or percussion over the lateral epicondyle.
- Pain occurs over the lateral epicondyle when the hand is dorsiflexed at the wrist against resistance (Figure 7.8). This sign alone is sufficient to justify a diagnosis of 'tennis elbow'.
- A positive middle finger test: there is pain over the lateral elbow when the middle finger is extended against resistance (Figure 7.9).

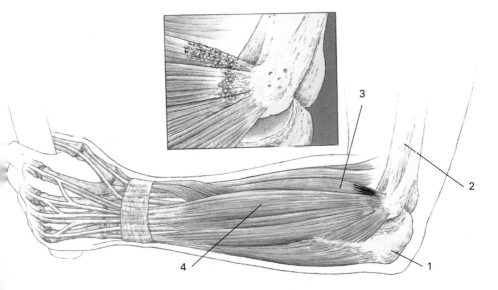

Figure 7.7 Tennis elbow with pathology in extensor carpi radialis brevis. 1, Ulna; 2, humerus; 3, extensor carpi radialis brevis; 4, extensor digitorum communis.

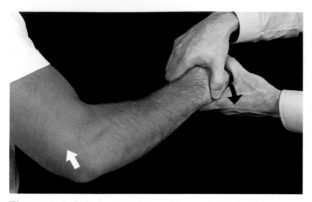

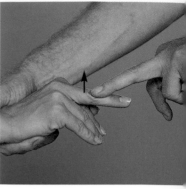

Figure 7.8 Pain is experienced in the lateral epicondyle (white arrow) when the wrist is dorsiflexed against resistance (dark arrow).

Figure 7.9 Pain is experienced in the lateral epicondyle when the middle finger is extended against resistance.

Involvement of the extensor carpi radialis brevis is typical in tenn[?] players. In lateral elbow tendinosis due to other causes, e.g. industri[?] work, it seems that the extensor digitorum communis is typicall[?] involved. This also leads to a positive middle finger test. In other word[?] there may be two different etiologies of lateral elbow tendinosis wit[?] different locations of the problem.

An accurate diagnosis of tendinosis includes an evaluation of th[?] magnitude of pathological change, which is helpful as a prognost[?] predictor, as well as formulating the treatment protocol. The patient[?] description of time and intensity of pain is the best guide to evaluatio[?]

The elbow can be X-rayed to exclude a loose body in the joint or fracture. Other possible diagnoses are rheumatic disorders, trapping [?] a nerve (the deep branch of the radial nerve or the ulnar nerve), an[?] radiating pain caused by degenerative changes in the spine in the regio[?] of the fifth and sixth cervical vertebrae.

Preventive measures

– Correct playing and working techniques are the most importa[?] preventive measures.
– Sometimes a forearm brace or a heat retainer can be used as a mea[?] of dissipating the forces outwards before they reach the epicondyle.
– Asymmetrical training techniques should be avoided.

In tennis, the following points should be emphasized:
1. Good footwork so that the player approaches the ball correctly.
2. The ball should be hit correctly with the racket and at the right momen[?]
3. The shoulder and the whole of the body should take part in eve[?] stroke so that 'braking' does not occur when the ball is hit. The stro[?] should be followed through and the wrist should be firm.
4. The court surface should be slow in order to decrease the velocity of t[?] ball. Fast surfaces such as grass or concrete cause the ball to hit the rack[?] with increased force, resulting in increased load on the player's arm.
5. The balls should be light. Wet or dead balls become heavy.
6. The correct equipment should be used. The racket should be individ[?] ally selected with regard to playing technique. A casual player should u[?]

a light racket, as a heavy racket causes greater load. The racket should be well-balanced and easy to handle, e.g. when making angled dropshots.

7. A tightly strung racket increases the impact and tension forces. The stringing of the racket should be individually adjusted and should not be too taut. Anyone troubled by tennis elbow should have the racket strung more loosely. Gut strings give more resilience and less vibration than nylon ones.

8. The size of the racket grip should be carefully chosen in order to fit the hand comfortably. A simple method of determining the appropriate size of grip is to measure the distance between the midline of the palm of hand and the tip of the middle finger; this distance should equal the grip's circumference (Figure 7.10).

9. A large 'sweet spot' (center of percussion, the area of the racket face where minimal torsion occurs on impact) is probably an advantage. Hits outside this spot will increase torsion and unwanted forces and vibrations.

The treatment should follow the healing response; this includes three phases: (1) an acute inflammatory phase; (2) a collagen and ground substance production phase; and (3) a maturation and remodeling phase. The *athlete* should:

– reduce pain and inflammation when the injury is in its acute stage by the use of cooling for about 2 days (elevation and compression are not needed, as swelling is not a problem);
– rest actively—that is, rest the injured area and avoid movements that trigger pain, but continue with conditioning activity such as running or cycling;
– continue with tennis but avoid the strokes that cause pain;
– apply local heat and use a heat retainer when the injury is no longer in its acute stage;
– treat with ice massage, perhaps alternating with heat treatment;
– try taping the wrist to support the elbow joint under load;

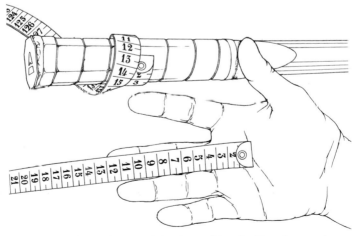

Figure 7.10 Measuring the right size racket grip. The distance between the mid-line of the palm and the tip of the middle finger is equal to the correct size of the grip.

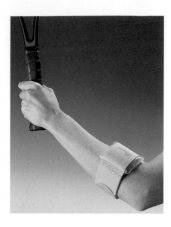

Figure 7.11 Bracing for tennis elbow.

– reduce the load on the extensors with the help of a brace, which shoul
be applied when the arm is relaxed and kept in position until th
rehabilitation period is over.

Counterforce bracing constrains key muscles groups. An air-filled bladd
has been developed as a counterpressure element (Figure 7.11). Th
constrictive band caused a significant reduction in integrated EMG
the extensor carpi radialis brevis and the extensor digitorum commun
when compared with controlled values and a standard band. Mo
research is needed to confirm the effect of braces for the treatment
tennis elbow. Clinical experience indicates, however, that the use of suc
braces is a valuable complementary tool in the treatment of tennis elbo
The elbow bands can be combined with heat-retaining Neoprene sleev
to add the positive effects of heat in stimulating healing.

Strength, stamina, and mobility should be improved by exercises on
the pain and inflammation are under control, i.e. the athlete can tolera
the pain of a handshake. The training program should follow the guid
lines set out below.

1. Isometric training of the wrist extensors (see pp. 497, 503). The trai
   ing is carried out with the wrist in three positions: first fully flex
   downwards, then in a neutral position, and finally flexed upwards. T
   joint should not be under load and the exercise should be carried o
   30 times a day. The wrist is flexed for 10 seconds at a time. Wh
   these exercises can be carried out without any pain, a load of 0.5
   (1 lb) can be introduced.
2. Dynamic training. An elastic band is slipped over the ends of t
   fingers, and then an attempt is made to spread the fingers against
   resistance. Another method is to extend (concentric) and flex (ecce
   tric) the wrist with a load of 1–2 kg (2–4 lb) 20 times a day.
3. Flexibility training (static stretching) of the wrist. The joint is bent
   an angle of 90° and the opposite hand is used to provide counte
   pressure. The elbow of the injured arm should be held complete
   extended and the forearm should be rotated inwards (pronated). T
   bent wrist is stretched to its outer range and is held there for 4
   seconds. After 2 seconds rest it is subjected to stretching for anoth
   6–8 seconds. The exercise is repeated 15 times a day.

4. Training of strength and mobility in shoulder and arm (p. 498).

The *doctor* may:
– prescribe anti-inflammatory medication;
– prescribe ultrasound treatment, high-voltage galvanic stimulation, or/and transcutaneous nerve stimulation. There is no agreement on which treatment is most appropriate for this common condition;
– prescribe acupuncture;
– administer local steroid injections in persistent cases and if pain interferes with the exercise program.

Injections should be given subperiosteally to the extensor brevis origin. These injections have an early and beneficial effect. During the initial 24–28 hours, increased pain may be experienced. A steroid injection should be followed by 1–2 weeks' rest and should not be repeated more than 2 times. Steroid injection seems to be effective for about 3 months, indicating that the patient must continue with the exercise program.

Failed healing is considered to have occurred if there are chronic symptoms of tendinosis pain for more than 6–12 months. If there is poor response to a rehabilitation program, if there is a history of persistent pain, or if the patient has not been able to return to an acceptable quality of life, surgery may be indicated. In patients undergoing surgery it has been found that in 100% the tissue involved was extensor carpi radialis brevis; extensor digitorum communis, especially the anterior edge, was involved in 35%, and there was osteophyte formation of the lateral epicondyle in 20%. Surgery consists of resection of damaged tissue. The attachment of normal tissues should be maintained and the healthy tissues protected. There should then be quality postoperative rehabilitation. The elbow is protected at 90° for 1 week in a counterforce elbow immobilizer. Strength and endurance resistance exercises usually start 3 weeks after surgery. Postoperatively, 85% experience complete pain relief and full return of strength.

A recurrence rate of 18–66% is reported. The degree of pain prior to treatment is the most important predictor of complete recovery: the greater the pain, the more likely is the treatment to be completely successful. Arthroscopic treatment of this condition is now being developed.

ealing A genuine tennis elbow often heals spontaneously and the prognosis is generally good. The symptoms can, however, persist for anything from 2 weeks to 2 years, especially if the athlete continues to load the arm. Strenuous activity can be resumed when the arm is fully mobile, has regained normal strength, and is pain-free. After surgery, 8–10 weeks should elapse before tennis is resumed.

Osteochondritis dissecans (loose bone cartilage)

In throwing movements the lateral part of the elbow joint is exposed to considerable loads, because of compression due to valgus loads. This can cause the convex upper articular surface of the radius in the forearm to

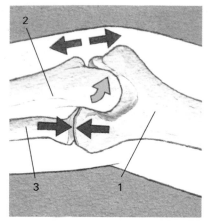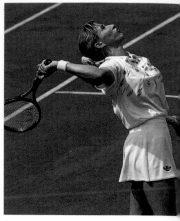

Figure 7.12 Mechanism behind elbow injuries: valgus overload of the elbow causes lateral compression and medial traction. 1, Humerus; 2, ulna; 3, radius.

come into violent contact with, and even to injure, the lateral out
portion of the articular surface of the humerus at the elbow. Cartila
from the articular surface, together with a fragment of the underlyi
bone, may become detached and form a loose body in the joint (Figu
7.12). Osteochondritis dissecans (loose bone cartilage) (p. 23) occurs mc
commonly in teenage boys.

<table>
<tr>
<td>Symptoms
and diagnosis</td>
<td>
– Pain is felt in the upper outer aspect of the elbow, triggered mair
   by throwing movements.
– Difficulties in straightening and bending the elbow joint are experience
– Locking of the joint occurs during elbow movements. The loose bo
   prevents completion of the intended movement, and such an occu
   rence is always painful. Muscle cramp and swelling follow.
– Swelling develops around the elbow.
– Tenderness can be felt, mainly on the outer aspect of the elbow joi
– Both elbow joints should be X-rayed, especially when the injured pers
   is young and still growing. On the X-ray of the injured elbow joint t
   osteochondritis, the defect, or loose bodies (calcifications) can be see
– MRI or arthroscopy will confirm the diagnosis.
</td>
</tr>
<tr>
<td>Treatment</td>
<td>See p. 24.</td>
</tr>
<tr>
<td>Healing</td>
<td>The injured athlete can usually resume sporting activity 2–3 months af
surgery.</td>
</tr>
</table>

Fracture of the head of the radius

The radius is thick and strong at the wrist, but considerably smaller
circumference and more fragile at the elbow. When the arm is stretch
out to break a fall, the forces imposed are distributed through the forea

to the upper part of the radius. The radial head, which forms part of the elbow joint, can be fractured with the possibility of chronic problems.

- Instant pain is felt when the injury occurs. This increases as the joint becomes swollen due to bleeding.
- Limitation of movement increases with the swelling. The elbow is usually held flexed at an angle of 90°.
- An X-ray confirms the diagnosis.

The *doctor* may:
- aspirate the blood from the injured joint with a syringe if severe swelling is causing pain;
- apply a brace which is worn for 1–2 weeks (after that the arm muscles should be strengthened by training);
- operate if the radius is badly fragmented or displaced.

A properly reduced fracture of the radial head heals in 6–8 weeks. Conditioning can be carried out through the rehabilitation period.

Medial elbow injuries

Thrower's elbow or golfer's elbow (medial epicondylitis, medial elbow tendinosis)

Thrower's or golfer's elbow is similar to tennis elbow, but the symptoms are located over the inner (medial) epicondyle of the elbow. A right-handed golf player may well suffer from tennis elbow in the (leading) left elbow and golfer's elbow in the (following) right elbow. Thrower's elbow is most common in javelin throwers, but also occurs in cricket and baseball players.

The primary pathological changes involved in medial tennis elbow are present in the origin of the pronator teres, palmaris longus, and flexor carpi radialis, close to the attachment of the medial epicondyle. Occasionally pathological changes also occur in the flexor carpi ulnaris.

The etiology of medial elbow tendinosis is the same as for lateral tendinosis. The majority of cases are due to faulty technique (Figure 7.13); however, top-level tennis players may develop medial epicondylitis owing to a serving action during which the wrist is bent at the same time as the forearm is turned inwards. Those who hit an exaggerated 'top spin' serve and in so-doing rotate the forearm vigorously inwards (excessive pronation) can also be affected. The flexor muscles that are principally responsible for these movements have their origins at the medial epicondyle of the elbow.

The symptoms are similar to those of tennis elbow (p. 162) but are located on the inner aspect of the elbow. There is pronounced tenderness when

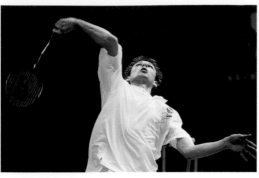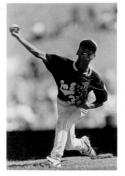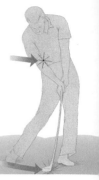

Figure 7.13 (Left) The shot in badminton or **(middle)** pitching in baseball can cause elbow problems. (By courtesy of All Sport: photographer, Doug Pensinger.) **(Right)** Poor technique in golf can also cause injury.

the medial epicondyle is subjected to pressure, and flexing the han downwards (palmar flexion) at the wrist joint against resistance cause pain.

Treatment

The treatment is the same as for tennis elbow. However, rehabilitatio can sometimes take a little longer after surgery.

Healing

The prognosis for medial elbow tendinosis is worse and the healing tim is longer than for the lateral side. It can sometimes take 6–12 month before a return to tennis is possible. Patients should be told this so th: their expectations are realistic.

Elbow instability (rupture of the medial collateral ligaments)

The valgus stress overload syndrome can cause medial tension resultir in torsion of the medial (ulnar) collateral ligament (MCL). This ligamen especially its anterior band, is of great importance for elbow stability. is composed of two parts: the origin of the anterior band is posterior the axis of elbow rotation, while the origin of the posterior band is ju posterior to the axis. The posterior portion of the MCL contributes litt to valgus stability. The radial head contributes significantly to stabili at 0°, 45°, and 90° of flexion, but the MCL is the most important stab lizer except at full extension. The anterior band is the major stabiliz from 20° to 120° of flexion.

Symptoms and diagnosis

- Pain on the medial side of the arm occurs during throwing (cocki phase) or serving.
- Tenderness if felt on the ligament.
- There is a sensation of the elbow 'opening' or 'giving way'.
- A valgus instability is tested with a valgus stress test. The shoulder then externally rotated, the elbow flexed 30° and a valgus load is appli (Figures 7.14 and 7.15). An opening of the joint indicates instability.

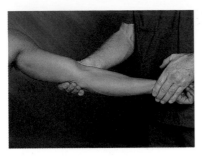

Figure 7.14 Testing for elbow instability with the arm extended.

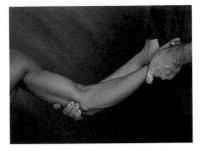

Figure 7.15 Testing for elbow instability with the arm flexed 30°.

- A valgus instability test can be performed arthroscopically with the elbow flexed 60–70°. An opening of the joint between the ulnar and humerus can be seen. An opening of more than 0.04 in (1 mm) indicates a complete tear of the ulnar collateral ligament.
- The pathophysiology involves edema (swelling) and inflammation or scar formation within the ligament. There can also be calcific densities within the scar or ossifications within the ligament. Ruptures can also occur. These changes can be verified by an MRI.

Treatment

The treatment includes rest and ice, generally followed by rehabilitation with strengthening exercises as the main focus. Surgery is indicated if 6 months of conservative therapy is unsuccessful, and occasionally in acute ruptures.

Return to sport after surgery is a test of the athlete's patience. Although some throwing is possible after 3–4 months, competitive throwing must be delayed for 9–12 months, and professional pitchers may need 12–18 months before reaching full capacity.

Entrapment of the ulnar nerve (ulnar neuritis)

If the medial posterior aspect of the elbow is accidentally hit, pain can be felt radiating to the fourth and fifth fingers of the hand. The ulnar nerve runs along the medial edge of the elbow just behind the epicondyle to which the flexor muscles of the wrist are attached. In throwing or racket sports the nerve can be stretched or slid out of its groove with subsequent mechanical irritation.

The majority of nerve lesions in athletes can be described as neuropraxia, the mildest form of nerve injury. It is characterized by a conduction block along a nerve where all nerve elements, axons, and connective tissue remain in continuity. The prognosis for complete recovery may be good, provided no irreversible tissue damage has occurred due to long-standing compression.

The nerve can be injured by friction, compression, contusion, tension (traction), or a combination of these. The ulnar nerve is also susceptible to stretch injury, although it may stretch up to 20% before damage occurs. Valgus extension overload during serving and pitching creates significant tensile overload on the medial elbow ligament structures, and compressive loads laterally. The medial part of the ulnar nerve can elongate 0.2 in (4.7 mm) during extension to full flexion. It can be moved 0.3 in (7 mm) medially by triceps. These tensile loads also affect the ulnar nerve as it crosses through the cubital tunnel, causing nerve friction, irritation, and compression. The nerve may become unstable as the elbow is flexed.

Ulnar nerve entrapment was found in 60% of surgical cases of medial tennis elbow. These entrapments were found distal to the medial epicondyle at the medial and muscular septum, as the nerve enters the flexor carpi ulnaris. The nerve entrapment may be secondary to elbow instability, spurs, synovitis, and more proximal compression.

Symptoms and diagnosis

- Pain arises from the medial aspect of the elbow, typically after long tennis or golf matches, or throwing the javelin.
- Pain may increase and radiate to the fourth and fifth fingers of the hand.
- Numbness and impaired sensation may be present in the little finger and half the ring finger.
- Tenderness may occur over the nerve on the medial dorsal side of the elbow (Figure 7.16).
- In serious cases even tapping the ulnar nerve lightly can cause pain extending as far as the ring finger.
- Dislocation of the nerve from the cubital tunnel on palpation (that is the nerve moves over the medial epicondyle during activity).

Treatment

The *athlete* should rest the arm.

The *doctor* may:
- prescribe anti-inflammatory medication;
- operate if the injury persists in order to free the nerve or move it to a position in which it is subjected to less tension. Surgery usually gives good results. In a chronic phase, especially if the nerve is subluxated, the nerve can be treated surgically with transposition of the nerve in front of the epicondyle and decompression for at least 2 in (5 cm) distal to the epicondyle.

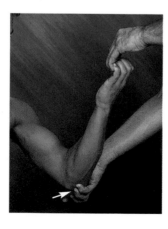

Figure 7.16 The ulnar nerve on the medial dorsal aspect (arrow) may be tender.

Little Leaguer's elbow

When a ball is thrown in baseball, the wrist and the fingers are vigorously pronated. The muscles responsible for this movement are all located in the inner (medial) compartment of the forearm. The force of the throw is transmitted up through the arm to the weakest part of the muscle group, which is the medial epicondyle from which the muscles originate. In growing adolescents these muscle origins are attached to a growth area that is considerably weaker than the adjacent bone, and problems are caused by the increased traction on the epiphyseal junction.

Symptoms and diagnosis
- Pain in the elbow often starts gradually. If the pain appears suddenly the epiphysis may have been torn off, which sometimes necessitates surgery. The pain can be induced when the elbow joint is flexed.
- There is stiffness in the elbow.
- Local tenderness is felt directly over the medial epicondyle.
- Both the elbows should be X-rayed. A fissure in the epiphysis can be seen if present.

Treatment
The *athlete* should
- rest from painful activity;
- give up throwing movements completely until the pain has resolved (usually after 8–9 weeks);
- continue with conditioning and general strength training.

The *doctor* may:
- prescribe rest and sometimes immobilize the elbow. If there is a fissure in the epiphysis, a cast may be used;
- operate if displacement is significant. Neither steroid injections nor anti-inflammatory medicines should be given to growing adolescents.

Healing
If the epiphysis has been injured, throwing training can be resumed at the earliest 8 weeks after the injury occurred. Prior to that, careful rehabilitation should aim to maintain muscle function.

Posterior elbow injuries

Posterior tennis elbow

Posterior tennis elbow, also known as posterior olecranon impingement or hyperextension elbow injury, is associated with aggressive elbow extension during the follow-through phase (Figure 7.17). The olecranon can impinge on the posterior aspect of the humerus and cause problems, such as triceps tendinosis. Osteophytes can form on the olecranon by forced hyperextension of the olecranon into the olecranon fossa, or by shear forces between the posterior medial aspect of the olecranon and the olecranon fossa secondary to the valgus movement placed on the elbow during the serve.

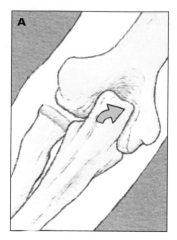
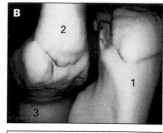
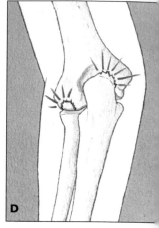
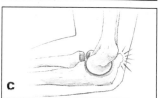

Figure 7.17 (A) Bone movements involved in elbow extension; **(B)** CT scan reconstruction of posterior elbow (1, ulna; 2, humerus; 3, radius); **(C)** formation of osteophytes; **(D)** formation of osteochondral fragment.

Pathological changes in the posterior compartment can be evaluate arthroscopically through a posterior lateral portal. The osteophytes ar usually located on the posterior medial aspect of the olecranon. Trea ment is usually conservative, but surgery is increasingly used to remov osteophytes and/or loose bodies. Return to sport is possible within 2– months.

Strain of the tendon of the tricep muscle

Falling on the hand when the arm is flexed or forceful throwing ca cause a rupture in the tendon of the triceps, and sometimes the tendo attachment can be torn away from the tip of the elbow.

Symptoms and diagnosis
– Pain occurs in the tip of the elbow where a gap can be felt in th tendon.
– There is impaired power in the arm or inability to straighten the ar at the elbow. An X-ray is needed to exclude bony injury.

Treatment
– In cases of minor ruptures no treatment, apart from rest, is necessar
– Surgery should be carried out when young, active athletes hav suffered a total rupture of the tendon or the tendon attachment.

Bursitis (student's elbow)

Just below the tip of the elbow (olecranon) there is a bursa into whic bleeding can occur following an accidental blow to the area or a fall c the elbow (Figure 7.18). In many sports, including orienteerin wrestling, volleyball, basketball, soccer, rugby, and team handball, th

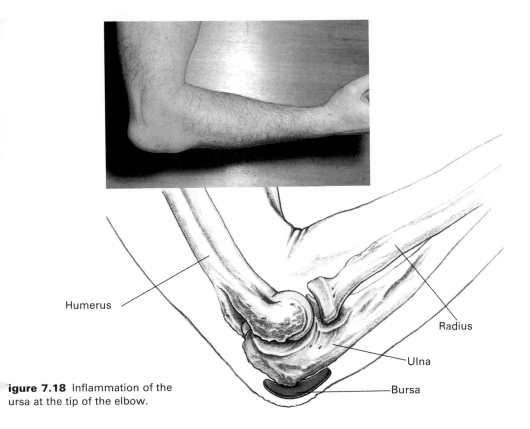

igure 7.18 Inflammation of the ursa at the tip of the elbow.

Humerus

Radius

Ulna

Bursa

injury is common as the participants wear no elbow guards; in others, such as ice hockey, the guards may provide incomplete protection.

After bleeding into the bursa, and also after prolonged loading of the elbow, the bursa can become inflamed and swollen. The condition is often called 'student's elbow' since it was popularly supposed to have affected students who rested their elbows on the desk while supporting their head in their hands while studying.

ymptoms nd diagnosis

- Pain is felt at rest and during movement.
- Swelling and tenderness occur over the tip of the elbow after acute bleeding into the bursa following a violent impact. Sometimes the skin is broken.
- Small blood clots form in the bursa and cause irritation of the surrounding tissues. This results in inflammation and effusion of fluid.
- When there is inflammation of the bursa, or when it has been subjected to prolonged pressure, it becomes distended with fluid and the overlying skin becomes red and tender. The swelling can extend to the forearm.
- There is limitation of mobility in the elbow joint.

reventive 1easures

Elbow guards that protect the olecranon (p. 84) should be used, especially by goalkeepers in team handball and soccer.

The *athlete* should rest until symptoms have resolved.
The *doctor* may:
- puncture the bursa and drain out blood or fluid;
- apply a bandage to be kept in position for 4–7 days;
- administer a local steroid injection when inflammation is persistent;
- remove the bursa surgically if it has been affected by repeated inflammation, especially when loose bodies or adhesions are present. This can be done arthroscopically.

Healing

After an episode of mild inflammation of a bursa in the elbow, the athlete can return to training 1 week after medical treatment has started. A severe bursitis can force rest for a long period.

Fracture of the olecranon

A fracture of the olecranon process can be caused by a fall on a bent elbow during contact sports, or in speedway racing and horse riding. The symptoms are swelling and tenderness over the elbow and an inability to straighten the joint. Surgery is often required as the triceps tendon pulls the fractured surfaces away from each other. It is 2– months before sporting activity can be resumed after an injury of this nature.

Anterior elbow injuries

Rupture of the distal part of the biceps tendon

The biceps tendon inserts distally into the radial tuberosity in the proximal forearm. It is responsible for flexion in the elbow and also for some supination. The tendon is susceptible to degenerative changes and ruptures occur in athletes over 35 years old. The injury mechanism usually a sudden extension of the elbow when the elbow is forcefully flexed.

Symptoms and diagnosis

- There is a history of a sudden snap in the elbow region during eccentric, sudden load of the elbow.
- Moderate pain occurs over the anterior aspect of the elbow.
- Palpation reveals tenderness over the radial tuberosity and the anterior aspect of the elbow.
- Swelling occurs over the distal anterior aspect of the upper arm.
- It is difficult to contract the biceps against resistance at the elbow the acute stage.
- There is weakness of the elbow in flexion.

The *athlete* should consult a doctor for advice.

The *doctor* may:

- prescribe careful mobilization with strengthening and stretching exercises (conservative therapy may result in a strength deficit of about 20–40%);
- operate on a complete tear in a young active person. The indication for surgery is the need of the athlete to regain full strength. The procedure consists of reattaching the distal tendon to the radial tuberosity.

- Early mobilization with strength and stretching exercises can begin as soon as pain and inflammation start to subside.
- Following surgery, healing usually takes 6 weeks, but range-of-motion exercises should start after 2–3 weeks. Strength training can be resumed around 6–8 weeks. Throwing activities are usually not allowed until after 4–5 months. The prognosis and results are good.

Entrapment of the radial nerve

The posterior interosseous or superficial radial nerve branches just below the elbow in the lateral part. It can occasionally be subjected to compression when it passes through the arcade of Frohse in the supinator muscle, which supinates the forearm. The symptoms may be similar to those of tennis elbow.

- Point tenderness may be present below and slightly in front of the lateral epicondyle, directly over the area of nerve entrapment.
- Pain is felt and strength impaired when the wrist joint is extended and the forearm is supinated.
- Electromyographic and nerve conduction studies may be helpful in identifying which motor segment is involved.

The *athlete* should rest and gradually increase activities.

The *doctor* may:

- prescribe anti-inflammatory medication;
- operate to free the nerve and enlarge the canal in which it runs. Surgery usually gives good results.

Entrapment of the median nerve (pronator teres syndrome)

The median nerve runs in front of the elbow joint and past the pronator muscle. Entrapment of this nerve is a rare condition in sport.

- Pain and tenderness occur in the middle anterior aspect of the elbow.
- Numbness is felt in the second and third fingers, and in the radial half of the fourth finger.
- Pain can be elicited by pronation of the lower arm against resistance.

- Weakness is present in palmar flexion of the hand.
- Discomfort during resisted elbow flexion and forearm pronation ca
  support the diagnosis.

Treatment

The *athlete* should:
- rest from painful activity;
- use heat.

The *doctor* may:
- prescribe anti-inflammatory medication;
- immobilize the elbow for a short time;
- operate in chronic cases.

Fractures and dislocations

Dislocation

Dislocation of the elbow joint occurs mainly in athletes participating
contact sports, such as football, rugby, and ice hockey, but can also occ
in riders, cyclists, wrestlers, skiers, and squash players. A common cau
of this injury is falling on the hand with a bent elbow. A similar inju
can occur if the elbow is overstretched in a fall.

A backward (posterior) dislocation of the elbow joint is most common
seen (Figure 7.19) and may be combined with a fracture. Dislocatio
always involve injuries to surrounding soft tissues, such as the medial a
lateral collateral ligaments, so that even when the injured joint is realign
promptly it can take some time for complete healing to take place.

**Symptoms
and diagnosis**

- Intense pain, swelling, tenderness and limitation of mobility are exper
  enced.
- There is deformity of the elbow joint.
- An X-ray confirms the diagnosis.
- Stability testing of the collateral ligaments at 20-30° flexion and
  extension will show the extent of ligament injury.

Treatment

The doctor may
- after having checked nerve function and circulation, replace the jo
  to its normal position and test it for stability; the sooner this is don
  the easier the manipulation;
- X-ray the joint after it has been restored to its correct position;
- immobilize the elbow joint in a brace for a few days depending on t
  extent of the injury. Mobility training (p. 503) should start as early
  possible;
- operate if there are extensive ligament injuries and instability in t
  joint.

**Healing and
complications**

When the brace has been removed, the injured athlete can resume con
tioning exercises such as running. The athlete's usual sport should

178

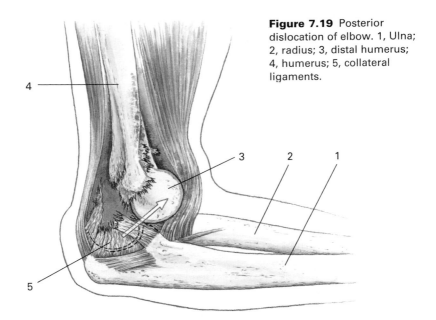

Figure 7.19 Posterior dislocation of elbow. 1, Ulna; 2, radius; 3, distal humerus; 4, humerus; 5, collateral ligaments.

be resumed until 9–10 weeks after the occurrence of the injury, when the ligaments have healed and full mobility is restored.

Nerve and circulatory injuries may occur and give permanent symptoms in the forearm and hand. If a dislocated elbow is treated inadequately, the result may be incomplete healing of the ligaments and joint capsule, and a susceptibility to recurrent dislocation.

Fracture of the lower end of the humerus (supracondylar fracture)

Children often sustain fractures of the lower part of the humerus because of falls from gymnasium apparatus, and in riding or cycling falls (Figure 7.20).

Symptoms and diagnosis
- Intense pain is felt during arm movements.
- There is tenderness on pressure.
- Swelling and bruising are noticeable.
- Contour changes.

Treatment
The injured person should be taken to a doctor as quickly as possible. Fractures of the lower part of the humerus very often require hospital treatment, especially in children or adolescents, as the important nerves and blood vessels situated near the broken ends of the bone can be affected by the resultant bleeding and are vulnerable to damage. Pulse and sensation below the injury should be checked.

The *doctor* will attempt to realign the fractured bones, and if this is not possible, surgery may be necessary.

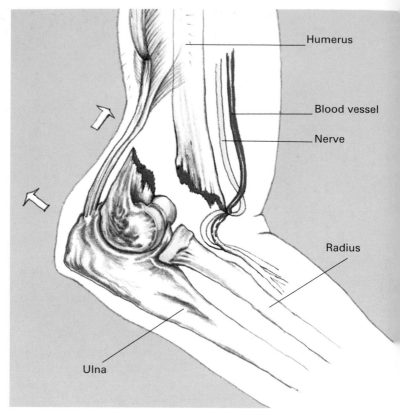

Humerus

Blood vessel

Nerve

Radius

Ulna

Figure 7.20 Fracture of the lower end of the humerus. Fractured bone fragments may press against and possibly damage blood vessels and nerves.

Healing

Mobility exercises (p. 503) are started at an early stage if the injury not too serious. After 8–10 weeks, when full mobility of the arm has bee regained, sporting activity can be resumed.

Arthroscopy

Arthroscopy is more and more commonly used for diagnosis and trea ment of many elbow injuries. By avoiding a large capsular excision, mai of the problems of postoperative scarring and capsular contraction of t elbow can be avoided.

Elbow arthroscopy should be performed slowly and deliberately, by surgeon who is experienced in sports medicine. Usually a 4 mm, 3 angle arthroscope provides optimal visualization of the elbow; sometim a 1.6 mm flexible arthroscope can be used (Figure 7.21). The anterol: eral portal, 2 cm distal and 3 cm anterior to the lateral epicondyle, commonly used. The lateral and posterior antebrachial cutaneous nerv must be avoided. The instrument should be directed toward the cen

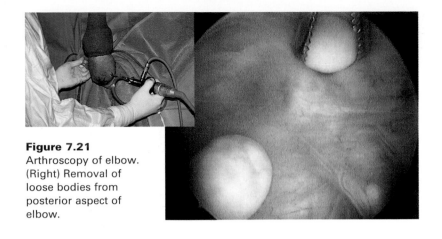

Figure 7.21
Arthroscopy of elbow.
(Right) Removal of
loose bodies from
posterior aspect of
elbow.

of the elbow with the elbow flexed at 90° at all times. The arthroscopic instruments pass within a mean distance of 4 mm of the radial nerve regardless of the flexion or extension of the elbow when the elbow is not extended with fluid. However, when 35–40 ml of fluid is inserted into the elbow capsule, the radial nerve moves an additional 7 mm anteriorly. The maximum distention of the elbow should be maintained at all times, particularly when established in initial arthroscopic portals.

Through a medial portal, 2 cm proximal and 1–2 cm anterior to the medial epicondyle, the radial head and the capitellum can be well visualized. The medial antebrachial cutaneous nerve should be avoided.

The posterolateral portal is sited 3 cm proximal to the olecranon superior and posterior to the lateral epicondyle. The olecranon fossa and tip of the olecranon can be seen as well as the distal humerus. It should be remembered that this portal is established with the elbow at 20–30° of flexion.

Bibliography

Elliott BC (1988) Biomechanics of the serve in tennis. A biomedical perspective. *Sports Medicine* 6: 285–294.

Kamien M (1988) Tennis elbow in long time tennis players. *Australian Journal of Science and Medicine in Sport* 20(2): 19–27.

Nirschl RP (1992) Elbow tendinosis/tennis elbow. *Clinics in Sports Medicine* 11(4): 851–870.

Forearm, wrist and hand

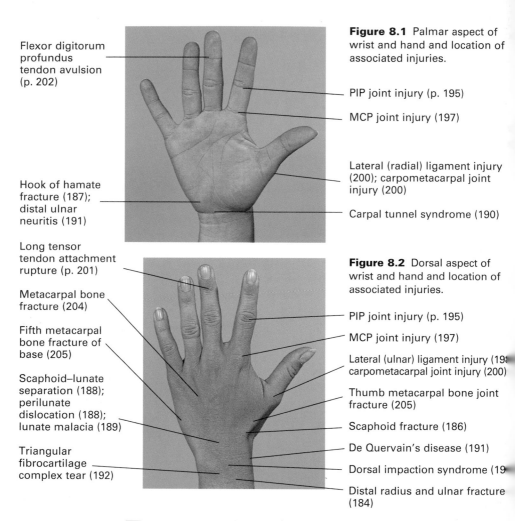

Flexor digitorum profundus tendon avulsion (p. 202)

Figure 8.1 Palmar aspect of wrist and hand and location of associated injuries.

PIP joint injury (p. 195)

MCP joint injury (197)

Lateral (radial) ligament injury (200); carpometacarpal joint injury (200)

Hook of hamate fracture (187); distal ulnar neuritis (191)

Carpal tunnel syndrome (190)

Long tensor tendon attachment rupture (p. 201)

Figure 8.2 Dorsal aspect of wrist and hand and location of associated injuries.

Metacarpal bone fracture (204)

PIP joint injury (p. 195)

MCP joint injury (197)

Fifth metacarpal bone fracture of base (205)

Lateral (ulnar) ligament injury (19 carpometacarpal joint injury (200)

Scaphoid–lunate separation (188); perilunate dislocation (188); lunate malacia (189)

Thumb metacarpal bone joint fracture (205)

Scaphoid fracture (186)

De Quervain's disease (191)

Triangular fibrocartilage complex tear (192)

Dorsal impaction syndrome (19

Distal radius and ulnar fracture (184)

Forearm injuries

Forearm injuries are not common in sports but can occur from overu in racket sports or from high-energy falls in other sports.

The forearm serves as an anchoring point for the muscles and tendo that pass to the wrist and hand. The two bones of the forearm (radi and ulna) can rotate over each other. This provides power and allows precise hand positioning for specialized functions.

Overuse injury

As a result of external pressure or repetitive one-sided movements, the extensor and flexor muscles of the forearm and their tendons and tendon sheaths are subject to overuse injury. The injury occurs mainly in rowers and canoeists at the start of their intensive training periods at the beginning of the season, but tennis, squash, table tennis and badminton players, skiers and others can also be affected.

Symptoms and diagnosis
- Pain occurs when the hands are flexed and extended (Figure 8.3).
- Local swelling and tenderness occur over the affected muscle and tendon.
- Tendon crepitus (creaking) is felt over the affected tendons on the back of the hand and the forearm when movements are made with the fingers and wrist.

Preventive measures
Inflammation may be prevented by:
- rest from painful activities;
- gradually increasing training and load;
- varied training avoiding one-sided movements;
- correct technique and equipment.

Treatment
The *athlete* should rest from painful activities; the injury often heals spontaneously, though it can take a considerable time to do so.
The *doctor* may:
- treat with a brace or a splint for 1–4 weeks;
- prescribe anti-inflammatory medication.

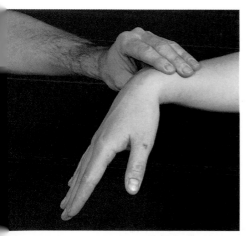 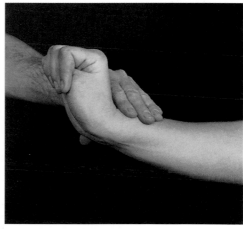

Figure 8.3 In overuse injury crepitation can be felt during motion of the wrist.

Compartment syndrome

Compartment syndrome (compare p. 334) is a rare injury, characterized by an exercise-induced ache or pain with a sensation of increased pressure or tightness. Intermittent weakness or numbness may be noted.

Because the causes of compartment syndrome are poorly understood, it is difficult to diagnose this injury. Direct evaluation of intramuscular pressure is helpful. As conservative treatment is rarely successful for these chronic conditions, treatment is usually surgical fasciotomy.

Fractures

Fractures of the forearm can occur after a fall or a direct blow and usually involve both the radius and the ulna. Fractures of the ulna alone can occur when parrying a blow with the forearm.

A fracture of the ulna can be combined with a dislocation of its articulation at the elbow joint (Monteggia's fracture). The elbow should therefore be examined and X-rayed when fracture of the ulna occurs.

Treatment It is important that the two bones, the ulna and the radius, are restored to their precise anatomical positions. Immobilization in a cast for 6–8 weeks is advisable, and surgery is frequently indicated, especially in cases of displacement.

When the cast is removed the arm should be strengthened by training for 6–10 weeks before the injured athlete can return to sporting activity.

Wrist injuries

Wrist problems are more common in hand-intensive sports and sports that entail gripping an object such as a tennis racket or golf club. Most injuries are due to repetitive overuse. Wrist fractures can occur in sports with high-energy falls, such as snowboarding, skiing, and skating.

The wrist and hand are complex anatomic structures that allow a wide variety of positions and functions. This is necessary to carry out the complex tasks that are required from the hand, such as writing, grasping, and picking up very small items.

The wrist is composed of seven carpal (mid-hand) bones that are joined together and stabilized by joint capsules and by ligamentous structures. Disruption of the ligaments generally requires high-energy trauma but when it does occur it can be very debilitating. An eighth carpal bone lies within one of the flexor tendons of the wrist and glides over another carpal bone as a 'sesamoid bone'.

Fracture of the distal radius and ulna

A fracture of the distal radius (Colles' fracture) is the most common of all fractures. It usually occurs as a result of a fall on the extended arm

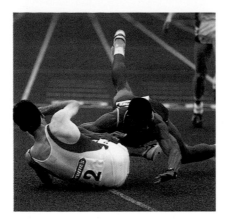

Figure 8.4 A fall on the wrist can injure it (by courtesy of All Sport).

(Figure 8.4), forcing the hand backwards and upwards. A less common injury is Smith's fracture where the mechanism is a forward flexion (palmar flexion) of the wrist. The injury is not uncommon among ice hockey, soccer, rugby, and team handball players, riders, wrestlers, alpine skiers, and others.

Symptoms and diagnosis

– 'Dinner fork' deformity of the wrist is characteristic of Colles' fracture (Figure 8.5). The position is caused by the fractured fragment of the distal radius being driven backwards (dorsiflexed) in relation to the

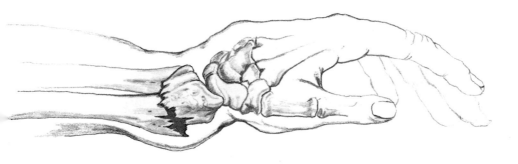

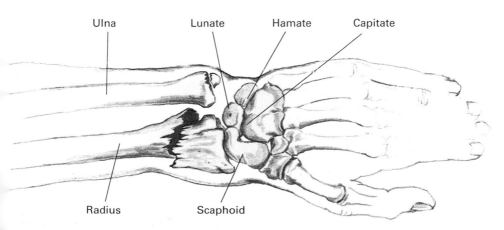

Ulna   Lunate   Hamate   Capitate

Radius   Scaphoid

Figure 8.5 Typical distal radius fracture (**top**) seen from side; (**bottom**) seen from above.

forearm. In Smith's fracture a forward (palmar flexion) dislocation of the distal radius is present.
- Swelling and tenderness occur in the wrist.
- Pain is felt on wrist movements.
- In milder cases, swelling and displacement may be minor. The injury may then be mistaken for a sprain, but when this is so, the wrist should be X-rayed to reveal any bony injury.

Treatment

The *doctor* may:
- restore the fractured ends of the bone to their correct position;
- apply a plaster cast (usually a splint or brace which can be removed after 4–5 weeks if the fracture is uncomplicated). The wrist is later strengthened by training;
- operate in cases of more serious fractures.

Healing

Conditioning can often be maintained during immobilization of the wrist. Other forms of sporting activity involving the wrist can be resumed after 8–12 weeks.

Fracture of the scaphoid

A fracture of the scaphoid bone in the wrist can result from a fall with the wrist bent backwards on an extended arm (Figure 8.6). The injury is particularly common in contact sports such as soccer, American football, rugby, ice hockey, and team handball, but can also occur in skiers and others.

The blood flow to the scaphoid is easily compromised, especially in fractures of its middle portion, and this slows the healing process. Athletes often find it difficult to accept the prolonged treatment that is needed for this injury to heal.

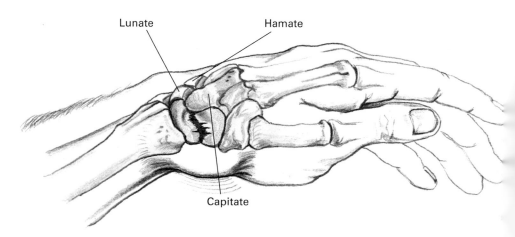

Figure 8.6 Fracture of the scaphoid.

Symptoms and diagnosis	– Moderate pain is felt with tenderness and swelling in the scaphoid region (the hollow formed at the base of the extended thumb: the anatomic snuffbox). – Power is moderately impaired during hand movements. – The injury is often disregarded and is looked upon as a sprain because of the apparent triviality of immediate symptoms. – An X-ray and bone scan or MRI will confirm the diagnosis.
Treatment	The *athlete* should consult a doctor for an X-ray in the case of any hand injury that could involve a fracture of the scaphoid. The *doctor* may: – apply a plaster cast or a brace when there is a suspected fracture, even if the early X-ray does not show one. A further X-ray should be taken 2–3 weeks later as it can take a long time for the bony changes to be revealed; a bone scan can, in some cases, be carried out earlier; – when a fracture is present, apply a plaster cast. Immobilization of the wrist should continue for at least 3 months, with serial X-ray examinations to monitor healing; – operate, in cases with any displacement of the fracture.
Healing and complications	– It is not unusual for the injured athlete to fail to consult a doctor and for the early symptoms to disappear. In these circumstances, healing may not occur and a false joint can be formed. This may ultimately cause degenerative changes in the wrist with discomfort, pain during movement, stiffness, and impaired function. – Premature cessation of treatment, or sometimes even adequate treatment, can be followed by formation of a false joint (pseudarthrosis). A pseudarthrosis of the scaphoid should have surgical fixation. – Athletes can, in spite of a fracture of the scaphoid, continue with acceptable conditioning activity.

Fracture of the hook of the hamate

The hook of the hamate bone projects anteriorly on the lateral side of the palm. A compression fracture of this bone is a rare injury, but it may occur in racket sports, baseball, ice hockey, and cycling if the handle of the racket, bat, club, stick or handlebar is compressed on to the hook of the hamate.

Symptoms and diagnosis	– Pain and tenderness are felt on the little finger side of the palm. – The grip has little power. – Numbness of the little finger is caused by irritation of the ulnar nerve. – An X-ray with a carpal tunnel view, or a CT scan, is necessary to verify the diagnosis.
Treatment	The *athlete* should: – rest and cool the injury; – consult a doctor.

The *doctor* may:
- verify the diagnosis with X-ray or CT scan;
- recommend a period of rest to allow symptoms to decrease;
- operate and remove the hook in some displaced fractures or when nonunion remains symptomatic.

Healing and complications
- This fracture is easily overlooked.
- Healing of this fracture is rare even with internal fixation, but nonunions of hamate fractures are often not painful.
- Distal ulnar neuritis.
- Flexor tendon injury.

The athlete can usually return to sport as soon as symptoms allow.

Dislocations around the wrist

Dislocations around the wrist are rare in sports, but are important to recognize because a good recovery depends on early and correct diagnosis and treatment. Even with proper treatment, these injuries often have long-term residual symptoms.

Separation between the scaphoid and lunate

Scapholunate dissociation may occur in forced dorsiflexion of the wrist. Ligamentous disruption between the scaphoid and lunate bones will cause the two bones to separate. This injury is felt to be a less severe form of the same mechanism that causes perilunate dislocation.

Symptoms and diagnosis
- Pain is felt on movement.
- There is swelling of the wrist, and tenderness over the lunate and scaphoid (see Figure 8.2).
- An X-ray shows an increased joint space between the scaphoid and the lunate and/or an abnormal angle between the scaphoid and lunate.

Treatment
The *athlete* should:
- cool, compress, and elevate the wrist;
- consult a doctor.

The *doctor* may:
- verify the diagnosis by X-ray;
- surgically reduce the displacement, suture the ligament and joint capsule, and hold the reduction with Kirschner wires;
- immobilize the joint for 8–12 weeks.

Perilunate dislocation

Perilunate dislocation is a dorsal dislocation of the capitate (see Figure 8.6) in relation to the lunate bone, which may sometimes be dislocated anteriorly at the same time. It may occur in association with a dislocation or fracture of the scaphoid and is caused by forced dorsiflexion or axial compression of the wrist.

Symptoms and diagnosis
- Changed contour is visible on the dorsal aspect of the wrist.
- Swelling and tenderness are present.
- Movements are painful and restricted.
- X-rays show the posterior dislocation of the capitate.

Treatment
The *athlete* should:
- cool, compress, and elevate the wrist;
- consult a doctor immediately.

The *doctor* may:
- verify the diagnosis by X-ray;
- operate to reduce the dislocation and hold it in position with Kirschner wires;
- in addition, repair the torn ligaments.

The lunate (see Figure 8.6) can dislocate both posteriorly (in a dorsal direction) and anteriorly (in a palmar direction). This injury is really just a continuation of the perilunate dislocation and scapholunate dissociation. With increasingly severe trauma, the injury progresses from scapholunate dissociation to perilunate dislocation and then to true lunate dislocation.

Malacia of the lunate (Kienböck's disease)

Lunatomalacia may occur as a result of repeated trauma or impacts. The circulation of the lunate is disturbed, and the bone softens and becomes devascularized. This injury is associated with a slightly shortened ulna in relation to the radius at the wrist (this is called negative variance).

Symptoms and diagnosis
- Movements are painful and restricted.
- Swelling and tenderness occur over the lunate.
- Weakness of the hand.
- Decreased size and sclerosis (increased bone density) of the lunate are seen on X-ray.

Treatment
The *athlete* should:
- rest the wrist;
- consult a doctor.

The *doctor* may:
- verify the diagnosis by X-ray or bone scan;
- immobilize the wrist in the acute stage;
- resort to surgery to relieve stress on the lunate in mild cases, or perform fusions for advanced cases.

The decision to return to sport will depend on individual circumstances.

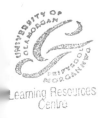

Carpal tunnel syndrome

Carpal tunnel syndrome is most often caused by overuse of the wrist which in turn causes narrowing and inflammation of the tunnel that houses the nerves and tendons that lead from the forearm to the wrist. Compression of the median nerve causes the symptoms. Overuse is common in hand-intensive activities, particularly when the wrist is used for support, as in cycling.

Symptoms and diagnosis
- Tenderness over the palmar aspect just distal to the wrist (Figure 8.7).
- Athletes with this injury may have intermittent tingling and numbness in the thumb and the next two and a half fingers. The tingling will be more prominent with the wrist in hyperflexion or hyperextension.
- The athlete will sometimes complain of clumsiness and loss of dexterity.
- In prolonged severe cases there may be loss of grip strength and hypotrophy of the thumb muscles.
- Holding the wrist in hyperflexion (Phalen's maneuver, Figure 8.8) for a 30 second period causes numbness in the hand.
- Electromyographic studies may be helpful to confirm the diagnosis but they are not always positive.

Treatment
The *doctor* may:
- advise a change in training;
- apply a splint to rest the wrist and avoid extremes of range of motion. Depending on the degree of symptoms the splint or brace may be worn only at night, during activities, or continuously;
- give anti-inflammatory medication;
- inject steroid into the carpal tunnel in refractory cases;
- operate to release the ligament overlying the carpal tunnel in cases refractory to the above measures (this increases the space available for the nerve). This surgery can be 'arthroscopic' (endoscopic).

Healing
The athlete may return to sports as soon as symptoms allow, often within 2-4 weeks of surgery. Taping, bracing or splinting may be helpful during activities.

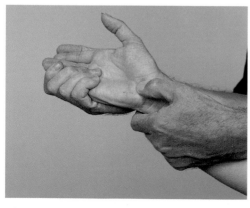

Figure 8.7 Distal palmar tenderness.

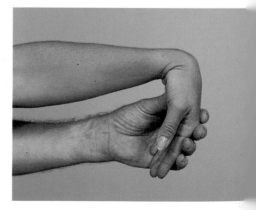

Figure 8.8 Phalen's maneuver.

Distal ulnar neuritis (Guyon's canal syndrome)

The ulnar nerve can be subjected to pressure where it crosses the wrist on the inner aspect of the hand (Figure 8.9). The pressure is caused by friction or impingement of the local tissues against the nerve causing mechanical irritation, as can happen during cycling (Figure 8.10). The symptoms of ulnar neuritis are pain and numbness in the little finger and half the ring finger, with muscular weakness on attempting to spread the fingers. The initial treatment is rest from painful activities and anti-inflammatory medication, but if this fails, surgery to decompress the nerve gives good results.

De Quervain's disease

Inflammation of the sheath of the short extensor tendon (extensor pollicis brevis) and long abductor tendon (abductor pollicis longus) to the thumb can occur. This is most commonly caused by repetitive thumb and wrist movements.

Symptoms and diagnosis
- Pain and tenderness are located at the base of the thumb where the tendons cross the wrist.
- Pain occurs with active thumb extension and abduction against resistance.
- Pain is elicited by placing the thumb in the palm followed by ulnar deviation of the wrist (Finkelstein's test).

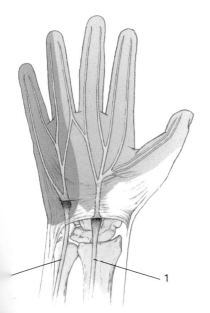

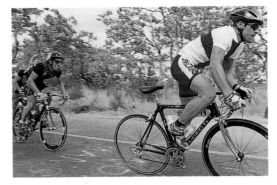

Figure 8.9 Carpal tunnel syndrome caused by entrapment of the median nerve (1), and distal ulnar neuritis caused by entrapment of the ulnar nerve (2).

Figure 8.10 There is often pressure on the wrist in cycling (by courtesy of All Sport: photographer, Mike Powell.)

Treatment	The *doctor* may:

The *doctor* may:

- advise a change in training;
- apply a splint to rest the thumb (depending on the degree symptoms, the splint may be worn only at night, during activities, continuously);
- give anti-inflammatory medications;
- inject steroid in the sheath around the tendons;
- operate to release the sheath covering the tendons in cases refractor to the above measures.

Healing

The athlete may return to sports as soon as symptoms allow. Tapin bracing or splinting may be helpful during activities.

Triangular fibrocartilage complex tears

The triangular fibrocartilage (TFC) is a cartilaginous disk, much like th meniscus cartilage of the knee, which overlies the distal aspect of the ul in the wrist joint. It is part of the TFC complex (TFCC) which suppor the carpal bones on the ulnar side of the wrist and provides some stabi ity for the distal radioulnar joint (part of the wrist). Tears of the TFC can occur from trauma, overuse, or tissue degeneration. Tears are ofte associated with a long ulna in relation to the radius at the wrist joi (positive ulnar variance). The traumatic tears are caused by injuries wi impaction, rotation, and ulnar deviation.

Symptoms and diagnosis

- Symptoms are often vague.
- Ulnar-sided wrist pain is felt (Figure 8.11).
- Pain is elicited when testing with compression, ulnar deviatio (Figure 8.12), and circumduction. A painful click or clunk may be f during this maneuver and on anterior-position movement of the ul (Figure 8.13).
- An MR arthrogram of the joint and arthroscopy will secure th diagnosis.

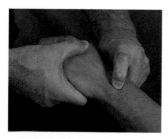

Figure 8.11 Ulnar-sided wrist pain in TFCC tears.

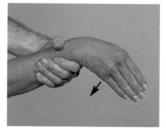

Figure 8.12 Ulnar deviation causes wrist pain in TFCC tears.

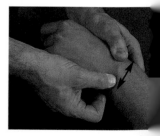

Figure 8.13 Anterior movement of the ulna caus wrist pain in TFCC tears.

The *doctor* may:
- immobilize the wrist for 4–6 weeks;
- operate if symptoms persist after immobilization and a rehabilitation program. Surgical options include repair or excision of tissue. The arthroscope has been useful in the diagnosis and treatment of TFCC injuries. Return to sports such as tennis may be possible in 3–4 months.

Dorsal impaction syndrome

Dorsal impaction is a chronic pain syndrome caused by repetitive axial loading of the wrist in dorsiflexion. This injury is common in young gymnasts.

- Pain is felt on the back of the wrist.
- The pain is increased with dorsiflexion and loading of the wrist.

Treatment should include:
- modification of training programs;
- wrist strengthening exercises;
- the use of wrist guards or a brace to prevent excessive dorsiflexion;
- for more severe pain, complete rest and immobilization.

Weakness in the wrist

Women about 20 years old of slender build sometimes complain of pain in the wrist with exertion (often disappearing at rest) which radiates along the upper side of the forearm. On examination, a degree of hypermobility and laxity of the wrist may be noticed, but often no significant abnormality can be found. Sometimes a small swelling, or ganglion, can be found on the back of the hand. This should not prevent training, but a support bandage should be applied around the wrist and strength training carried out in parallel with the usual training. The symptoms often disappear in time.

Bibliography
See p. 206.

Hand injuries

The hand is one of the most common sites of injury during athletic competition. The palm consists of five metacarpal bones, one for each digit. The metacarpals in the middle of the hand have very little motion and provide a stable palm, while the little finger and especially the thumb have significantly more motion to allow the hand to grasp objects. Without the large motion allowed by the joints of the thumb metacarpal we would be unable to oppose the thumb to the palm for grasping. Fortunately severe injuries to the thumb are rare, but they can be devastating.

Each of the four fingers has three phalangeal bones: a proximal phalanx (closest to the palm), a middle phalanx, and a distal phalanx. The proximal interphalangeal (PIP) joint lies between the proximal and middle phalanges, and the distal interphalangeal (DIP) joint lies between the middle and a distal phalanges. The thumb has only two phalangeal bones, a proximal and a distal phalanx. Between the fingers and palm are the metacarpophalangeal (MCP) joints: these are almost exclusively for bending and straightening the fingers and have very little side-to-side movement; this allows the hand to conform to objects for better grasping and allows precise finger placement during detailed work.

Contusions and lacerations

Contusions are the most common injury in the hand. Principles for their treatment are described on p. 35. Care must be taken to rule out more serious injuries such as fractures and ligamentous or tendinous injuries. A contusion can lead to trauma-induced tendonitis; however, the majority of these, too, can be treated with time and conservative measures.

Lacerations of the hand also are very common in sports. They require thorough evaluation of the tendons, nerves, and blood supply, with particular attention to the nerves of the fingers. Simple lacerations can be treated with irrigation, loose closure, and protection as necessary. Lacerations over the joints require careful evaluation of extension into the joint. The position of the hand when the injury occurred is important: with a clenched fist laceration the lesion may appear not to have penetrated the joint when the hand is flat—this is the so-called 'tooth injury' which is often overlooked. If there is extension into the joint, or an associated fracture, a doctor should be consulted immediately. The doctor will perform a thorough irrigation and debridement, and prescribe antibiotic prophylaxis for at least 48 hours. For all lacerations the athlete should ensure that antitetanus vaccination is up to date.

If lacerations are neglected and not properly cleaned, bacterial infection may ensue, necessitating prolonged treatment. If an infection does occur, a doctor should be consulted immediately. Treatment includes antibiotics and possibly surgical drainage to clean out the wound and prevent further spread. Infected wounds on the hand must never be neglected, since the consequences can be catastrophic.

Ligamentous injuries and dislocations

Injury to the ligamentous structures surrounding the fingers and thumb common during sports activities, especially those that involve ball handling

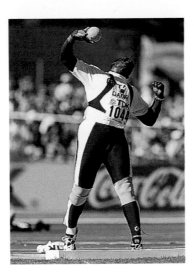

Figure 8.14 Sports involving ball handling may result in injury to the fingers (by courtesy of All Sport: photographer, Gary Prior).

or heavy physical contact (Figure 8.14). The key to the treatment of hand injuries is to make an accurate diagnosis through careful history and examination. Failure to recognize the importance of these injuries leads to poor outcomes. The majority of these injuries can be treated nonoperatively, and they rarely result in prolonged loss of participation.

PIP joint injuries

The proximal interphalangeal (PIP) joint (of the two finger joints, this is the joint nearest to the palm) is the most commonly injured joint in the hand. Loss of motion is common following injury to the joint and may even be seen in uninjured joints that have been immobilized for other reasons. Any fixed deformity of the joint causes significant disability.

Collateral ligament injuries
Injuries of the collateral ligaments (the side ligaments of the PIP joints) are quite common in athletics. They often occur in sports such as team handball, volleyball, basketball, and rugby.

Symptoms and diagnosis
- Pain and distinct tenderness occur in the injured area at the side of the joint.
- Mobility is impaired.
- Instability (increased side-to-side movement of the joint) can be present if the tear is complete.

Treatment
Collateral ligament injuries can be treated by bandaging or taping the injured finger to an adjacent finger for support ('buddy taping'). Active motion exercises of the injured finger can then start without any side-to-side loading. The bandage is worn for about 2 weeks for minor injuries and longer for complete tears. Buddy taping should be used during athletic competition for several months. As a rule, surgery is not needed except for injuries to the ligaments of the thumb.

195

Healing
- Residual effects with slight swelling and stiffness of the injured finger can continue for a long time (6–9 months) after the injury has occurred.
- Protected early return to sport is usually possible.

Dislocation of PIP joint

Dislocation of the PIP joint (Figure 8.15) is a common injury which often affects team handball, basketball and volleyball players, and cricketers. In 80% of cases it is the little finger that is damaged. The most common mechanism of injury is axial loading and hyperextension of the joint causing dorsal dislocation (dislocation upwards and backwards). The dorsal dislocation always results in disruption of the anterior capsular ligaments and volar plate. Lateral dislocation (dislocation to the side) of the PIP joint occurs when a single collateral ligament ruptures with a portion of the volar (palm) plate. The rare volar (forwards into the palm) dislocation of the PIP joint is a more serious injury. This dislocation results in disruption of the extensor tendon and one of the collateral ligaments. Because of rupture of the extensor tendon this injury can result in a deformity. Many dislocations of the PIP joint go untreated by a physician because they are reduced by the athlete or coach on the sideline. Lack of treatment can cause permanent disability, particularly in the case of a missed fracture/dislocation.

Symptoms
- Pain is accompanied by tenderness and impaired function.
- Deformity of the joint outline can be seen.

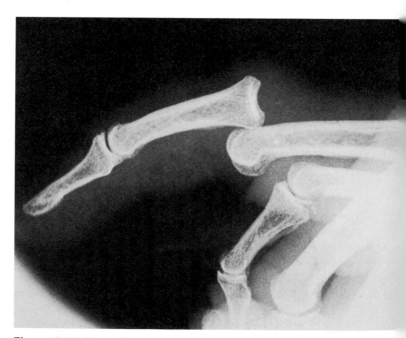

Figure 8.15 X-ray of a dislocated finger joint.

196

The *doctor* may:
- reduce the joint back into its normal position. The sooner this is done after injury, the easier the procedure. If manipulation is carried out within a few minutes, severe pain is not generally experienced;
- tape the digit to the adjacent finger (buddy tape) or, in severe injury, immobilize by applying a splint, which is worn for 1-2 weeks, to block extension. Buddy taping should be used during athletic competition for several months;
- splint only the PIP joint in continuous extension for 6–8 weeks for dislocations toward the palm;
- X-ray the joint, as a bone fragment may have been torn loose;
- allow protected early return to sport, which is usually possible.

MCP joint injuries

Collateral ligament injuries

Collateral ligament injuries are occasionally seen in the metacarpophalangeal (MCP) joints (the joint between the palm of the hand and the fingers). The mechanism of injury is side-to-side force placed on a bent MCP joint.

- Pain and distinct tenderness occur in the injured area at the side of the joint in the web space.
- Mobility is impaired.
- Instability (increased side movement of the joint) can be present if the tear is complete. In the MCP joint, this is tested with the joint flexed.

- Splinting and/or taping to the finger beside it (buddy taping) are usually sufficient treatment. Active motion exercises without any side-to-side load can begin immediately. The bandage is worn for about 2 weeks for minor injuries and longer for complete tears. Buddy taping should be used during athletic competition for several months.
- X-rays should be taken to be sure no bone fragments are lodged in the joint.
- Pain can persist for up to a year following the injury.
- Protected early return to sport is usually possible.

Dislocation of MCP joint

Dislocation of the MCP joint is a rare injury. When it does occur the border digits (the index and little fingers) are most commonly affected. Dorsal dislocation of the MCP joint occurs following forced hyperextension (bending backwards) of the fingers. The volar (palm) plate is ruptured and the head of the metacarpal can sometimes be buttonholed through the volar plate and surrounding structures (complex dislocation). This can make reduction difficult. A characteristic dimple in the palm is often seen in this variety of dislocation.

- Pain occurs together with tenderness and impaired function.
- Deformity of the joint outline can be seen.
- For complex dislocations, a characteristic dimple may be present in the palm.

Treatment

The *doctor* may:
- reduce the joint back into its normal position. Failure of attempt closed reduction is typical of the complex dislocation;
- operate: open reduction is usually required for the complex disloc tion;
- apply a splint to stop the finger from straightening all the way. Th is worn for 2–3 weeks. Active motion in the splint should begin early as possible to avoid stiffness. Buddy taping should be used duri athletic competition for several months;
- X-ray the joint to make sure there is no fracture.

Protected early return to sport is usually possible.

Thumb ligament injuries

Thumb IP joint injuries

The thumb interphalangeal (IP) joint (thumb tip joint) is similar to t PIP joint of the fingers, and injuries should be treated in the same wa Mild stiffness of the IP joint of the thumb is generally well tolerated. the injured thumb IP joint with hyperextension laxity and a suspect volar (palm) plate injury, it is important to rule out a rupture of t flexor pollicis longus tendon. A tendon rupture should be surgica repaired. Less frequently, rupture of the extensor pollicis longus m occur; this also requires surgical reconstruction.

Thumb MCP joint dislocations

The MCP joint is capable of a large degree of motion. The supporti structures of the thumb–MCP joint are uniquely developed. Dor (backwards) dislocation of the thumb MCP joint is a similar clini entity to dislocation of the MCP joints of the fingers, with volar pla disruption and possible entrapment of the metacarpal head by the butto holed tissue. Closed reduction by gentle manipulation is possible mc often than in similar injuries to the finger joints, though surgical op reduction is still sometimes necessary. If closed reduction of the disloc tion is possible and the collateral ligaments are stable, then 4 weeks immobilization to block the thumb from straightening and to allow acti bending should be adequate.

Lateral ulnar ligament injuries (skier's thumb, gamekeeper' thumb, Stener's lesion)

Around 10% of all injuries in alpine skiing involve the ulnar collate ligament complex of the thumb (the side ligament at the thumb w space), making this the second most common injury sustained by skie Its incidence in skiing has been estimated to be between 50 000 a 200 000 per year.

Lateral ulnar ligament injuries occur from a side stress placed on t thumb while the MCP joint is straight (Figure 8.16). This can occ when a skier falls on an outstretched arm, and in so doing, forces t thumb upwards (abduction) and backwards (extension) against the pole. This injury is also not uncommon in crosscountry skiing. In t

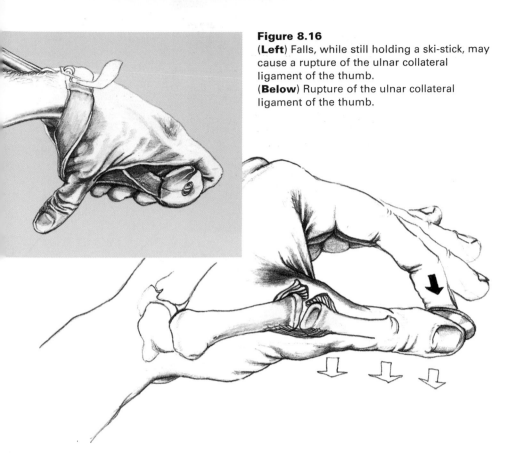

Figure 8.16
(Left) Falls, while still holding a ski-stick, may cause a rupture of the ulnar collateral ligament of the thumb.
(Below) Rupture of the ulnar collateral ligament of the thumb.

sport the strap is grasped between the palm of the hand and the pole grip, so injury can occur when carrying out a forceful pole-plant (compare Figure 4.10); it also occurs in ice hockey when a player's stick becomes trapped and forces the thumb backwards.

Symptoms and diagnosis	– Pain occurs in the thumb web space.

– Pain occurs in the thumb web space.
– Tenderness is noted when pressure is applied to the thumb web space at the side of the MCP joint.
– Bruising and swelling can be seen in the thumb web space.
– Instability of the joint is found when the thumb is tested in abduction (movement away from the palm) at an angle of 20–30° (Figure 8.17). The critical degree of laxity (i.e. the degree of laxity that indicates a total rupture has occurred) is 30° greater than the normal opposite thumb. In total rupture, the ligament can be displaced to such an extent that the ulnar extension of the adductor aponeurosis becomes lodged between the ruptured end of the ligament and its attachment to the base of the first phalanx (Stener's lesion).
– An X-ray may demonstrate a collateral ligament bone fragment off the ulnar side of the proximal phalanx.
– Stress films, arthrograms or an MRI may assist with diagnosis of complete tears with Stener's lesions (adductor aponeurosis interposition).

199

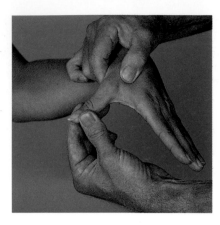

Figure 8.17 Testing the stability of the ulnar collateral ligament of the thumb.

Treatment

The *athlete* should:
- cool the injury with ice packs, apply compression, and keep the thumb elevated;
- consult a doctor.

The *doctor* may:
- carry out a thorough stability examination;
- for partial ruptures, apply a thumb spica cast for 4 weeks;
- operate; because of the frequency of Stener's lesion in complete tears, surgical repair is recommended for acute complete ruptures of the lateral ulnar ligament.

Healing and complications

Rehabilitation is similar for both surgically and conservatively treated injuries. The thumb is immobilized in 20° of flexion in a cast for 4 weeks. The IP joint is left free to allow for active motion to prevent scarring of the extensor tendon. A removable splint is fabricated at 3–4 weeks, and active exercises are allowed several times a day. The splint may be removed at 5–6 weeks for normal activity. For participation in sports, the thumb is protected for 3 months either by taping it to the index finger or by a silicone cast.

If this injury is inadequately treated, there is a risk of permanent instability, resulting in weak grasp and arthritis. Surgery on a neglected injury can often be effective.

Lateral radial ligament injuries

The lateral radial ligament of the MCP joint of the thumb (the side ligament away from the palm) is less commonly injured. The mechanism of injury is usually a forceful rotation of a bent MCP joint. Injuries to this ligament are treated in a similar fashion to those of the ulnar ligament. The conservative regimen and indications for surgery are identical.

Carpometacarpal joint injuries

The biconcave shape of the carpometacarpal (CMC) joint of the thumb (the joint of the extension of the thumb to the wrist) makes it anatomically different from the other hand joints. This saddle joint permits special function of opposition of the thumb to the little finger. The volar oblique ligament is the most important structure in maintaining stability. Complete dislocations of the CMC joint without associated fracture are relatively rare. The most common mechanism of injury is a fall on the outstretched hand.

Symptoms

- Pain occurs together with tenderness and impaired function.
- Deformity of the joint outline can be seen.

Treatment

The *doctor* may:
- reduce the joint back to its normal position;
- immobilize the joint for 4–6 weeks in a cast or splint;
- recommend surgery when the stability of the joint is in doubt, surgically inserting a wire through the joint to hold it in position.

Healing and complications

In cases of chronic instability, surgical reconstruction of the volar ligament may be indicated. In cases of recurrent laxity following reconstruction, or where joint changes are present, removal or fusion of the CMC joint may be the ultimate treatment.

Tendon injuries

Closed injuries to tendons of the hand and wrist are common in the athlete. These problems are often neglected and may not be seen by a physician until the end of the season, when the athlete notes a significant disability. Failure to initiate treatment in the acute stages may jeopardize the final result. Every effort should be made to ensure early evaluation and treatment of these injuries.

Attachment rupture of the long extensor tendon (mallet finger, mallet thumb)

The extensor tendon of the finger is attached to the terminal phalanx (distal end of the finger). Disruption of the extensor tendon at this insertion (mallet finger) is one of the most common tendon injuries in sports. It is especially common in ball-handling sports. The usual mechanism of injury is that of a forceful bending applied to an actively straightening joint, typically when a ball unexpectedly hits the fingertip and forces the finger to bend. A small bone fragment may sometimes be torn loose together with the tendon. The bone fragment will show up on X-rays.

Mallet thumb is much less common than mallet finger. It is diagnosed from the inability to actively straighten the tip of the thumb. Symptoms and treatment are identical for both conditions.

Symptoms

- Slight tenderness is found between the nail and the first joint (DIP) of the finger.
- The fingertip is slightly bent, and the first (distal) joint cannot be actively extended.

Treatment

The *doctor* may:
- X-ray the finger to evaluate for fracture fragments or malalignment o the joint;
- treat with a splint to keep the first (distal) finger joint extended. The splint should keep the first joint completely straight while allowing free motion of the PIP joint (Figure 8.18). The splint should remain in place continuously for a minimum of 6 weeks;
- operate, if a large bone fragment has been torn away and there i malalignment of the joint.

Healing and complications

- Participation in sports is allowed during treatment of mallet finger a long as the finger is continuously splinted in extension.
- Splinting has been shown to be effective in injuries left untreated fo 3 months after injury.
- Chronic mallet injuries, if left untreated, may progress to a flexio deformity at the DIP joint, and hyperextension deformity at the PI joint (swan-neck lesion).

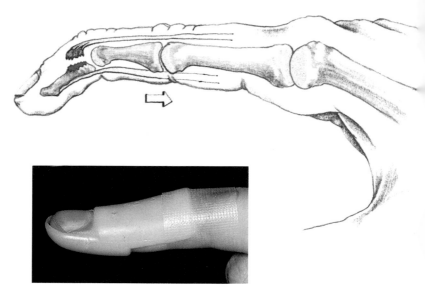

Figure 8.18 (Top) Rupture of the attachment of the long extensor tendon of the finger.
(Bottom) The injured finger can be easily immobilized in a plastic finger-splint.

Avulsion of the flexor digitorum profundus tendon (jersey finger)

Avulsion of the flexor digitorum profundus tendon (the tendon th bends the tip of the finger) at its insertion on the distal phalanx is injury often seen in athletes. The injury occurs most often during footb. or rugby, and usually results from grasping the jersey or shirt of opposing player. As the player pulls away, the finger is forcibly straigh ened while the profundus flexor tendon continues to try to bend t finger. Although any digit may be involved in profundus avulsion, the ring finger is most commonly affected. Profundus avulsion injuries frequently go undetected in the acute stages.

Symptoms
- Athletes with this injury will be unable to bend the tip of the finger.
- Tenderness is felt at the ruptured insertion site at the distal finger crease.
- Tenderness occurs elsewhere along the finger or in the palm. The precise localization of tenderness is important in order to identify the level of retraction of the avulsed tendon.

Treatment

The *doctor* may:
- X-ray the finger: plain X-rays may show an avulsion fracture, which can help to show where the end of the tendon is located;
- operate. Urgent open repair restores tendon and joint function. The operation should be performed within a few days, as the healing potential reduces dramatically beyond that time.

Healing and complications
- Following repair, the wrist and hand are splinted. Passive range-of-motion exercises may be started within the first few days but splinting is continuous for 4 weeks. At 4 weeks, intermittent splinting begins. The individual should not be allowed maximum gripping activities for 10–12 weeks after repair.
- In sports in which grasping is not essential, return to competition within 2 weeks is possible with use of a 'mitten' splint or playing cast.
- In considering treatment options for athletes during the playing season, all should be informed that best results are obtained from early repair regardless of the level of tendon retraction.
- For chronic injuries, treatment options include: (1) neglect, in cases in which symptoms are minimal; (2) excision of the retracted tendon in the palm, if painful; (3) fusion of the joint at the tip of the finger. Independent profundus function in the ring finger is necessary for musicians and certain other highly skilled professions; most others do well without active fingertip flexion and the majority do not need late surgical procedures.

Fractures

The fingers

Fractures of the phalanges are not particularly common, but may occur in team handball, volleyball, basketball, soccer, cricket, and other sports. Rotational alignment is critical when treating phalangeal shaft fractures. Rotation may be difficult to judge because the finger may look straight when it is extended but may overlap an adjacent finger when a fist is made.

Symptoms and diagnosis
- Tenderness, swelling, and pain occur in the finger.
- There may be deformity.
- An X-ray will confirm the diagnosis.

Treatment	– Most phalangeal fractures may be treated with a plaster cast or splint for 2–4 weeks. Immobilization should not exceed 3–4 weeks owing to stiffness problems.
	– If the phalangeal fracture is displaced and unstable, or if the fracture involves the joint surface, surgery may be needed. One advantage of internally fixed fractures is that motion can begin earlier, this must be weighed against the risk that the greater trauma to the tissue may increase scarring and stiffness.
Healing	Sporting activity can resume if a splint can be worn and the finger can be adequately protected.

Metacarpal bones

Fractures of the metacarpal bones are particularly common among handball players, but also occur in volleyball, ice hockey, basketball, soccer, American football, and cricket. Such fractures can be caused by forcible straightening of the fingers (e.g. during shooting in team handball, when the hand hits the covering arm of the defensive player) or as a result of a direct blow. Even a blow to the end of the bones, as in boxing and ice hockey, can result in fractures of the metacarpal shaft (Figure 8.19).

Symptoms and diagnosis	– Tenderness, swelling, and pain occur in the hand.
	– There may be deformity or loss of prominence of the knuckle.
	– An X-ray will confirm the diagnosis.
Treatment	– In most cases, treatment with a plaster cast or splint for 3–4 weeks sufficient.
	– In cases with severe angulation or shortening, or with rotation malalignment, surgery may be indicated.
Healing	The athlete can return immediately to participation in sports that do not require grasping, provided a splint is used for protection. Team handball and other hand-intensive sports may be resumed 6–8 weeks after injury.

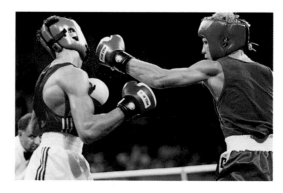

Figure 8.19 Blows in boxing can result in injury to the hand (by courtesy of All Sport; photographer, Mike Powell).

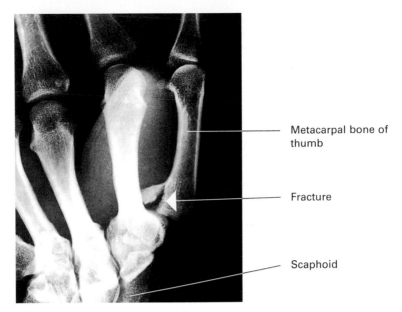

Metacarpal bone of thumb

Fracture

Scaphoid

Figure 8.20 X-ray of Bennett's fracture.

Joint fractures of the thumb metacarpal bone (Bennett's fracture)

A Bennett's fracture is a fracture of the joint surface at the proximal end of the thumb metacarpal (Figure 8.20). The significance of this fracture is that the deep ulnar ligament which stabilizes the carpometacarpal joint is attached to the small nondisplaced fragment and the abductor pollicis longus tendon is attached to the metacarpal shaft. The pull of the abductor causes displacement of the metacarpal shaft, resulting in significant fracture displacement and joint malalignment. Surgery is needed to reduce the fracture and hold it with wires. If good fixation is obtained, casting can be discontinued after the incision has healed. Protection in a splint is needed during sports participation for at least 6–8 weeks—longer for a contact sport. Failure to obtain adequate reduction of the fracture can result in post-traumatic arthritis of the thumb CMC joint.

Fractures of the base of the fifth metacarpal bone ('baby Bennett')

Fractures of the base of the fifth metacarpal are similar to the Bennett's fracture at the base of the thumb metacarpal, but are much less common. The metacarpal shaft angulates backwards and away from the palm, with the small fracture fragment being held in place by ligaments attaching it to the fourth metacarpal and wrist bones. The main problem with these fractures is recognition of the backward displacement of the metacarpal shaft. Careful examination of the X-rays is needed to detect this. If the

joint malalignment is undetected and untreated, chronic pain and insta
bility can result. The principles of treatment are the same as those fo
the Bennett fracture. Surgery is usually needed to reduce the fractur
and hold it with wires.

Bibliography

Culver JE (1992) Injuries of the hand and wrist in the athlete. *Clinics i*
   Sports Medicine. 11:101–28.
McCue FC, Mayer VA (1989) Rehabilitation of common athletic injurie
   of the hand and wrist. *Clinics in Sports Medicine* 8: 731.
Stener B (1962) Displacement of the ruptured ulnar collateral ligamen
   of the metacarpophalangeal joint of the thumb: a clinical and anatomi
   study. *Journal of Bone and Joint Surgery* 44B: 869.

9 Back

Back problems affect 80% of all people at some time in their life. There is no specific category of subjects who suffer back pain more frequently than others—labourers are affected as often as clerks, men as often as women. Important contributory factors are hard physical work, lifting, static working postures, and vibration. In spite of the fact that the heaviest industrial tasks are now carried out by machines, the number of people seeking advice for back pain does not seem to have decreased. Of all sufferers, 70% return to work within a week and 90% within 3 months, regardless of the treatment they receive.

Functional anatomy and biomechanics

The spine is composed of 7 cervical (neck) vertebrae, 12 thoracic (chest) vertebrae and 5 lumbar (lower back) vertebrae, plus the sacral and coccygeal vertebrae. Each vertebra consists of a body from which a dorsal arch of bone arises. On each arch there are articular processes which allow limited mobility between adjacent vertebrae. Between the vertebral bodies are flexible plates of fibrocartilage, the disks, which facilitate movements of the spine and act as shock absorbers. Intervertebral disks have no blood or lymph supply and only a limited nerve supply (Figure 9.1).

The spinal column has supportive, protective and locomotive functions. The neck region is very mobile and the lower back region is fairly mobile, with most movement between the fifth lumbar vertebra and the first sacral vertebra. The chest region, on the other hand, is less mobile because the ribs are attached to their corresponding vertebrae. The regions of the spine that have most mobility generally give rise to most problems.

There is an anterior and an posterior longitudinal system of ligaments along the spine. In addition there are smaller ligaments around the joints and between the vertebrae and their spinous processes. These ligaments are responsible for the passive stability of the back. Active stability is contributed by the muscles of the back and the abdomen and is of great importance. These muscles can be divided into an anterior group, which includes the abdominal and psoas musculature, and posterior deep and superficial groups.

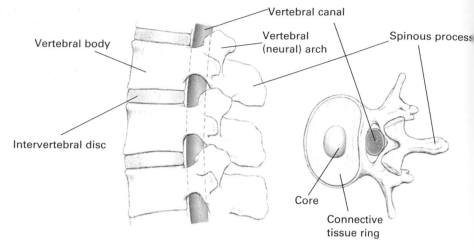

Figure 9.1 Schematic diagram of the anatomy of the spine.

The spine is exposed to a heavy load when the body is bent forward or turned, and the activity of the muscles of the back increases notic ably when the body is bent forwards at an angle of 30°. The san muscles have to work harder when the body is sitting rather than stand ing and this exposes the disks to increased pressure. In general, injud cious flexing of the spine, side bending, excessive twisting or loadin asymmetrically should be avoided. During lifting, the load should be placed as near to the body as possible.

Investigation of back pain

Diagnosis of back problems depends on the expert evaluation of pair physical examination results, back function, constitutional factors, and ray findings. The location, intensity, duration, and quality of pain shou be considered, as well as factors that precipitate or relieve it. Th function of the back should be studied with regard to its range ar pattern of movements, posture, muscle tone and control, and constit tional factors should be evaluated. Changes in the shape of the spine, e. an exaggerated S-shaped curve (scoliosis), can, like the overall physiqu be of importance.

A number of skeletal changes such as slipping of one vertebra o another, stress fractures, bony outgrowths along the edges of the vert bral bodies, and degenerative joint changes, can be identified by ordina X-ray examination, while a 'slipped' disk can be seen with the help of contrast medium. Computerized serial X-rays (tomography) can gi additional information about the various tissues making up the spir column.

Radiography should be performed in maximal flexion, extension, or any other position that evokes pain. Magnetic resonance imaging (MRI) gives both soft tissue and skeletal information, which can reveal instability or other causes of pain.

The injured person's social situation and psychological mood can be important when a history of back problems is given, and should be evaluated by enquiring into family circumstances, education, working conditions, and so forth.

Neck

The two uppermost cervical vertebrae bear the brunt of turning (rotatory) movements while flexion and extension occur predominantly at the occiput and at the first cervical vertebra. Injuries that may affect this area include fractures and dislocations with ligamentous damage. Degenerative changes can affect the disks and give rise to bony outgrowths (osteophytes) along the edges of the vertebral bodies, resulting in pressure on nerve roots and thus pain. Injuries and diseases of the cervical spine can cause pain which not only affects the neck but can radiate to the back of the head, the shoulders, arms, and hands, as well as the lower body parts.

Traumatic injuries

Blows to the head and cervical region can fracture the cervical vertebral column and also cause dislocations with simultaneous injuries to the joint capsules, ligaments, and disks. The injuries can be either stable or unstable. The most common modes of injury are bending backwards (extension) or forwards (flexion), rotating too violently, or hitting the head so that the impact is transmitted to the cervical region (axial compression).

Bending forwards can cause a compression fracture at the front, and ligament injuries at the back, of a vertebral body. Sometimes fractures of the joint processes and injuries to the joint capsule also occur, and ligament injuries may be present without any visible injury to the skeleton. After an injury associated with flexion it is essential to decide, with the help of X-rays, whether the injury is stable or unstable. Extension (bending backwards) produces similar injuries, with disk and ligament damage at the front and compression damage at the back of the vertebral bodies. A twisting impact can occur in isolation or in combination with flexion or extension. Unilateral damage to joint processes and ligaments can occur with a resultant dislocation.

A fracture and/or ligament injury of the cervical spine result from violent collision with an opponent or with surrounding objects, e.g. a goal post, and can be serious. Within the cervical vertebral column, the vertebral canal contains the spinal cord, which, together with its nerve roots, can be subjected to pressure and damaged by bone and ligament injuries.

Whiplash

Another important cause of cervical spine trauma is the 'whiplash' injury which occurs when the neck is rapidly extended and then flexed, typically in a road traffic accident when one vehicle is run into by another from behind (Figure 9.2). Ligament, bone, and muscle injuries, which may result in chronic pain, can occur, and anyone who has suffered a whiplash injury should be X-rayed.

Symptoms and diagnosis
- Pain is felt in the cervical region, especially during movements.
- Radiating pain occurs with numbness in the arms.
- There is impaired sensation in the skin below the level of the injury.
- Muscle weakness or paralysis may be present below the level of injury.

Treatment
The *athletic trainer or coach* should:
- arrange transport of the injured athlete to hospital for examination;
- delegate further handling to expert staff if available.

The injured athlete needs to be placed carefully on a stretcher in such a way that the head and body are lifted simultaneously and the position of the cervical vertebrae is not disturbed. Clothing, cushions, or similar supports are placed on each side of the neck during the journey to hospital, to splint the neck and prevent further injury.

The *doctor* may carry out a careful examination of the nervous system and arrange for an X-ray (and if needed an MRI or CT scan) of the cervical vertebral column in order to assess its stability and the extent of damage. Depending on the severity of the injury, treatment may consist of use of a neck collar, traction, external fixation with a halo-west, or open surgery.

An unusual lifethreatening injury to the cervical vessels can occur in ice-hockey and other skating sports. An opponent's skate may cut vessels in the anterior part of the neck. Lifethreatening bleeding can be prevented by wearing a protective neck collar (see Figure 4.4).

Figure 9.2
Neck injury may occur in body contact sports such as rugby (by courtesy of All Sport: photographer, Stu Forster).

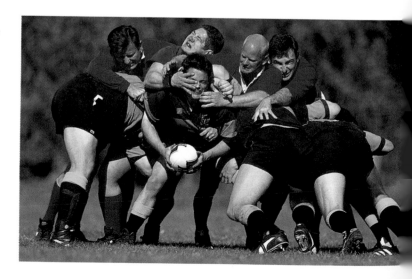

Pain radiating from the neck (cervical brachialgia, cervical rhizopathy)

Pains in the cervical region can be caused by disk degeneration, herniation, or osteophyte formation. The changes affect nerve roots, which can produce waves of pain. Even a temporary strain or trapping of a nerve can produce similar symptoms. It is usual to distinguish between pain confined to the nape of the neck and back of the head, and pain radiating into the arms with either a widespread (cervical brachialgia) or clearly defined (cervical rhizopathy) distribution (Figure 9.3).

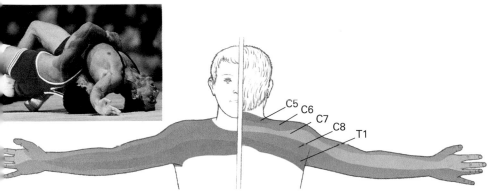

Figure 9.3 Schematic diagram of pain radiation from trapped nerve roots. (**Inset**) Nerves in the neck can be at risk in some sports (by courtesy of All Sport: Photographer, David Cannon).

Symptoms and diagnosis
- Pain radiates from the nape of the neck into the shoulder, arm, and/or fingers. The pain is usually deep and widespread (brachialgia), but it can have clearly defined limits with intense, sharp pain following the distribution of the affected nerves (rhizopathy). The pain is felt more acutely during neck movements than during shoulder movements.
- Pain radiating up the neck and into the back of the head can cause headaches, insomnia, and sometimes dizziness.
- Numbness and weakness are felt in the arm and fingers. There may be areas of complete anesthesia.
- An X-ray examination should be carried out, especially if pain is caused by movement. The examination should elicit those positions that provoke the pain in order to detect any abnormal mobility.
- Magnetic resonance imaging (MRI) may show the effects on soft tissues, e.g. by pressure of osteophytes on herniated disks.

Treatment
Treatment consists of:
- rest;
- neck collar and a heat retainer;
- analgesic and anti-inflammatory medication;
- physiotherapy with or without traction.

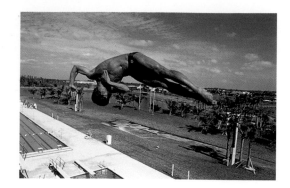

Figure 9.4 There are often twisting movements of the neck by divers (by courtesy of All Sport).

Pain in the neck (cervicalgia), torticollis (wry neck)

Pain located in the neck that does not radiate into the arms is called *cervicalgia* (see lumbago, p. 217). *Torticollis* is a painful condition that can occur in young athletes after violent turning movements of the neck, e.g. when diving and when heading or jumping in soccer (Figure 9.4). It is probable that the nerve roots arising from the cervical spinal cord are affected by, for example, a momentary compression or stretching, causing a reflex spasm in the neck muscles.

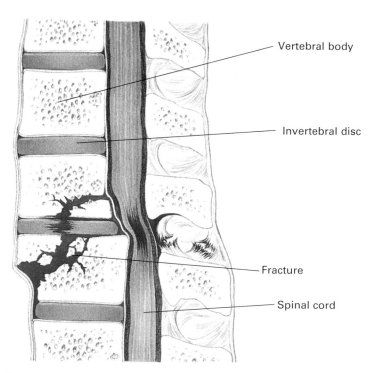

Vertebral body

Invertebral disc

Fracture

Spinal cord

Figure 9.5 Fracture of vertebrae with displacement and pressure on the spinal cord.

- Vice-like pain is felt in the neck and in the angle between the nape of the neck and the shoulder, never extending below the shoulder joint. The pain is triggered by neck movements. The musculature is tender and tense.
- Twisting of the head is painful.
- Mobility of the back of the neck is impaired.

Treatment consists of:
- local heat treatment;
- analgesic and anti-inflammatory medication or muscle relaxants;
- rest from painful activities;
- traction;
- neck collar or heat retainer.

The condition often improves within a week. If this is not the case, a doctor should be consulted.

Thoracic and lumbar spine

Fractures of thoracic and lumbar vertebrae

Fractures of vertebrae in the thoracic and lumbar regions are uncommon in sports, but can occur in riders, alpine skiers, ski-jumpers, and participants in contact sports (Figure 9.5).

- Severe pain is felt at the site of the fracture.
- Pain is triggered by any back movement.
- If pain radiates into the legs it must be assumed that the spinal cord or its nerve roots have been affected.
- Loss of sensation and paralysis are signs of a serious injury.

- The injured person must be taken to hospital for a neurological examination and an X-ray (and if needed a CT or MRI scan) to assess the stability of the vertebral column and other damage.
- When thoracic and lumbar vertebrae have been damaged during sporting activity, compression of the damaged vertebral body is usually only moderate and heals after a period of rest.
- In extreme cases, severe compression of the vertebrae may occur, and injury may also be caused to the spinal cord and nerve roots. These injuries are treated with bed rest, perhaps with a stabilizing brace or other immobilization, for 2–3 months, or with surgery.

Fractures of the transverse processes of the lumbar vertebrae

Fractures of the transverse processes of the vertebrae can result from direct violent impact to the side of the vertebral column, or from tearing in cases of muscle injury, especially in the lumbar region.

Symptoms and diagnosis
- Tenderness is felt over the transverse processes at the side of the vertebral column.
- Pain occurs on movement, especially when the back is bent sideways.
- An X-ray examination confirms the diagnosis.

Treatment
The athlete should rest until the pain has resolved. The injury is benign and heals in 6–8 weeks.

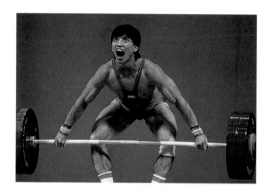

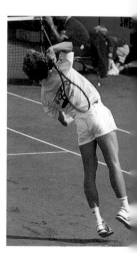

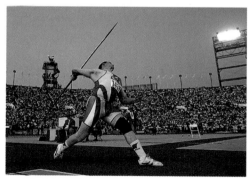

Figure 9.6 The back muscles are in danger of rupture in many sports (by courtesy of All Sport photographers, Simon Bruty, Mike Powell, and Gray Mortimore).

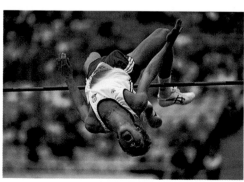

Muscle ruptures

Ruptures of the back muscles occur in weightlifters; javelin and discus throwers; pole-vaulters; football, handball, basketball, and volleyball players, wrestlers and boxers; and many others (Figure 9.6). The injury usually consists of minor ruptures and is most often located in the long back extensors and the large, flat back muscles (Figure 9.7).

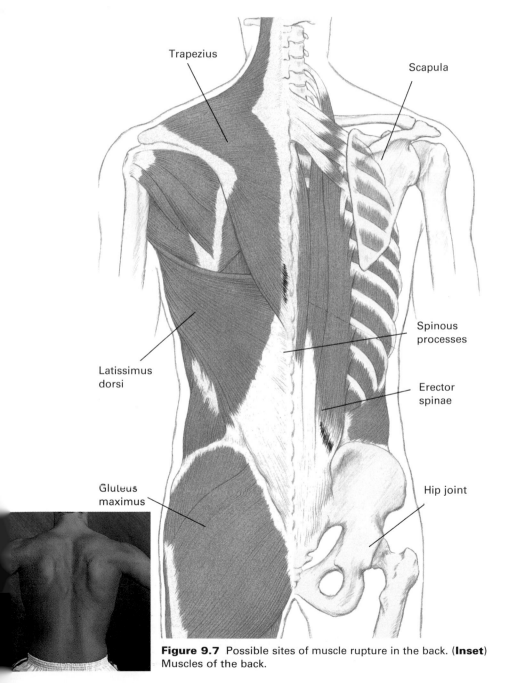

Figure 9.7 Possible sites of muscle rupture in the back. (**Inset**) Muscles of the back.

| Symptoms | – Piercing pain is felt on flexion, extension, and rotation. |
| | – Local tenderness is found over the area of rupture. |

Treatment	The *athlete* should:
	– begin controlled muscle training after a few days;
	– mobilize as tolerated with pain as a guide;
	– apply local heat and use a heat retainer, though not until 2–3 days aft
	the injury has occurred.

The *doctor* may give analgesic and (perhaps) anti-inflammatory medicatio

| Healing | If training and competition are resumed before the injury has heal |
| | completely there is a risk of renewed bleeding and delayed healing. |

Inflammation of muscle attachments

The muscle attachments around the spinous processes of the thoracic a
lumbar spine can become inflamed as a result of overuse (Figure 9.8). Su

Figure 9.8 (**Main**) Sites of inflammatory reactions in attachments to muscles and tendons. (**Inset**) Example of a heat retainer that can be of value in the treatment of injuries in the lower back.

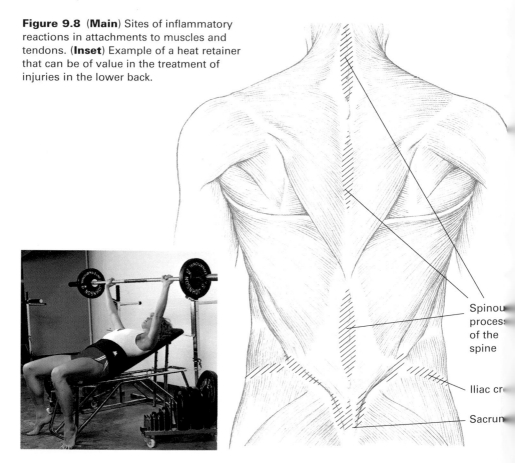

Spinou
proces
of the
spine

Iliac cr

Sacrun

injuries are most common among crosscountry skiers, javelin, discus and hammer throwers, weightlifters, and players of racket sports (Figure 9.9).

The athlete experiences:
- pain during exertion;
- aching after exertion;
- tenderness on pressure over the spinous processes;
- pain in the attachment of the muscle in question, which is triggered by its contraction.

The *athlete* should:
- mobilize as tolerated;
- apply local heat and use a heat retainer.
- exercise with a large ball before return to sport (Figure 9.10).

The *doctor* may:
- prescribe anti-inflammatory medication;
- administer local steroid injections followed by 1–2 weeks' rest from explosive and heavy weightlifting activities.

The inflammation often heals after a few weeks.

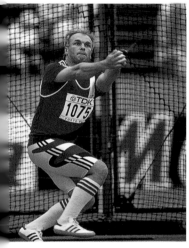

uro 9.9 Muscle attachments can become nful as a result of overuse (by courtesy of Sport: photographer, Gray Mortimore).

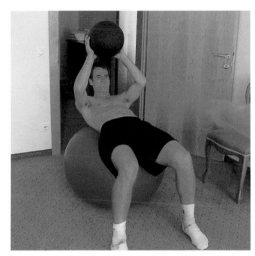

Figure 9.10 Exercise with a physical therapy ball is very useful for all planning to return to sport after back and shoulder problems.

Low back pain (lumbago)

Low back pain can occur in connection with most sports, and its precise cause is unknown. Acute lumbago mainly affects those aged 30–40 years.

- The symptoms often appear after lifting a heavy object or turning rapidly, but can also occur without previous exertion.
- The pain is usually located in the lower back and does not radiate down into the legs (Figure 9.11).

217

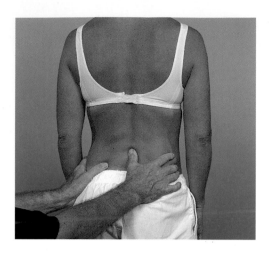

Figure 9.11 One possible location of low back pain.

- Stiffness occurs in the back.
- The posture may appear asymmetrical, with the back bent to one si
  as a result of muscle spasm inhibiting the movements of the back th
  trigger pain.

Treatment

The *athlete* should:
- adopt the position that causes the least possible pain;
- apply local heat, for example with a heat retainer and hot baths;
- avoid body movements that involve flexing or turning the spine.

The *doctor* may:
- give ergonomic advice;
- prescribe analgesic drugs in order to break the pain cycle which ari⃰
  from reflex muscle spasm impairing circulation and causing mus
  pain, which in turn precipitates more reflex spasm. Peripheral mus⃰
  relaxants can sometimes be of value;
- recommend rest several times daily in a psoas position, and give otł
  advice about ensuring good support when in the sitting position, a
  avoiding positions and movements that cause pain. When rising fr⃰
  a side-lying position the athlete should use the arms for suppc
  similarly, when rising from a chair, the chair arms can be used;
- prescribe a course of physiotherapy when symptoms are recurrent (2
  visits may speed return to work and sport in acute cases);
- prescribe manipulation;
- prescribe a corset or body belt which gives temporary support and ⃰
  be worn when the patient carries out activities that usually trigger
  problem. A corset can be of value in the acute stage of lumbago ⁙
  should be used for the shortest possible time if muscle hypotrophⁿ
  to be prevented;
- arrange a CT or MRI scan of the lumbar region if pain has b⃰
  present for more than 1–2 months or if symptoms are recurrent
  raised erythrocyte sedimentation rate (ESR) may be a sign of inł
  tion, tumor, or inflammatory disease;
- prescribe preventive and rehabilitative training (p. 506) as early
  possible. Jogging has been shown to be beneficial.

Lumbago is often benign and as a rule the symptoms disappear spontaneously within 1–3 weeks. In certain individuals, however, symptoms may be prolonged.

People with back complaints should lead physically active lives. Their activities, however, should be tailored to suit the symptoms in question.

Sciatica, herniated disk ('slipped disk')

Pain that radiates from the lower back down one or other leg is known as sciatica. It is often exacerbated by exertion, coughing, sneezing, or straining. One of its most common causes is a 'slipped disk' which exerts pressure on one of the roots of the sciatic nerve, and it can also be triggered by a temporary local trapping or straining of the nerve or its

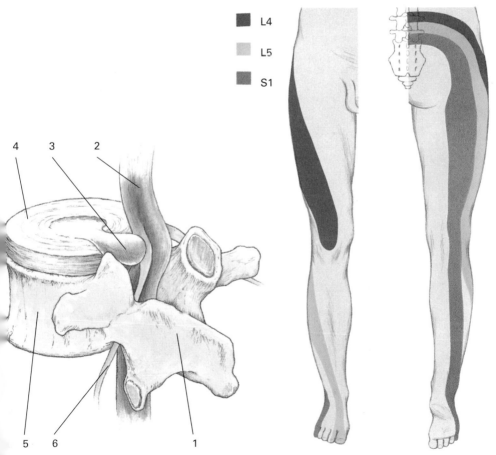

Figure 9.12 Nerve root being pressed upon. 1, vertebral arch; 2, spinal cord; 3, herniated disk; 4, disk; 5, vertebra; 6, nerve root.

Figure 9.13 Schematic diagram of pain radiation with a slipped disc showing L4, L5 and S1 syndromes.

roots. Rarer causes include tumors, bony deposits, spondylolysis, spondylolisthesis, and infections which can affect the sciatic nerve throughout its course.

The intervertebral disks are composed of a connective tissue ring and a core of a pulpy, semifluid substance. Slipped disks often show signs of degenerative changes, even in relatively young individuals. Cracks form in the connective tissue ring of a disk, allowing the pulpy substance to seep through and cause pressure on the adjacent nerve roots (Figure 9.12). The prime cause of a slipped disk is bending forwards and to the side to lift a heavy object. Athletes who suffer slipped disks have often had previous attacks of acute lumbago. Depending on where the slipped disk is located in relation to the nerve root, different syndromes occur (Figure 9.13):

- *L4 syndrome* when the nerve root adjacent to the disk between the third and the fourth lumbar vertebrae is affected;
- *L5 syndrome* when the nerve root adjacent to the disk between the fourth and fifth lumbar vertebrae is affected;
- *S1 syndrome* when the nerve root adjacent to the disk between the fifth lumbar vertebra and the first sacral vertebra is affected.

Symptoms

As a rule, the S1 syndrome affects people up to about 40 years of age, while the L5 syndrome is more common in older individuals. Each syndrome has a characteristic pain radiation pattern and affects sensation, reflexes, and muscle power.

A combination of lumbago and sciatica occurs in which pain is felt mainly in the lumbar region but also radiates into one leg and increases on exertion. There may be numbness in the area of distribution of the nerve, weakness in the leg, and diminution of the reflexes. The pain can be triggered by coughing or straining and can be so severe that the lumbar region becomes locked into a position of lateral flexion (scoliosis).

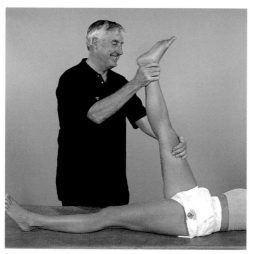 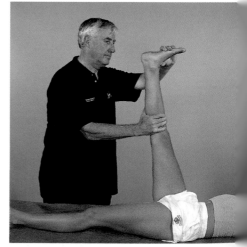

Figure 9.14 (**A**) Straight-leg raising test for sciatica. (**B**) Passive dorsiflexion of the foot is additional provocation in the test.

- The diagnosis is confirmed by the characteristic history of the pain.
- Examination of the spine may reveal a scoliosis caused by strong muscular contraction in the lumbar region.
- Mobility is impaired and the musculature is tender and tense.
- Straight-leg raising (Lasègue test): that is, with the patient lying supine. The passively extended leg is raised by the examiner, and at some point the patient experiences pain radiating down the leg (Figure 9.14).
- Neurological examination may reveal diminished reflexes, weakness or paralysis, and impaired sensation.
- In serious cases, disturbance of the nerve supply to the bladder results in difficulty in passing urine. If this occurs, a doctor should be consulted immediately.
- A diagnosis of slipped, herniated disk is confirmed by a CT or MRI scan.

The *athlete* should:
- rest from painful activities; the psoas position may help (Figure 9.15). As rest causes rapid wasting of the back muscles, special training exercises should be started as soon as possible;
- apply local heat and use a heat retainer.

The *doctor* may:
- advise rest, and increase of activity as tolerated for 8–12 weeks;
- prescribe analgesics, anti-inflammatory medication, or muscle relaxants;
- start gentle traction treatment under the supervision of a physiotherapist when the condition has passed its acute stage;
- prescribe transcutaneous nerve stimulation (p. 100) in persistent cases;
- perform emergency surgery in cases of bladder function impairment;
- operate when acute pain persists in spite of analgesic drugs, when paralysis occurs, and/or when a disabling postural defect resulting from reflex muscle spasm fails to correct itself or deteriorates further. A preoperative CT or MRI scan is needed so that the surgeon can identify and locate the slipped disk.

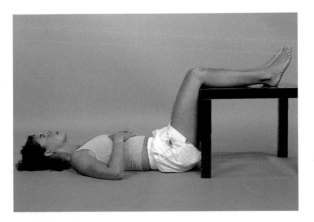

Figure 9.15
The psoas position allows the muscles to relax and gives some pain relief.

- Most individuals who suffer from a slipped disk recover gradually ov
time with rest and exercises alone.
- Following surgery, depending on the technique and extent of injur
the athlete can return to active sport or heavy work in 6–10 weeks.
- The results of surgery are good: 95% of patients make a comple
recovery.

Spinal stenosis

The vertebral column can be affected by stenosis (narrowing of the vert
bral canal) from causes other than a slipped and protruding disk, inclu
ing wear of the facet joints and osteophyte formation. This conditio
which is not common, mainly affects those over 60 years old, especial
middle-aged former wrestlers and weightlifters who have sustained stre
uous loads to the back, mainly in the lower back (Figure 9.16).

**Symptoms
and diagnosis**
- The symptoms are often indeterminate, with vague discomfort.
- Pain starts in the back, especially when it is straightened from t
flexed position.
- Pain and weakness are felt in the legs after walking a short distanc
The pain recedes at rest, especially if the patient is sitting down, b
returns after further brief exertion.
- An X-ray examination and a CT or MRI scan (Figure 9.17) confir
the diagnosis.
- Other possible causes of the pain, for example arteriosclerosis, have
be eliminated.

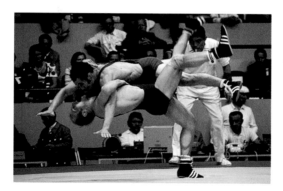

Figure 9.16
Strenuous loads to th
back may cause
problems later in life
(by courtesy of All
Sport: photographer,
Tony Duffy).

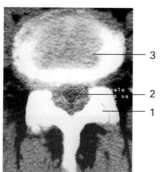

Figure 9.17 CT scan of lumbar spinal
stenosis. The space remaining for nervou
tissue in the spinal canal is shown inside
the dotted line. 1, Vertebral arch; 2, space
3, vertebral disk.

The *doctor* may:
- prescribe physiotherapy;
- prescribe a corset;
- operate in exceptional cases and remove the cause of the narrowing. It is, however, a major operation and there is the risk of relapse.

Facet joint syndrome

The joints between the vertebral arches, the intervertebral facet joints, are oriented in such a way that they reduce the rotation capability of the vertebrae. If there were no facet joints the disks would wear out more quickly as a result of rotatory movement in the spine.

When the disks are affected by age-related degenerative changes, increased compression and displacement of the vertebrae occur, and the possibility of disk compression is increased. This can lead to increased load on the joints, causing osteoarthritis. The cartilage of the articular surface is destroyed, and the resulting osteophytes then press on the nerves so that radiating pain is experienced without a disk having slipped.

Symptoms and diagnosis
- Facet joint syndrome affects those aged 40 years and over and manifests itself as a sudden pain in the lumbar region.
- Rest makes the pain worse, but it is helped by movement and training, a feature that distinguishes this type of osteoarthritis from others.
- Stiffness and a limited range of movement are found in the back.
- Tenderness occurs beside or along the spinous processes and pain is experienced when straightening the back.
- Pain in the back and buttock is felt on lifting the extended leg.
- An X-ray and a CT or MRI scan confirm the diagnosis.

Treatment

The *doctor* may:
- prescribe physiotherapy;
- prescribe analgesic medication;
- prescribe a lumbar heat retainer;
- inject local anesthetic solution into the area of the affected joint (under fluoroscopic control);
- operate in a few cases.

'Weak back' (lumbar insufficiency)

Some people have a 'weak back', which means that they show symptoms such as fatigue, stiffness, and weakness, accompanied by aching, during or after slight loading of the back.

Treatment

The *athlete* should:
- improve technique or change working posture in order to relieve the symptoms;
- strengthen the back muscles by comprehensive training (p. 506) which should be a part of all training programs.

The *doctor* may prescribe physiotherapy with a back muscle program and give advice on lifting technique.

Juvenile kyphosis
(Scheuermann's disease)

Scheuermann's disease is a hereditary condition which produces progressive rounding of the back (kyphosis) and can sometimes hinder sportinactivity (Figure 9.18). The complaint mainly affects adolescent boy Usually three to five thoracic vertebrae are involved, which becom wedge-shaped.

Symptoms and diagnosis

– Slight fatigue in the thoracic region is present on exertion after th affected person has (for example) been sitting in school all day.
– Weakness and pain are felt in connection with strenuous back exercis or loading the back.
– The complaints is often brought to medical attention by parent coaches, or trainers when they notice changes in the shape of th child's back.
– Increased breathing capacity is found in, for example, swimmers an skaters.
– An X-ray examination or a CT or MRI scan confirms the diagnosi Adolescents who have long-standing back complaints of this type ca

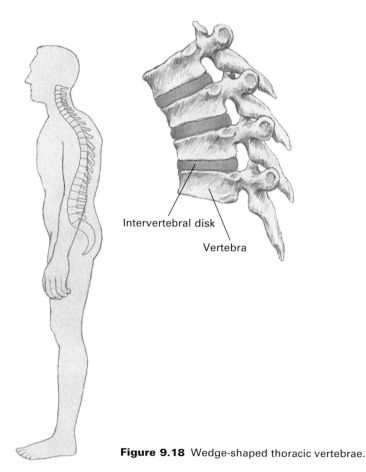

Intervertebral disk

Vertebra

Figure 9.18 Wedge-shaped thoracic vertebrae.

be X-rayed so that infectious diseases and tumors of the vertebral column can be ruled out.

Treatment – In cases of weakness of the back, physiotherapy and muscle strength training may be of help.
– The disease progresses relatively slowly until the skeleton has stopped growing. In cases of exceptionally rapid progression, a corset, brace, or support is prescribed.

Healing and complications – The disease seldom causes any further symptoms once the growth of the skeleton has ceased.
– Individuals who suffer this back deformity have, as adults, a lower rate of absenteeism from work because of back problems than other people.

Scoliosis

In scoliosis, lateral curvature to the left or right of part of the spine renders the vertebral column S-shaped (Figure 9.19). The cause of this complaint, which affects growing children, is unknown. It is often discovered by the physical education teacher, coach, or parents, and should lead to a visit to the doctor.

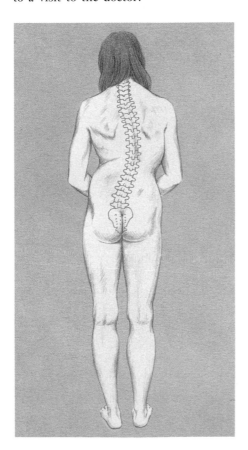

Figure 9.19 Scoliosis.

Scoliosis occurs in about 5% of all children in a normal population but a mild form is more common than that among athletes who pursu asymmetrical training, e.g. tennis players and javelin throwers. Javeli throwers who have been training for more than 8 years can develop type of scoliosis which appears to cause them no problems in the sho term. The explanation may be found in the throwing mechanism: durin the throw the body is bent towards the throwing arm and is twisted the same time as the back becomes more lordotic (sway-backed Repeated training with throwing movements results in the upper bac muscles becoming more highly developed on one side of the body..

Symptoms

Scoliosis hardly ever causes discomfort or pain and does not preclud physical activity. The most important sign is the curvature of the spin which is established by X-ray. Severe scoliosis can cause complication involving the heart and lungs in middle life.

Treatment

– All children and young people with scoliosis should be managed by a orthopedic specialist.
– In mild cases the patient should be kept under observation, while more severe cases a brace or surgery may be needed.

Spondylolysis and spondylolisthesi:

A defect in the vertebral arch is called spondylolysis. The defect can congenital, or may be caused by injury or overloading resulting in stre

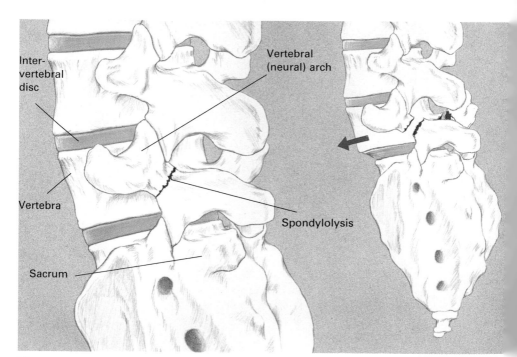

Inter-
vertebral
disc

Vertebral
(neural) arch

Vertebra

Spondylolysis

Sacrum

Figure 9.20 (Left) Spondylolysis. **(Right)** Spondylolysis with spondylolisthesis. Vertebral anterior displacement is indicated by an arrow.

fracture. Spondylolysis creates the necessary conditions for one vertebra to be able to slip forwards in relation to the one below it. Once this has occurred the condition is called spondylolisthesis (Figure 9.20). The younger the individual in whom the arch defect occurs, the greater the risk of the vertebral body slipping forwards; the risk of slippage is very small after the age of 25 years.

The problems that arise are determined partly by the speed with which the slippage takes place and partly by its extent. Spondylolysis can in itself cause problems, including pain in the back and sciatica. These are precipitated by a local effect on the nerves due to changes around the defect without any slippage having occurred. The symptoms of spondylolisthesis begin as the vertebral body slips forwards and begins to exert traction and compression on the nerve roots. In growing adolescents the symptoms often appear after physical exertion.

Spondylolisthesis may occur in about 3–7% of the population, and it is usually the fifth lumbar vertebra that is involved. In sports in which the back is exposed to heavy shear loads, for example gymnastics, diving, javelin throwing, wrestling, weightlifting, and golf, a comparatively larger proportion of participants is affected. The injury occurs above all in growing adolescents taking part in sports involving frequent bending of the spine to extreme extended positions, e.g. in gymnasts and linemen in American football (Figure 9.21).

Symptoms and diagnosis

- Fatigue is accompanied by aching in the lumbar region in young people, most frequently after physical exertion.
- Sometimes sciatic symptoms develop in both legs, in which case pain on straight-leg raising is often seen in both right and left legs. Sometimes a step-off notch can be felt in the spine during examination.

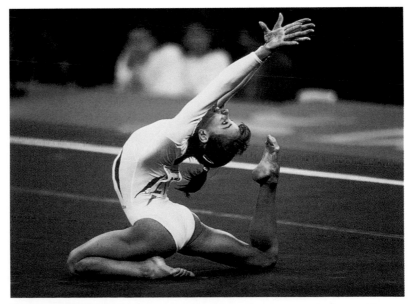

Figure 9.21 Bending of the spine is common in some sports (by courtesy of All Sport: photographer, Yann Guichaoua)

- An X-ray examination should be done with the athlete in a position that triggers the pain.
- An early bone scan may show signs of tissue damage such as a stress fracture.
- A CT or MRI scan (Figure 9.22) confirms the diagnosis.

Treatment

The *athlete* should:
- rest from painful activities until symptoms have resolved;
- consult a doctor for an opinion;
- continue training, in most instances, provided that the back is protected from overexertion, sciatic symptoms are absent, and the symptoms do not become worse. Exercises emphasizing flexion should be prescribed. Extension exercises should be avoided since they will increase shear stress across the defect. Young people below 16–18 years of age should avoid extreme movements in the lumbar region.

The *doctor* may:
- recommend a change of sport;
- prescribe rest when the injury is in its acute stage;
- prescribe physiotherapy with a back muscle program, give advice on lifting technique;
- prescribe a soft brace and a lumbar heat retainer (see Figure 9.8);

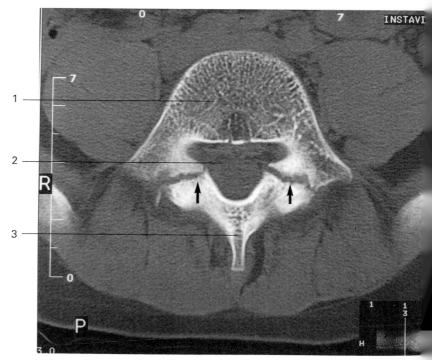

Figure 9.22 CT scan showing spondylolysis of fifth lumbar vertebra. Note the defect in the vertebral arch (arrows). 1, Vertebral body; 2, spinal canal; 3, vertebral arch.

- prescribe a rigid lumbar support such as the Boston brace for fatigue fractures;
- operate when other treatment has not been successful;
- keep growing adolescents who have had this condition under observation with annual X-ray examinations.

Ankylosing spondylitis

Ankylosing spondylitis, also known as Bechterew's disease or pelvo-spondylitis ossificans, mainly affects the sacroiliac joint, the joints between the vertebral arches and the anterior long ligament of the spine, which may gradually ossify. It usually afflicts young and middle-aged men and should be suspected in cases of chronic, but not severe, pain in the lumbar region. The condition is always associated with other disorders. Of the men who suffer from this disease, about 75% have chronic inflammation of the prostate gland (chronic prostatitis), 20% have intestinal inflammation, and 5% have psoriasis. In women, ankylosing spondylitis is connected with intestinal disease in 80%, with recurrent urinary tract infection in 15%, and with psoriasis in 5%.

Symptoms and diagnosis
- Stiffness and pain are felt in the morning.
- Aching in the back disturbs sleep at night.
- Pain radiates out towards the groin and down into the legs.
- Other joints can also be affected, e.g. hip, shoulder, and toe joints. Increasing kyphosis may appear.
- Recurrent eye inflammations (iritis) may occur.
- Special blood tests may confirm the diagnosis.
- An early bone scan is valuable.
- An X-ray examination of the sacroiliac joint can show irregularities in the joint. When the thoracic and lumbar regions are X-rayed, early ossification of the anterior long ligament can be identified as well as an increase in the angularity of the shape of the vertebrae.

Treatment
The *athlete* should:
- relieve stress on the affected joints;
- avoid rapid twisting movements;
- avoid cold and drafty conditions;
- use a heat retainer;
- consult a doctor.

The *doctor* may:
- prescribe exercises and physiotherapy to counteract incorrect posture and increase mobility in back, shoulders, and hips;
- prescribe anti-inflammatory medication;
- treat other associated diseases.

Healing and complications
Active mobility training should be commenced at an early stage, but the disease from which the patient suffers in addition to ankylosing

spondylitis should be treated before training and competition ar
resumed. In the early stages and during symptom-free periods, sportin
activities can be continued without major limitations, though a docte
should be consulted. During active exacerbation sporting activity shoul
be limited.

Bibliography

Keen JS, Albert MG, Springer SL, Drummond D, Clancy WG (198?
Back injuries in college athletes. *Journal of Spinal Disorders* 2: 190–19

Marks M, Haas H, Wies SW (1988) Low back pain in competitive tenn
players. *Clinical Sports Medicine* 7: 277–287.

Micheli LJ (1985) Back injuries in gymnastics. *Clinical Sports Medici*
4: 85–93.

Groin and thigh

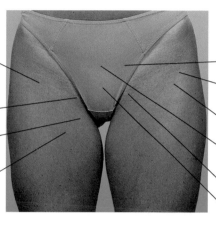

Figure 10.1 Anterior aspect and location of associated injuries.

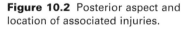

Incipient abdominal hernia (p. 250)

Rectus femoris muscle–tendon unit rupture and overuse injury (241)

Femur neck or upper shaft fracture or stress fracture (247, 248); epiphysiolysis (258)

Abdominal muscle overuse injury and rupture (243)

Adductor muscle–tendon overuse; adductor rupture (234, 237)

Osteitis pubis (245)

Figure 10.2 Posterior aspect and location of associated injuries.

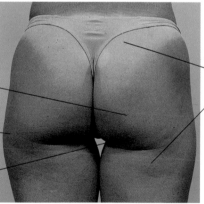

Sacroiliac dysfunction (p. 254)

Hamstring rupture (263)

Figure 10.3 Lateral aspect and location of associated injuries.

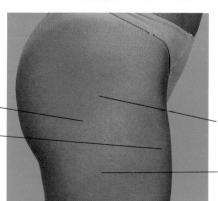

Snapping hip (p. 241); trochanteritis (255)

Traumatic myositis ossificans (260)

Groin pain

Groin pain in athletes is a common problem: it occurs in soccer in 5–13%
of injuries in men and in 4–5% of injuries in women. It is one of the mo
difficult problems in sports medicine. A groin injury may be acute but
often leads to chronic pain with diffuse symptoms that are difficult to chara
terize, and these injuries are therefore often difficult to locate and to diagnos
Successful management, however, depends on correct diagnosis. The exami
ing physician, physical therapist, or trainer must have a thorough knowled
of the differential diagnostic possibilities in the groin area. Teamwork is oft
necessary for a successful outcome: ideally this team should include not on
an orthopedic surgeon and a primary physician, but also an experienc
radiologist, a general surgeon, a gynecologist, and a neurologist. An expe
enced trainer and physical therapist should also be included.

The most common location for groin pain is the adductor muscl
tendon region, and the pain is usually caused by overuse injuries invol
ing the adductor longus muscle–tendon junction. These injuries occ
mostly in soccer and ice hockey, but are also seen in many other spo
(Figure 10.4). Another common cause of groin pain is a hernia. In athle
with diffuse groin pain which is difficult to diagnose, the doctor shou
reasonably suspect a hernia. Hernia-related pain usually is centered on t
inguinal region and spreads laterally along the inguinal ligament pro
mally in the muscles and to the opposite side. This pain can cause rema
able chronic discomfort. Radicular pain occurs in about 30%. The
patients should be examined by a general surgeon. Herniography h
shown to be successful in diagnosing intra-abdominal hernias. T
syndrome of posterior inguinal wall weakness without a clinically obvic
hernia causing chronic pain is increasingly recognized by practitione
Other reasons for groin pain are osteitis pubis, hip pain of different etio
gies, bursitis, snapping hip, nerve compression injuries, stress fractur
infections such as prostatitis and urinary infections, and tumors.

Information about chronic groin pain problems is still limited a
mostly based on clinical experience. Groin injuries may in themselves
be serious. They may, however, lead to chronic pain and impair athle
ability and performance, if not correctly diagnosed and promptly treat

Functional anatomy

The anatomy of the hip and groin is complex (Figure 10.5). In addit
to numerous muscles and tendons, there are also glands, bursae,
other soft tissue areas that can be inflamed and involved in the injur

The bones are the pelvic and the hip bones, the sacrum, and
coccyx. There is little movement across the joints of the pelvis and
muscles act on these joints. The pelvis serves as a weightbearing conn
tion between the lower extremities and the trunk. The hip joint is v
stable. The force transmitted across the hip is 2.6 times body wei
Running increases the force to 5 times body weight during the sta
phase and 3 times body weight during the swing phase.

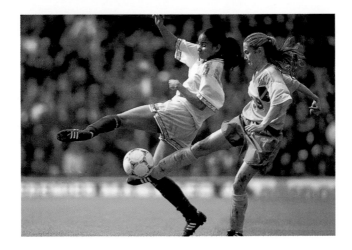

Figure 10.4
Groin pain can
arise in soccer
(by courtesy of
All Sport:
photographer,
Mike Powell).

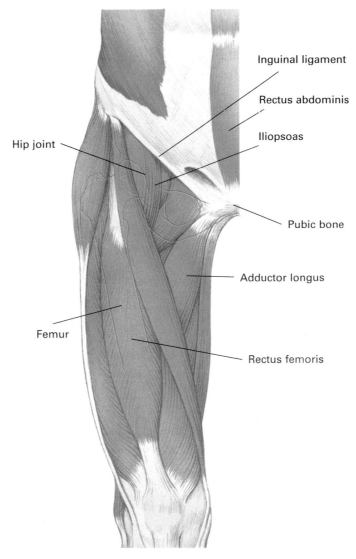

Figure 10.5
Diagram of the
muscles in the
groin region.

Inguinal ligament

Rectus abdominis

Iliopsoas

Hip joint

Pubic bone

Adductor longus

Femur

Rectus femoris

Groin injuries

Overuse of the adductor muscle–tendon unit

The muscles that draw the leg inwards (adduct at the hip joint) are primarily the adductor longus, the adductor magnus, the adductor brevis and the pectineus muscles. The gracilis muscle and the lower fibers of the gluteus maximus also work as adductors. However, it is usually the adductor longus that is damaged during sporting activity.

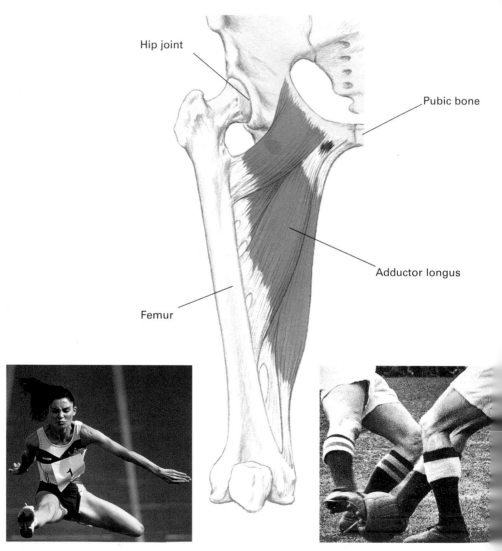

Hip joint

Pubic bone

Adductor longus

Femur

Figure 10.6 A common seat of overuse and rupture of the muscle that draws the leg inwards. (**Insets**) A sudden strain on the abductor muscles may occur in many sports (by courtesy of A Sport).

The adductor longus muscle tendon arises from the pubic bone and is inserted into the back of the midshaft of the femur (Figure 10.6). Overloading can be caused by sideways kicks in soccer, hard track training, and drawing the free leg inwards when skating. It is also common in team handball and ice hockey players, skiers, weightlifters, hurdlers, and high-jumpers. The symptoms may begin insidiously, perhaps at a training camp or during other intensive training periods.

Symptoms
and diagnosis

- Pain can often be located in the origin or at the junction of the muscle–tendon unit and may radiate downwards into the groin. The pain often decreases after initial exertion and can disappear completely, only to return after training with even greater intensity. There is a risk that athletes will enter a cycle of pain in which case the condition is difficult to treat.
- Tenderness is felt at one particular point on the pubic bone over the origin of the muscle. This tenderness is distinct.
- The pain can be triggered by pressing the legs towards each other against resistance (Figure 10.7).
- Functional impairment is common. Sometimes the athlete cannot run but can manage to cycle. The athlete should not participate in explosive sports.
- An X-ray examination may show calcification around the origin of the muscle on the pubic bone.
- An MRI or ultrasound can be helpful.

The distance between the origins of the adductor longus and the rectus abdominis muscles is small, and inflammatory changes probably affect both muscles simultaneously.

Preventive
measures

Preventive training with specially designed strength and flexibility exercises (p. 507) is essential and should be included in every training program as an integral part of the warm-up and cool-down. The coach should be aware of the training levels of the different athletes and should,

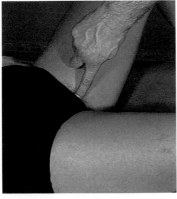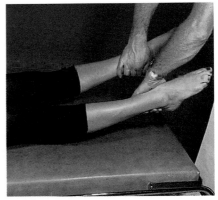

Figure 10.7 (Left) Tenderness in one area over the origin of the muscle in the pubic bone. **(Right)** Pain can be triggered in the injured area by pressing the leg inwards against resistance.

if possible, vary the training individually with this in mind. Athletes wh
undergo good basic fitness training are injured less often than others, an
this is especially true of muscle injuries.

Treatment

The *athlete* should:
- rest from painful activities as soon as pain in the groin is felt; th
  condition will then resolve relatively quickly without any other trea
  ment (this is based on the assumption that the injured athlete does n
  return to training and competition until there is no tenderness or pai
  when making movements with the leg under load);
- use general heat treatment in the form of hot baths;
- maintain basic fitness by cycling (preferably on an exercise bicycle) c
  swimming, using a crawl stroke, but only if these activities are pain-fre
- apply local heat and use a heat retainer in chronic conditions (Figure 10.8

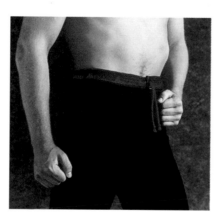

Figure 10.8 A heat retainer fo
groin pain.

The *doctor* may:
- prescribe anti-inflammatory medication;
- prescribe a special program of muscle training, preferably under t
  supervision of a physical therapist or athletic trainer (see below);
- administer a steroid injection around the muscle attachment or tend
  attachment in question, and also prescribe 1–2 weeks' rest from exce
  sive exercise after the injection (the injection should only be giv
  when there is distinct tenderness over the attachment into the bon
- prescribe local heat or other treatment;
- operate in cases of delayed resolution. Surgery often consists of tend
  release and/or local removal of damaged tendon tissue.

The following training and rehabilitation program is suitable f
anyone who has injured the adductor longus muscle.
1. Warm-up: a light dynamic training program, such as using an exerci
   bicycle, for 5–10 minutes.
2. Isometric training without loading the adductor muscle, at differe
   joint angles up to the pain threshold.
3. Dynamic training without resistance.
4. Isometric training, gradually increasing the external load.
5. Stretching (p. 508).
6. Dynamic training with gradually increasing load.

7. Technique-specific coordination or proprioceptive training.
8. Sport-specific training.

The exercises and movements that caused the inflammatory condition in the adductor muscle should not be resumed until the pain and tenderness have disappeared. If the affected athlete rests immediately pain begins, the condition will heal in 1-2 weeks, but if training is resumed too early treatment can be much more difficult. If the condition is not managed properly there is a risk that it will become prolonged or chronic. Return to sport is often possible within 1-3 months but chronic cases may take a long time if not handled properly after surgery; a return to sport may be possible after 3–5 months.

Rupture of the adductor muscles

Ruptures of the adductor longus can be partial or complete. Complete ruptures are usually located at the muscle's insertion into the femur, but can also occur at its origin in the pubic bone. Partial ruptures usually occur in the muscle–tendon junction (Figure 10.9). A rupture of the adductor longus muscle can occur when the muscles of the adductor group are tense and overused, for example in soccer, when the ball and an opponent's foot are kicked with the inside of the foot at the same time, or when a fast start, a gliding tackle, or a sudden turn is made.

Symptoms and diagnosis

- Sudden momentary stabbing pain in the groin region is experienced. When attempts are made to restart activity, the pain returns.
- Local bleeding can cause swelling and bruising, which may not appear until a few days after the injury has occurred.
- If the muscle cannot contract there is reason to suspect a total rupture.
- When the rupture is in the muscle–tendon junction a defect can be felt at the site of injury, and the muscle is also most tender there.
- A clinical examination should be performed when the muscle is in a relaxed state as well as in a contracted state with resistive tests.
- An X-ray should always be taken in athletes with groin pain. If a swelling is present, as in complete rupture, an MRI or ultrasound scan should be performed.

Treatment

The *athlete* should:
  treat the injury immediately with cooling, compression, bandaging, and elevation;
- rest initially (crutches may be helpful);
- avoid pain causing activities;
- start careful exercises and keep up range of motion.

The *doctor* may:
- treat a partial rupture as described on p. 32. A partial rupture will heal with scar tissue and a subsequent inflammatory reaction after the acute stage;
- operate in cases of complete rupture;
- operate in cases of an incomplete rupture with chronic pain after unsuccessful conservative treatment;

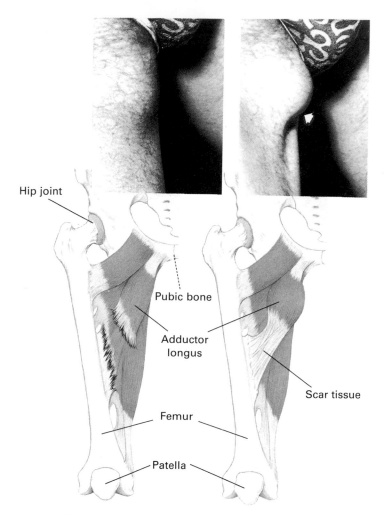

Figure 10.9 Example of a total rupture in the attachment of the muscle th~~~ draws the leg inwards (the adductor longus muscle). (**Top left**) The muscl~ in a relaxed state. (**Top right**) The muscle in a contracted state. (**Lower left**) Rupture in the attachment of the muscle to the thigh bone (femur). (**Lower right**) Healing with scar tissue.

Healing and complications

During the rehabilitation period the injured athlete should contin~ muscle training (p. 509), cycling, light jogging, swimming and gradual~ increased conditioning. Not until the athlete is completely free fro~ discomfort when the injured muscle group is subjected to a load c~ regular training be resumed. Its intensity should at first be limited a~ then increased gradually. Matches and competition should be avoid~ until recovery from the injury is complete, and the fully trained athl~ has been tested under competition conditions.

Complete rupture of the adductor longus muscle can occur witho~ great discomfort. It can, however, cause the affected individual to suspe~ the presence of a tumor, as the belly of the muscle increases in size owi~ to compensatory growth.

Overuse injury of the iliopsoas muscle

The iliopsoas muscle is by far the strongest flexor of the hip joint. It arises from the lumbar vertebrae (psoas) and the inner aspect of the hip bone (iliac muscle) and is inserted into the lesser trochanter (the inner aspect of the femoral shaft). Load on the muscle essentially means load on the insertion. Overuse injury of the iliopsoas muscle can occur during strength training with weights and simultaneous knee-bending, sit-ups, rowing, plowing through snow for conditioning, running uphill, intensive shooting practice in football, badminton, long jump and high jump, hurdling and steeplechasing.

Behind the iliopsoas muscle tendon lies the iliopectineal bursa, which semicircles the tendon and can become the location of inflammation, either in isolation or simultaneously with the tendon of the iliopsoas muscle (Figure 10.10). These conditions can be difficult to distinguish, and in the following section they are treated together.

Symptoms and diagnosis
- As a result of this injury the athlete can enter a cycle of pain.
- Tenderness at the insertion of the tendon into the femur may be present but can be difficult to demonstrate in a muscular individual.

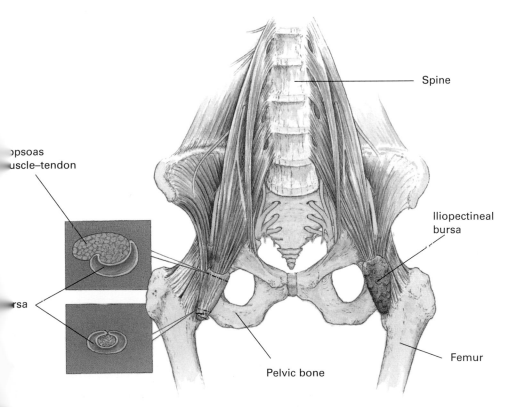

Figure 10.10 The iliopsoas muscle–tendon unit and iliopectineal bursa.

239

- Pain in the groin may occur on flexing the hip joint against resis
  tance.
- When the bursa as well as the tendon of the iliopsoas muscle
  inflamed, a sensation of tension and swelling can arise in the groin. I
  spite of the fact that the bursa is distended with fluid, it can still b
  difficult to feel in a muscular individual.

The *athlete* should:
- initially rest; a gradual increase in activity is tolerated;
- apply local heat and use a heat retainer.

The *doctor* may:
- prescribe anti-inflammatory medication;
- prescribe a muscle training program (p. 509);
- administer a steroid injection into the muscle insertion to t
  followed by 1–2 weeks' avoidance of explosive and strenuo
  activities;
- aspirate the bursa to confirm the diagnosis. This may be difficu
  and should therefore be done under fluoroscopic control. After t
  bursa has been drained 1 ml of a steroid preparation can be inject
  into it.

Healing and complications

When there are signs of recurring injury in the groin muscles the athle
should rest and avoid painful activities, otherwise the condition can eas
become prolonged and chronic.

Rupture of the iliopsoas muscle–tendon unit

Rupture of the iliopsoas muscle–tendon unit is rare; it occurs usually
the muscle–tendon junction or at the tendon insertion at the less
trochanter, and sometimes with avulsion of a bony fragment.

Symptoms and diagnosis

- Pain occurs suddenly, like a stab in the groin, and returns as soon
  the injured athlete tries to flex the hip joint.
- When rupture is partial, deep pain is felt at the iliopsoas inserti
  into the inner aspect of the femur when the hip joint is flexed agai
  resistance.
- Swelling and local tenderness may be present at the tendon inserti
- A definite weakness in flexion of the hip joint is apparent in cases
  total rupture.
- Sometimes a bone fragment may be torn away, so an X-ray exami
  tion is required, particularly in a growing individual.

Treatment

- A partial rupture of the muscle–tendon unit should be treated in
  same way as a rupture of the adductor muscles.
- Complete rupture of the iliopsoas muscle requires surgery.

Snapping hip

'Snapping hip' syndrome can be caused by injuries both within the joint and outside the joint. The condition is not well defined. Causes are as follows.

1. Lateral snapping: the thickened iliotibial band riding over the greater trochanter or a thickened bursa.
2. Anterior deep snapping:
   - the iliopsoas tendon passing over the anterior aspect of the hip joint (the iliopectineal eminence) and through the iliopectineal bursa, which may be inflamed and thickened.
   - the iliofemoral ligament passing the femoral head.
   - intra-articular pathology: loose bodies, labrum tears, etc., inside the joint.

The snapping associated with hip motions is the reason for complaint. Occasionally pain is associated with this syndrome, which is predominantly seen in women. Tenderness and pain may be an indication for more active therapy. The biomechanical reasons for the snapping should be investigated. Occasionally, surgical treatment is indicated in patients with continued symptoms.

The snapping caused by the iliopsoas tendon when it rides over the iliopectineal eminence and through the bursa occurs when the hip is abducted (away from the body) and externally rotated. Iliopsoas bursography can be carried out to demonstrate bursitis. An MRI scan can be used to substantiate this finding. Surgical treatment in these cases includes lengthening or sectioning of the iliopsoas tendon with reasonably good effects, and/or excision of a thickened bursa.

Overuse injury of the upper part of the rectus femoris muscle–tendon unit

The rectus femoris muscle arises above the articular cavity of the hip joint. The muscle flexes the hip and extends the knee joint (Figure 10.11). After intensive shooting practice in soccer, repeated fast starts, strength training, and similar activities, pain can be felt just above the hip joint.

Symptoms and diagnosis
- Pain occurs during and after exercise.
- Pain is triggered by flexing the hip joint or extending the knee joint against resistance.
- Local tenderness is felt at the origin of the muscle above and anterior to the hip joint.

Treatment

The treatment is the same as that for overuse injuries of the adductor muscle–tendon unit (p. 236).

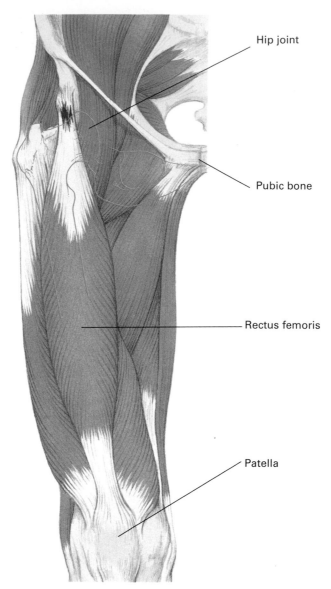

Hip joint

Pubic bone

Rectus femoris

Patella

Figure 10.11 Location of a rupture and inflammation in rectus femoris. T injury in this example is located in the origin of the muscle–tendon unit.

Rupture of the upper part of the rectus femoris muscle–tendon un

Pain in the groin can be caused by a rupture in the origin or the up third of the rectus femoris muscle–tendon junction. This rupture usually partial, but complete rupture may occur. The rupture can oc during shooting and tackling in football and also during fast accelerat in general.

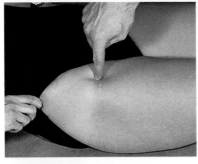
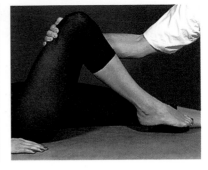
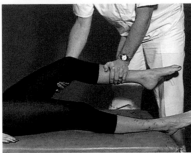

Figure 10.12
(**Above left**) Local tenderness around the origin of the muscle.
(**Above right**) Pain when bending the hip joint against resistance.
(**Left**) Pain when straightening the knee joint against resistance.

<table>
<tr><td>

mptoms
d diagnosis

</td><td>

- During vigorous flexing of the hip joint or extension of the knee joint a sudden stabbing pain is felt in the groin (Figure 10.12).
- In cases of complete rupture it is impossible to contract the muscle.
- A defect and tenderness can often be felt in the belly of the muscle.
- An X-ray examination is needed since a fragment of bone may have been torn away from the origin, especially in growing adolescents. At a later stage there may be residual calcification following bleeding.

</td></tr>
<tr><td>

reatment

</td><td>

- Partial rupture: see p. 33.
- In complete rupture, surgery is probably preferable, especially if the origin of the muscle has been torn away from the skeleton near the joint, taking with it a fragment of bone.

</td></tr>
</table>

Overuse injury and rupture of the abdominal muscles

In cases of ruptures and overuse injury of the abdominal muscles it is usually the rectus abdominis muscle that is damaged, but the oblique and transverse muscles of the abdomen can also be affected. The rectus abdominis arises from the sternum and the fifth, sixth and seventh costal cartilages, and inserts on the upper part of the pubic bone at the symphysis. Overuse injury and partial rupture of this muscle are usually located at its insertion to the pubic bone (Figure 10.13). Ruptures can also appear in the transverse (oblique) muscles towards the sides of the abdomen and can confuse the diagnosis if they are located over the appendix.

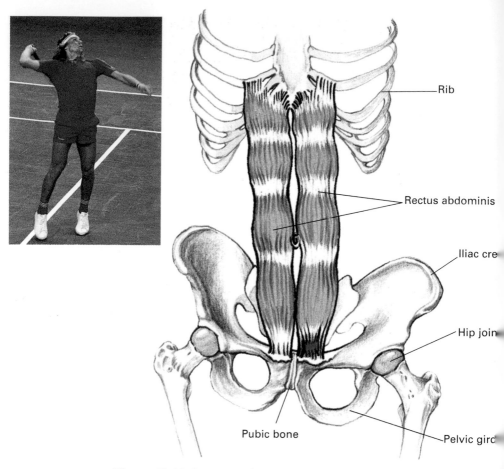

Figure 10.13 Rupture at the origin of rectus abdominis in the pubic bone (**Inset**) This can be a problem for tennis players while serving.

Ruptures of the abdominal muscles occur in weightlifters, throwe gymnasts, rowers, wrestlers, pole-vaulters and others. Inflammation often triggered by exertion, such as strength training, sit-ups, shooti practice in soccer, and serving and smashing in tennis and badminton

Symptoms and diagnosis

– On forceful use of the abdominal muscles a sudden stabbing pain m indicate that a rupture has occurred.
– There may be tenderness and/or inflammation over the area in wh the rupture has occurred.
– There is impaired function affecting, for example, forceful forwa thrust in walking and running.
– A rupture of the abdominal muscles can be difficult to distingu from inflammation of the internal abdominal organs such as appe dicitis. It is typical of a rupture that the tenderness and the pain more pronounced when the abdominal muscles are contracted th when they are relaxed.
– Pain can be elicited if the injured athlete lies flat and lifts legs agai resistance (Figure 10.14).

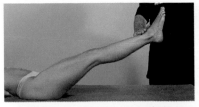
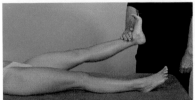
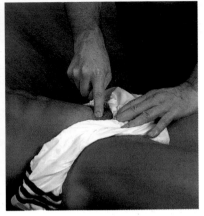

Figure 10.14 Eliciting pain in cases of abdominal muscle overuse or rupture. (**A**) Both legs resisted; (**B**) one leg resisted; (**C**) tenderness on palpation.

- In cases of overuse injury of the abdominal muscles there is often tenderness and pain over the insertion of the rectus abdominis muscle into the pubic bone. The symptoms are triggered by contraction of the abdominal muscles.

Treatment

The *athlete* should:
- initially rest; gradually increase activity as tolerated;
- apply local heat and use a heat retainer.

The *doctor* may:
- prescribe anti-inflammatory medication;
- prescribe an exercise program (p. 506);
- administer a local steroid injection followed by 2 weeks' avoidance of strenuous and explosive activities when there are signs of inflammation of the tendon attachment;
- operate when there is prolonged pain.

Healing and complications

If the athlete rests immediately when there are signs of overuse of the abdominal muscles, healing takes only 1–2 weeks. In muscle ruptures the healing time varies according to the extent of the injury. The injured athlete should not return to training and competition until healing is complete, otherwise new ruptures may ensue and delay the healing process. Large muscle ruptures can lead to hernia formation in the abdominal wall.

Most athletes train their abdominal muscles by sit-ups. In order to protect the iliopsoas muscle during the rehabilitation period, the hip joint should be held bent so that this muscle does not contract. The best method of training the rectus abdominis muscle is half sit-ups, done slowly with bent knees.

Osteitis pubis

Some athletes are afflicted by pain located in the anterior aspect of the pubic bone. Inflammation of the pubic bone occurs in soccer, ice hockey and American football players, as well as in long-distance runners an weightlifters. There is usually no trauma involved, instead there is gradual onset with pain centrally localized in the groin, often radiatin either up to the abdomen or down to the medial aspects of the thigh The precise cause of this injury is unclear, but muscle strain or stre fractures have been suggested. Pubic instability secondary to adducte imbalance, trauma or overuse may contribute to osteitis pubis. Ruling o disease of the bladder or prostate gland is important.

<table>
<tr><td>Symptoms
and diagnosis</td><td>

– Gradual onset of pain, centrally localized in the groin with radiatic to the sides and distally, is typical.
– Tenderness is felt over the symphysis pubis.
– Passive abduction (away from the body) and active adduction (towar the body) and internal rotation of the hip are painful.
– Pain may often be more intense the morning after a training event, when changing position in bed at night.
– A bone scan may show an increased uptake early in the course of t disorder.
– Typical radiographic findings may be present after 2–3 weeks, such erosion or sclerosis (hardened bone) of the symphyseal junction.
– MRI and CT scans can give valuable information.

</td></tr>
</table>

It should be pointed out that X-ray changes resembling those of ostei pubis can sometimes be incidental findings, causing the athlete problems whatsoever.

<table>
<tr><td>Treatment</td><td>

The condition is self-limiting, and the athlete should be informed of th The problem is that the condition is sometimes long-lasting and difficu to manage.
– Pain-causing situations should be avoided.
– Anti-inflammatory treatment and physical therapy may help.
– Heat retaining pants may help.
– A steroid injection may be given under fluoroscopic control (Figure 10.1
– Surgery is rarely indicated; in extremely resistant cases with instab ity it may be tried, but results are debatable.
– Return to sport is on average possible after 9 months of conservati treatment. Occasionally symptoms may last more than 2 years.

</td></tr>
</table>

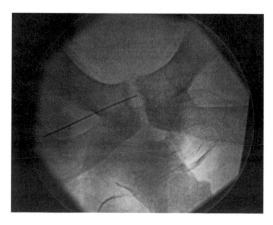

Figure 10.15 Injecti of cortisone may occasionally be given under fluoroscopic control for osteitis pubis. Observe the bony erosions.

Other causes of pain in the hip and groin

Overuse injury or rupture of other groin muscle–tendon units

A number of muscles and tendons affecting the groin region, including the pectineus, the sartorius, the tensor fasciae latae, and the gluteus medius, can be damaged during sporting activity. The precise location of the pain, together with an assessment of muscle function, can elucidate the diagnosis.

Symptoms and treatment are in principle the same as those described for overuse injuries of the adductor muscle–tendon unit (p. 236).

Hip joint changes

Pain in the groin may be referred from the hip joint and can be an early symptom of changes due to wear (osteoarthritis, p. 25), rheumatoid arthritis (p. 27), or osteochondritis. Loose bodies can occur in the joint, formed by a release of fragments of bone and cartilage (osteochondritis dissecans, p. 23). In exceptional cases the edge (limbus) of cartilage that surrounds the joint cavity may have been displaced and driven into the joint. These conditions cause pain on exertion and loading, and also sometimes locking of the hip joint. Continuous and persistent aching discomfort is often precipitated by exertion. Pain during movements of the hip joint, especially during extension, should motivate an X-ray examination or MRI. This MRI can sometimes be carried out, with a contrast medium (arthrogram), with the hip held in the position which triggers the pain. Arthroscopy may also be considered.

Dislocation of the hip joint

The hip joint is extremely stable under normal circumstances, but can be dislocated (usually backwards) by very violent impact (e.g. in American football or motorsport). The injury is serious because the femoral head can be damaged permanently through impairment of its circulation. Dislocations of the hip joint rarely occur without simultaneous skeletal injuries, and prolonged follow-up treatment is needed before a return to sporting activity can be made. This injury may result in necrosis (tissue death) of the femoral head, which may cause permanent dysfunction.

Fracture of the neck or upper shaft of the femur

Fractures of the neck of the femur and of the upper part of its shaft are comparatively common injuries in the elderly. The former, however, also occurs in younger individuals who have fallen directly on the hip while

skating or skiing, for example. It is typical of fractures of the neck of t
femur that the injured leg is shortened and rotated outwards (externall
after the injury. These fractures are nearly always operated on, a
healing and rehabilitation are a slow process. Return to pounding acti
ities is often possible.

Stress fracture of the neck of the femur

Stress fractures (p. 8) can occur in the upper femur, in the neck of t
femur, and in the pelvis bone, typically in long-distance runners, as
result of prolonged and repeated load. Women with the female triad (
470) are liable to this injury.

**Symptoms
and diagnosis**

- Pain occurs during loading of the hip joint and also aching in the jo
  after exertion.
- Pain is felt in the hip joint on movement.
- When there is persistent pain in the hip region, X-rays should
  carried out.
- A bone scan or an MRI can be useful, particularly in cases where the
  is a high risk of stress fractures.

Treatment

- Rest the leg until the fracture has healed, which usually takes 5
  weeks, depending on the location of the fracture and the age of
  injured athlete. Unloading with crutches may be necessary. No retu
  to sport until complete healing is secured.
- If the fracture is on the upper outside portion of the femoral ne
  surgical placement of screws over the fracture may be the best tre
  ment. This is because of the high incidence of complete fractu
  following this type of stress fracture.

Hernia

Inguinal and femoral hernias are not uncommon and can be symptom
producing radiating pain diffusely in the groin area. In athletes w
persistent pain, 'sports hernia' can be a cause of problems: this i
syndrome of weakness of the posterior inguinal wall causing chronic gr
pain, but without a clinically recognizable hernia.

Inguinal hernia

An inguinal hernia is a protrusion of the contents of the abdom
through the peritoneal lining resulting from a weakness of the mus
and connective tissue layers of the abdominal wall (Figure 10.16). Of
hernias, 80% are inguinal and appear as swellings at some point al
the inner half of a line between the pubic tubercle and anterior supe
iliac crest. They can be the cause of pain in the groin which is trigge
by exertion or even by coughing, sneezing, and straining. When

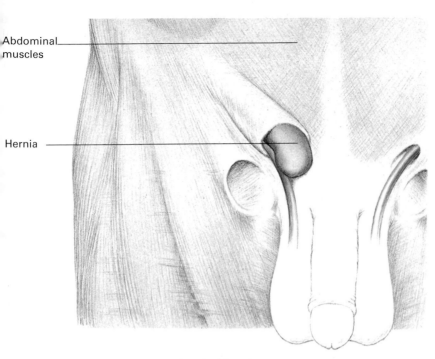

Abdominal muscles

Hernia

Figure 10.16 Inguinal hernia.

causes of vague pains in the groin are sought, the doctor usually checks for the presence of an inguinal hernia.

These hernias are treated by surgery, which may be endoscopic. The patient can often resume muscle exercises 1–2 weeks after the procedure. Return to strength training, however, should be postponed for 6–10 weeks, depending on the surgery.

Femoral hernia

Almost 10% of all hernias are femoral hernias, which protrude on the front of the upper thigh below the groin fold. The treatment is similar to that of inguinal hernia.

'Sports hernias'

Hernias are increasingly recognized as a cause of persistent groin pain, in the absence of other pathological findings. Sports hernia syndrome is assumed to be caused by a congenital weakness of the posterior wall of the inguinal channel, causing chronic groin pain, but without a clinically recognizable hernia. Initially it results in a symptomatic bulging in active athletes, and probably later in life forms a fully developed hernia. The pain of this injury is located deeply in the groin area. The pain may progress and the discomfort may become more severe, making it impossible to stride properly during running or turn quickly without a stab of pain. The pain is often worse on one side, but may radiate laterally and across the midline down the inside of the thigh into the adductor area and into the scrotum and testicles. About half the athletes give a history of pain when coughing. Physical examination reveals the main tenderness to be worse over the pubic tubercle of the affected side. The scrotum is then invaginated and the inguinal rings palpated from the inside. The area around the external ring is tender. Since this condition is difficult to detect by clinical examination, a herniogram or a modified CT herniogram may be used for diagnosis.

The treatment of these hernias is surgical repair to the posterior inguinal wall. Reported results are excellent: 87% of athletes can return to full activity within 2 months and the remaining 13% are improved.

Incipient abdominal hernia

Pain with negative clinical findings is also associated with incipient hernias which sometimes correspond to sports hernias. These are hernias within the abdomen that can cause pain radiating out towards the groin. Soccer players can develop these incipient hernias on the side of the dominant leg. Herniography, in which contrast medium is injected into the abdomen and allowed to sink down into the hernia, may reveal this lesion (Figure 10.17). Herniography is very sensitive and the results must be carefully correlated with presenting symptoms. Operative treatment of these incipient hernias gives excellent results, with an early return to sports.

Hydrocele

A hydrocele is an accumulation of watery fluid around the testes. It does not usually cause serious problems and is treated by draining the fluid. Large hydroceles may sometimes need surgical treatment.

Figure 10.17
Herniography.
The white areas
are the injected
contrast
medium.

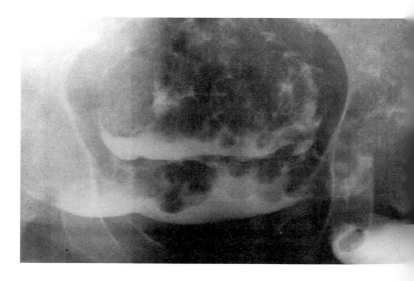

Other testicular conditions that can cause symptoms referred to the groin include tumors in the testes, inflammation of the tissues in the surrounding area, varicose veins in the scrotum, and torsion of the testes.

Inflammation of internal organs
Appendicitis

Appendicitis is characterized by aching pain in the lower right-hand side of the abdomen and mild fever. Nausea and vomiting often occur, and lifting the right leg exacerbates the pain. Symptoms that persist for more than a few hours should lead to urgent consultation with a doctor. Return to sport is possible 3–8 weeks after surgery.

Prostatitis

Inflammation of the prostate gland can cause pain radiating towards the groin. Difficulty in passing urine is common, and worse during cold weather. The condition should be investigated by a doctor and treated appropriately: rectal examination is required in athletes with groin pain.

Urinary tract infection

Urinary tract infections are characterized by burning pains on urination and frequent, urgent passage of urine which may smell unpleasant. Such infections can cause pain radiating into the groin region. Urinary tract infections should be investigated by a doctor and treated with antibiotics active against the particular types of bacteria present in the urine.

Gynecological disorders

Gynecological disorders can cause pain radiating to the groin. They may include inflammatory conditions, infections, and tumors.

Tumors

Tumors are not uncommon in the groin region and can cause pain and aching which may first appear during sporting activity. Other symptoms are similar to those caused by overuse injuries and ruptures of muscles and tendons, and when they are persistent investigation sometimes reveals a tumor as the cause. The rectum should also be examined carefully.

Persistent pain in the groin must be thoroughly investigated with the help of X-rays and MRI.

Sciatica

Pain radiating to the groin and down the thigh may be caused by the L
syndrome of sciatica (p. 219).

Nerve entrapment

Pressure on the nerves in the groin is usually due to local anatomica
conditions. The nerves in question are primarily the ilioinguinal an
iliohypogastric nerves, the genitofemoral nerve, and the lateral cutaneou
femoral nerve of the thigh, which all supply skin areas around the groi
folds, and also the anterior cutaneous femoral nerve of the thigh and th
obturator nerve (Figure 10.18).

The *ilioinguinal and iliohypogastric nerves* run zigzag through the thre
layers of the abdominal wall muscles. They supply the lower abdome
and the skin just above the penis and scrotum or labia, and the inside of
the thigh, and pain in these regions should lead to a suspicion of pressur
on the nerve. The intensity and character of the pain varies. Numbnes
or increased sensitivity in the area can be demonstrated by scratching
needle lightly over the skin from a painless to a painful area, and th
diagnosis can be confirmed by injecting local anesthetic solution arour
the nerve. When symptoms are severe and persistent, a local cortisor
injection and then surgery such as neurolysis are sometimes resorted t

The *genitofemoral nerve* supplies a skin area just below the groin fo
and also parts of the external sexual organs, while the *lateral cutaneo
femoral nerve* of the thigh, as its name suggests, supplies the anteri
lateral part of the thigh. Symptoms and treatment in cases of pressu
on these nerves are the same as those outlined above for pressure on th
ilioinguinal nerve. The rehabilitation time is 3–4 weeks.

Posterior pelvic region discomfort/piriform muscle discomfort

Pain can sometimes be experienced when the piriform muscle is stretche
Compression of the sciatic nerve as it passes the piriform muscle has be
suggested as a cause of groin pain. The patient will have discomfort wh
sitting and with activities that cause hip flexion and internal rotation. Pa
is experienced when the examiner internally rotates and extends the thi
forcefully (Pace sign). An MRI scan may show thickening of the inflam
nerve. The treatment is anti–inflammatory medication and occasionally
steroid injection. Physical therapy is often indicated. In chronic cas
surgery with sectioning of the piriform muscles has been reported to gi
acceptable results, despite the absence of any major pathological change

Hamstring syndrome

Pain localized to the distal part of the buttocks at the hamstring orig
can be caused by compression of the sciatic nerve by the hamstri

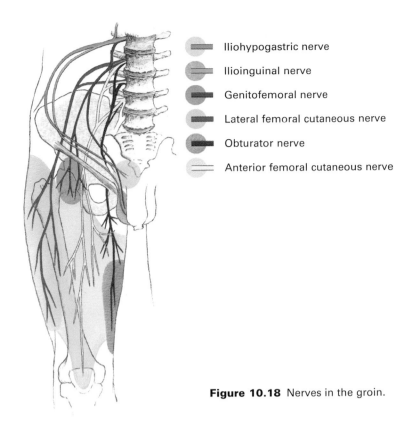

Iliohypogastric nerve

Ilioinguinal nerve

Genitofemoral nerve

Lateral femoral cutaneous nerve

Obturator nerve

Anterior femoral cutaneous nerve

Figure 10.18 Nerves in the groin.

muscles (hamstring syndrome). The characteristic complaint is pain in the sitting position. This syndrome has been found among runners, especially sprinters and hurdlers (Figure 10.19); long-distance runners seem to have no problems from this injury. Soccer players and active athletes in other explosive sports may have this syndrome.

The clinical findings include pain in the buttock, sometimes radiating down the leg, which is aggravated with activity. Resistive hamstring contraction will cause pain in the buttock. Sometimes tenderness is present. The treatment is conservative for a long time, using physical methods and stretching. Surgical excision of damaged tissue and freeing of the nerve may occasionally be indicated.

For hamstring ruptures, see p. 263.

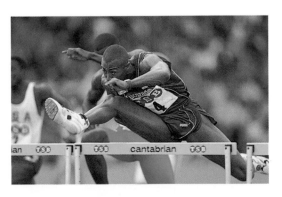

Figure 10.19
Hurdlers are at risk of developing hamstring syndrome (by courtesy of All Sport: photographer, Gray Mortimore.)

253

Sacroiliac dysfunction (inflammation of the sacroiliac joint)

Inflammation of the sacroiliac joints (the joint joining the pelvis and the spine) is not uncommon as an isolated condition among athletes who pursue winter sports. It can also be part of generalized disease, such as Bechterew's disease. In sports, sudden violent contractions of the hamstrings or abdominal muscles with severe direct load to the buttocks or forceful straightening from a crouched position, can generate forces the sacroiliac joints that may cause injury and pain at a later stage. The main symptom of this syndrome is pain in the region of tenderness.

Symptoms and diagnosis

There are several tests for sacroiliac joint pathology, one of which is the three-step test. During this test the examiner's hand moves proximally investigate first the hip and the iliopsoas muscle, then the sacroiliac joint and finally the lumbar spine. The patient lies face down. The first step is to extend the hip joint with the knee flexed combined with pressure on the buttocks. In the second step the examiner's hand moves to the sacrum (the lowest part of the spine), and further extension of the leg will affect the sacroiliac joint. The third step is examining the lumbar spine with the leg in the same position, but with the examiner's other hand fixing the lumbar junction. Discomfort or compression of the iliac rings when the patient is lying supine also indicates a pathological problem.

- Vague symptoms include aching and stiffness in the lower part of the lumbar region. These are most pronounced in the morning and after periods of inactivity. They come and go, and long periods free from problems are typical.
- The aching can radiate towards the back of the thigh, the hip joint or the groin. Changes in the sacroiliac joint can, however, be painless.
- Inflammation of the sacroiliac joint can sometimes be combined with inflammation of other joints, e.g. the knee and ankle.
- A raised erythrocyte sedimentation rate occurs along with other blood changes typical of inflammatory disorders.
- An X-ray or CT scan may show osteophytes, which can be a sign of pathologic motion.

Treatment

Many different treatments have been tried, but the success rate depends on whether the diagnosis is accurate or not. Anti-inflammatory medication and occasionally steroid injections may help. Rheumatoid spondylosis (Bechterew's disease) can also affect the sacroiliac joint causing vague and diffuse symptoms.

The *doctor* may:
- prescribe anti-inflammatory medication;
- prescribe physiotherapy;
- recommend a lumbar heat retainer.

Healing and complications

The symptoms are prolonged, but the condition is considerably more benign in women than in men.

Lateral hip discomfort trochanteritis (inflammation and calcification of the greater trochanter)

Some of the large muscle groups of the buttocks have their attachments to the greater trochanter of the femur in the upper, outer (lateral) part of the thigh. An irritant inflammatory condition can be initiated in the muscle attachment of the gluteal muscles in, for example, crosscountry runners and orienteers.

– Pain occurs over the upper part of the femur on the lateral aspect of the hip.
– Tenderness occurs on pressure over a small area around the greater trochanter.
– Pain is precipitated by pressing the leg outwards against resistance.
– An X-ray examination sometimes reveals calcification in the area in question.
– Ultrasound or MRI scans may show soft tissue pathological changes.

The *athlete* should:
– rest initially, and then gradually return to activity as tolerated;
– apply local heat and use a heat retainer.

The *doctor* may:
– prescribe anti-inflammatory medication;
– initiate a muscle exercise program (p. 508);
– administer a steroid injection combined with prescribed rest.

Trochanteric bursitis

Over the upper lateral part of the femur, beneath the fascia lata, lies a super-ficial bursa, with a deeper one between the tendon of the gluteus medius muscle and the posterior surface of the greater trochanter (Figure 10.20). In cases of falls or blows affecting the hip, the superficial bursa can become the site of bleeding, sometimes resulting in clot formation (p. 54). Clots are gradually transformed into loose bodies or adhesions which give rise to inflammation and accumulation of fluid.

Inflammation secondary to friction and overuse can affect either bursa, and is a more common cause of pain than hemorrhagic bursitis. An exces-sive pronation of the foot (and other malalignments) (p. 396) can contribute to overuse in this region, as can running on cambered roads.

– Pain is particularly pronounced during running.
– Intense pain is caused by swelling and inflammation; this rarely resolves spontaneously, so medical advice should be sought.
– Local tenderness occurs over the upper, lateral part of the thigh.

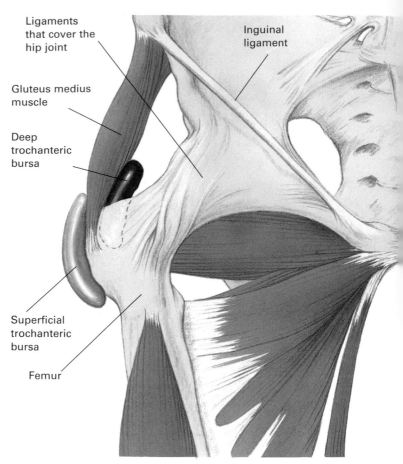

Ligaments that cover the hip joint

Inguinal ligament

Gluteus medius muscle

Deep trochanteric bursa

Superficial trochanteric bursa

Femur

Figure 10.20 Inflammation of the superficial and deep bursae of the greater trochanter.

- Pain can be elicited by passive adduction (of the leg) at 90° of h
  flexion.
- Impaired function and limping are caused by pain and discomfort.
- Pain radiates down the thigh at night.
- Loose bodies and adhesions in the bursa can give rise to crepit
  (creaking sensations) during hip movements and can sometimes ̇
  felt as small, mobile beads when the skin overlying the bursa
  palpated.
- To confirm the diagnosis the doctor may ask the athlete to lie dov
  on the healthy side and raise the leg on the tender side. Th
  compresses the bursa, resulting in severe pain. If the same moveme
  is carried out against resistance, the pain increases.

Treatment

The *athlete* should:
- rest the injured area;
- apply cooling to the area;
- run on even surfaces.

The *doctor* may:

– prescribe an orthotic device if, for example, excessive foot pronation is present;
– prescribe anti-inflammatory medication;
– aspirate and drain the bursa in cases of bleeding or extensive accumulation of fluid (Figure 10.21);
– administer a steroid injection;
– in cases of prolonged problems operate to remove loose bodies and any adhesions in the bursa. Usually the bursa itself is also excised.

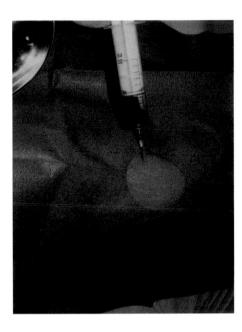

Figure 10.21 Aspiration of bleeding in the superficial trochanteric bursa after acute contusion.

Hip complaints in children and adolescents

Perthes' disease

Perthes' disease afflicts children between the ages of 3 years and 11 years. Its precise cause is unknown. The bone structure of the head of the femur becomes deformed and flattened due to osteonecrosis (death of bone). The child complains of tiredness and of pain in the groin and sometimes the knee, and a limp is present. The diagnosis is made by X-ray examination, bone scan, and MRI. Depending on the severity of changes in the femoral head, the treatment varies from surgery to none at all. The healing process is prolonged. Although Perthes' disease only affects the hip joint, pain is sometimes absent from that joint and is felt instead in the knee. Both joints should be X-rayed in cases of knee pain if Perthes' disease is not to be missed. Children with this condition usually have to avoid pounding activities.

Epiphysiolysis

Epiphysiolysis (slippage of the epiphysis at the neck of the femu occasionally affects boys aged 11–16 years. Pain begins in the gro region, but as is usual in hip disorders, is also felt in the knee. It can triggered by sporting activity. It is important that young people wl complain of this type of symptom should be X-rayed to exclude tl possibility of slipped epiphysis. Surgery is usually needed.

Synovitis of the hip

Acute pains in the hip in children are usually caused by synovitis (inflar mation of the tissues surrounding the joint). The pain increases wi time, and the child shows an aversion to hip movements and sometim has difficulty with walking—limping may be the result. Inflammation the hip joint is seen mainly in children below the age of 10 years; it considered to be a benign condition, which should be investigated by specialist but which resolves spontaneously.

The hip disorders in children and adolescents described above should distinguished from serious conditions such as bone infection (osteomyeliti tuberculosis, rheumatic diseases, and tumors.

> Pain in knee or hip joints, and limping in children and adolescents, should prompt medical examination. Pain localized by the child to the knee may originate from the hip condition.

Bibliography

Ekberg O, Person NH, Abrahamson PH, Westling N (1988) Gro pain in athletes. A multi-disciplinary approach. *Sports Medicine* 56–61.

Fricker PA, Taunton JE, Ammann W (1991) Osteitis pubis in athlet infection and inflammation of injury? *Sports Medicine* 12: 266–279.

Hackney RG (1993) The sports hernia: the cause of chronic groin pa *British Journal of Sports Medicine* 27: 58-62.

Renström PR, Peterson LP (1980) Groin injuries. *British Journal* *Sports Medicine* 14: 30–36.

Thigh injuries

Injuries to the thigh are relatively common in athletes. Muscle inju predominate, such as contusion injuries which often occur in soc Muscle strains are common in explosive sports such as sprinti involving especially the hamstring muscles. Other causes of pain are stress fracture, compartment syndromes, and referred pain. Vague pain in the thigh may be caused by stress fracture or by sciatica (p. 219).

Rupture of the quadriceps muscle

The quadriceps muscle group consists of four muscles on the anterior aspect of the femur: rectus femoris (Figure 10.22), vastus medialis, vastus lateralis, and vastus intermedius. These muscles contain predominantly type II muscle fibers and are best suited to rapid, forceful activity. Most quadriceps ruptures are of the compression-contusion type, but strains do occur.

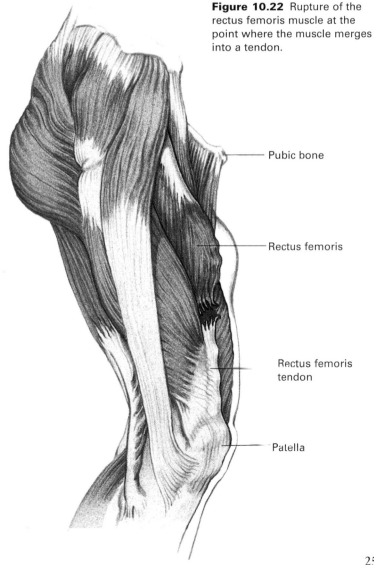

Figure 10.22 Rupture of the rectus femoris muscle at the point where the muscle merges into a tendon.

Pubic bone

Rectus femoris

Rectus femoris tendon

Patella

Ruptures of the quadriceps muscles can occur as a result of impa against contracted muscles, typically in soccer when one player's kn hits another's thigh, or from a sudden, vigorous explosive contraction the muscle such as a fast start or sprint. In cases of rupture caused external impact (contusion ruptures, p. 34), the muscles lying close the bone are most commonly affected. Superficial muscle ruptures a usually caused by overload and are usually located in the muscle–tend junction.

Symptoms and diagnosis
- The athlete often notices a stab of intense pain as the injury occu Similar pain recurs on exertion.
- The muscle may go into spasm.
- There is intense tenderness over the injured area.
- Increasing pain and swelling occur.
- Pain can be elicited by contracting the muscle against resistance.
- In cases of a complete or major partial rupture a defect can be felt the muscle.

Treatment
Ruptures of the muscles of the thigh are treated according to the gui lines on p. 35.

Healing and complications
- The healing time is 2–12 weeks depending on the extent of the ble ing and whether the rupture is partial or complete.
- Scar tissue in the muscles adds to the risk of a further hemorrhage rupture.
- Significant hematoma inappropriately treated can result in heterotor bone formation (see below).

Traumatic myositis ossificans

Traumatic myositis ossificans (heterotopic bone formation, 'charley hor can occur in the thigh muscles as the result of impact, particularly in con sports, such as soccer, rugby, American football, team handball, and hockey. Muscle function and mobility in the knee joint are impaired, there is a risk of recurrent injury in the same area.

Symptoms and diagnosis
- The patient can often recall a particular trauma initiating symptoms.
- The pain may be localized, with tenderness.
- Loss of knee flexion is typical. Bending the knee is often painful this can persist for 1–2 weeks.
- Active quadriceps contraction causes pain.
- The radiographic evaluation of heterotopic bone formation can be at 2–4 weeks. By the third or fourth week, small calcifications are s within the mass and start to show bone reactions. Between 3 we and 6 weeks the bone mass stabilizes in size. It may be joined to femur by a broad-based connection, or by a stalk; some have connection (Figure 10.23). A CT scan may determine the exact and location.

– At the time of injury the priority is to restrict bleeding and limit the hematoma. Compression is important. Knee motion must be restored; and supervised training is recommended.

– Careful isometric contractions combined with gentle, active flexion exercises can sometimes be started when the hemorrhage is under control. These activities should be comfortable for the athlete. No

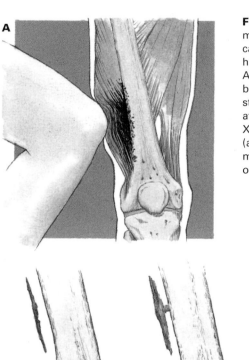

Figure 10.23 Traumatic myositis ossificans. (**A**) This can be caused by a knee hitting the thigh in soccer. (**B**) An ossification free from the bone. (**C**) Ossification on a stalk. (**D**) Ossification attached to the bone. (**E**) X-ray views of ossification (arrows) at 6 weeks and 12 months. (**F**) Removed ossification.

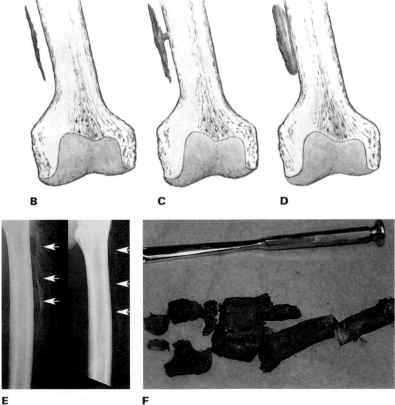

261

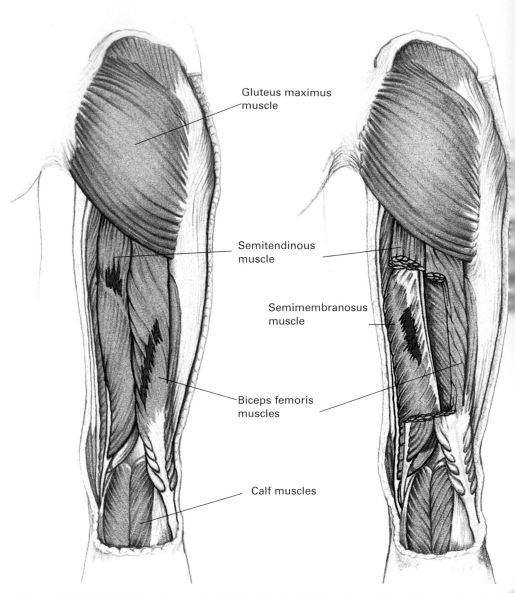

Gluteus maximus
muscle

Semitendinous
muscle

Semimembranosus
muscle

Biceps femoris
muscles

Calf muscles

Figure 10.24 (Left) The injury on the left-hand side of the leg is a rupture of the semitendinos
muscle at the back of the thigh. The injury on the right-hand side of the leg is a rupture of the
biceps femoris muscle. **(Right)** Rupture of the semimembranosus muscle at the back of the thig
The middle parts of the semitendinosus muscle and the biceps femoris have been removed to
show the rupture.

stretching is permitted at this stage. When 90° of knee motion
been achieved, a progressive resistive exercise program can start.

**Healing and
return to
sports**

Most athletes can be treated conservatively. The prognosis is good: i
possible to return to full activity 5–10 weeks after severe contusio
Occasionally surgery is needed if a good range of motion cannot
achieved in spite of lengthy conservative treatment. The bony mas
then excised as a whole.

Hamstring ruptures

Rupture of the hamstring muscles (biceps femoris, semimembranosus, and semitendinosus) which act as flexors of the knee joint and as extensors of the hip usually occurs at the muscle–tendon junction regardless of the strain rate, or at their insertion (Figure 10.24). The injury occurs as a result of overload forceful contraction during flexing of the knee joint or extension of the hip. Greater force and energy absorption occur prior to failure of the contracting muscle compared with a nonstimulated muscle. Sprinters, middle-distance runners, and participants in contact sports are especially susceptible to this type of injury, but long-jumpers, triple-jumpers, and players of badminton, tennis, team handball, volleyball, and other sports can be affected (Figure 10.25). The injury is most common, however, in water-skiing.

mptoms
d diagnosis
- The injury can be located anywhere along the whole hamstring muscle–tendon unit. There is a tendon overlap over the course of the muscle (with the exception of the semitendinosus); this means that almost any area along the muscle is a potential location for injury as there is a long musculotendinous junction following most of the muscle length.
- There is typically a history of sudden onset of pain in the posterior thigh associated with explosive activity. A 'pop' may have been heard.
- Local tenderness is found on palpation with the athlete prone.
- The hematoma may reach the skin, causing discoloration after a few days.
- Sometimes a palpable defect can be present, although it is not typical.
- The injured athlete has pain flexing the knee or extending the hip against resistance.
- An MRI scan can be helpful (Figure 10.26). Ultrasonography can give valuable information in experienced hands.

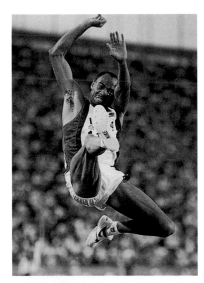

Figure 10.25 Long-jumpers can be at risk of hamstring ruptures (by courtesy of All Sport: photographer, Mike Powell).

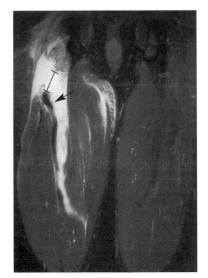

Figure 10.26 MRI of complete avulsion rupture of proximal hamstrings (arrow). Line shows the extent of the defect.

Treatment

– Rest, ice, compression, and elevation (and sometimes crutches) may be initially used for 3–5 days.
– After 5 days a gradual exercise program (including stretching) should start (Figure 10.27). Progression is based on gradual relief from pain and improvement of motion.
– Anti-inflammatory medication can be prescribed.
– Return to sports for most injuries is often possible within 2–4 weeks depending on the severity of the injury. Occasionally these injuries can become chronic, especially the more proximal hamstring injuries (hamstring syndrome), and may require months of rehabilitation. Occasionally surgery may be indicated.
– Complete proximal ruptures should be treated surgically.

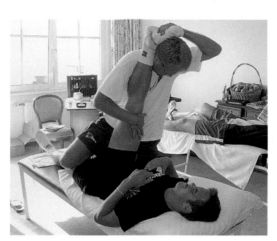

Figure 10.27 Passive hamstring stretching is important, but requires an experienced physical therapist.

Distal biceps femoris muscle–tendon injury

The biceps femoris muscle is the most commonly injured muscle of hamstrings. It acts as a knee flexor; it can be affected by partial or complete rupture and also by injuries due to overuse. The most frequent injury in the knee joint region occurs at the muscle–tendon junction or at the tendon insertion into the head of the fibula. Fragments of bone can sometimes be torn away. The injury may occur in combination with a tear of the lateral collateral ligament. It is seen in contact sports and also sometimes among wrestlers, track and field athletes, and others.

Symptoms and diagnosis

– Local tenderness and swelling occur at the insertion of the biceps in the posterior aspect of the head of the fibula and/or the muscle–tendon junction on the posterior distal aspect of the thigh (Figure 10.28).
– Pain starts when the knee joint is bent against resistance.

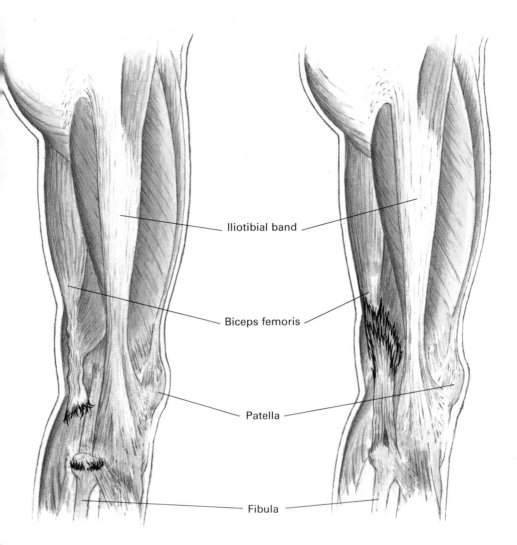

Iliotibial band

Biceps femoris

Patella

Fibula

Figure 10.28 Sites of distal biceps femoris muscle–tendon unit injury.

- Muscle function is absent in cases of complete rupture.
- In cases of injury due to overuse a typical pain cycle is present.
- An X-ray examination can sometimes show that fragments of bone have been torn loose. An MRI scan will secure the diagnosis.

Treatment
The *athlete* should:
- apply ice and a compression bandage in the acute phase;
- rest, apply local heat, and use a heat retainer until there is no pain under load;
- carry out strength and stretching exercises after the acute phase.

The *doctor* may:
- prescribe anti-inflammatory medication;
- apply a brace in cases of rupture;
- operate when there is a complete rupture.

Compartment syndromes

The muscles in the thigh are surrounded by fascias, but they are not a clearly confined to compartments as the lower leg muscles. Nevertheless some athletes, especially long-distance runners, crosscountry skiers, an ice hockey players who use their thigh muscles intensively, experienc thigh pain, weakness, and fatigue associated with sports activity. Th pain can arise within minutes, and may be bilateral. There is no assoc ated trauma. The pain can be anterior, lateral or posterior, or involve th whole thigh. There are usually no neurological symptoms, and intr muscular pressure measurements are often normal. Diagnosis is chief by exclusion. When physical therapy, including stretching, has been trie for a long time without improvement, fasciotomy (opening of the fasci anteriorly and/or posteriorly may give good relief. Usually the rectu femoris, vastus medialis, and vastus lateralis are involved, and should t fasciotomized separately.

Bibliography

Brunet ME, Hontas RB (1994) The thigh. In: DeLee JC, Drez D (ed Orthopaedic Sports Medicine: Principles and Practice, vol. 2, 1086–1112. Philadelphia: WB Saunders.

Ryan JB, Wheeler JM, Hopkinson WJ et al (1991) Quadriceps cont sions: West Point update. American Journal of Sports Medicine 1 299–304.

11 Knee

The knee is the most frequently injured joint in athletics (Figures 11.1–11.4). Most injuries are due to the extreme stresses of twisting and turning activities such as those found in skiing, soccer, and American football. Medial collateral ligament and meniscal injuries are in the majority, but anterior cruciate ligament ruptures are also common and are responsible for a considerable amount of lost time from sport. The most common overuse problems are patellofemoral pain syndromes and patellar tendinosis.

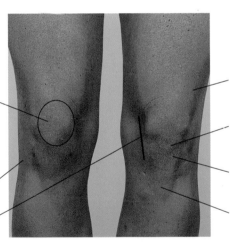

Figure 11.1 Anterior aspect of the knee and location of associated injuries.

atellofemoral
ain syndrome
. 310); patella
acture (320);
epatellar
ursitis (324)

ateral meniscus
jury (302)

ica syndrome
07)

Quadriceps tendon injury (p. 308)

Jumper's knee (321);
Sinding–Larsen–Johansson disease (322)

Patellar tendon rupture (320)

Osgood–Schlatter disease (323)

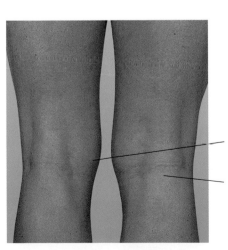

Figure 11.2 Posterior aspect of the knee and location of associated injuries.

Medial meniscus injury (p. 301)

Baker's cyst (326)

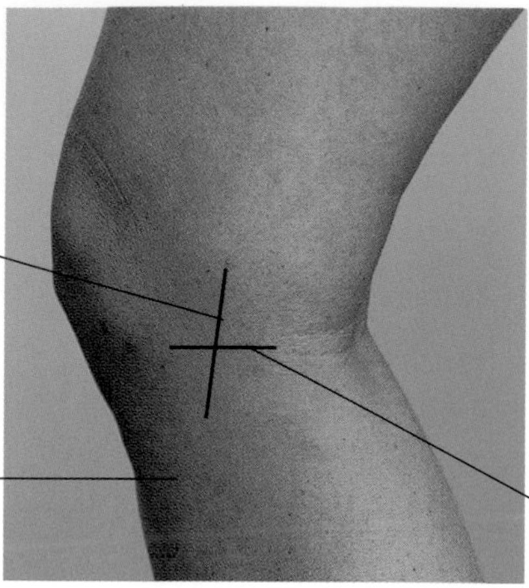

Figure 11.3 Medial aspect of the knee and location of associated injuries.

Medial collateral ligament injury (p. 282)

Pes anserinus bursitis (325)

Medial meniscus injury (p. 301)

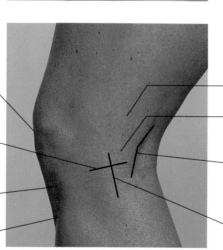

Figure 11.4 Lateral aspect of the knee and location of associated injuries.

Jumper's knee (p. 321); Sinding–Larsen–Johansson disease (322)

Lateral meniscus injury (302); discoid meniscus (304)

Infrapatellar bursitis (325)

Osgood–Schlatter disease (323)

Runner's knee (p. 327)

Popliteal tendon overuse injury (329)

Distal biceps femoris muscle–tendon injury at knee (330)

Lateral collateral ligament injury and posterior lateral instability (291)

Functional anatomy and biomechanics

The knee joint is formed by the femur and tibia. In addition, the pate lies within the patellar tendon and glides over a groove on the front the femur during knee motion. The patella provides a mechanical adva tage for the quadriceps muscle to straighten the knee. The contacti surfaces of the three bones are lined with articular cartilage, and the joi is surrounded by a layer of synovium. The joint is stabilized by fo strong ligaments: the medial collateral ligament (MCL); the lateral coll eral ligament (LCL); the anterior cruciate ligament (ACL), and the post rior cruciate ligament (PCL). The MCL and LCL prevent side-to-si motion, while the ACL and PCL limit abnormal front and back motio Twisting injuries that cause excess forces in these ligaments can tear t ligaments. The MCL and ACL are often injured together; the mana; ment of these injuries is improving, and athletes can often return participation in sports. Injuries to the PCL and LCL are more difficult to treat, especially those that involve the capsule and other structures on the lateral–posterior (outer-back) portion of the knee.

Investigation

Grading

Ligament injuries can be graded according to the severity of the injury, most commonly into three grades:
- grade I: there is tearing within the microstructure but no obvious stretching of the ligament;
- grade II: the ligament is stretched and there is a partial tear;
- grade III: a complete tear causing the ligament to separate into two parts.

History and clinical examination

A thorough examination of a knee injury is the basis for its diagnosis.

History

The history should include an analysis of the injury mechanism. The magnitude of the energy and the direction of impact at the moment of injury are important pointers to the severity and type of injury.

Inspection of the injured area

There may be swelling around as well as within the joint. Bruising over or around the knee indicates bleeding and a ligament injury. In case of effusion the swelling usually extends above the patella. The examiner can establish whether such an effusion is present by pressing the area above and below the patella at the same time as pressing the patella toward the femur with the thumb of one hand. When there is an effusion the patella meets a spongy resistance that ceases when the articular surface of the patella is compressed against the femur. When the pressure of the patella is released it can be seen to rise again because of the underlying fluid.

Palpation

The examining doctor should palpate the joint lines of the knee; tenderness indicates a meniscus injury. The palpation continues over the course of the collateral ligaments and the location of tenderness is noted since this may be the injury site. Swelling caused by an effusion can be felt.

Testing the range of movement

A restriction of extension and flexion of the knee should be looked for however, the patient rather than the examiner should move the knee in order to control the pain. Pain on movement or a decreased range of motion can be a sign of meniscus injury as well as ligament injury.

Stability examination

This examination is essential to decide whether a ligament injury has been sustained. Muscle relaxation is of great importance; sometimes pain can make adequate examination impossible. The following tests are indicated:

- anterior cruciate ligament: Lachman's test, anterior drawer test, pivot shift test (p. 276);
- medial collateral ligament: varus, valgus stress test (p. 283);
- posterior cruciate ligament: posterior drawer test, quadriceps active test (p. 288);
- lateral collateral ligament: see p. 292. Examination following posterior lateral instability uses the reverse pivot shift test (p. 292).

Aspiration

Aspiration of the joint (withdrawal of fluid through a needle) can be performed in cases of extensive swelling in order to decide whether an effusion of blood is present.

When bleeding has occurred in a knee joint, a serious injury must be suspected.

Radiology

Plain X-rays are essential in any serious knee injury, to exclude fracture or avulsions or to show defects of the bone lying beneath the articular cartilage. Views taken with the athlete weightbearing (standing) can show changes in the thickness of the articular cartilage. Thinning of the cartilage, which indicates early osteoarthritis, will make the femur and tibia appear closer together.

Magnetic resonance imaging (see Figure 11.7) is useful for evaluating the soft tissues (ligaments, tendons, muscles, capsule, meniscus) and can show swelling in the bone that accompanies fractures or 'bone bruises'. It shows PCL ruptures very well; although the sensitivity for detecting an ACL rupture is good, it is sometimes difficult to decide whether the injury complete or partial. In most situations an MRI is unnecessary because the diagnosis can be made by clinical examination. In unusual or difficult cases an MRI will show an ACL tear or meniscal tear with high sensitivity. Despite

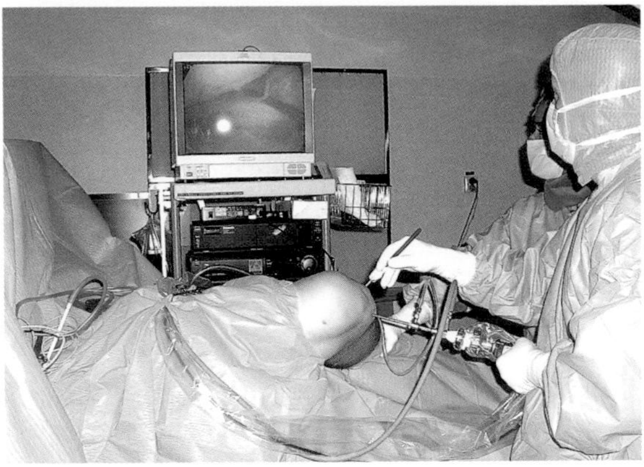

Figure 11.5
Knee arthroscopy.

recent advances, routine MRI is not very sensitive for evaluating articular cartilage damage. The use of contrast medium has improved the accuracy.

A bone scan will show areas of increased (or decreased) bone turnover. It is sensitive for stress fractures and osteonecrosis.

Arthroscopy

Arthroscopy is used in some countries as a routine diagnostic tool. This is probably unnecessary because the diagnosis is usually obvious from clinical examination and other noninvasive tests such as MRI. Where clinical examination and other tests are inconclusive, arthroscopy gives the best examination of the structures within the knee joint (Figure 11.5). It will not evaluate injury to structures outside the joint (skin, nerves, muscles, tendons). Arthroscopy is performed under local, spinal, or general anesthesia.

Anesthesia

Injections of local anesthetic solution can help to locate the problem, particularly in the case of a neuroma (an abnormal growth at the end of an injured nerve). An injection of local anesthetic solution at the neuroma will temporarily eliminate the pain.

Ligament injuries

Anterior cruciate ligament injuries

ACL injuries of the knee are the most common injuries to the knee; the loss of an ACL not only produces abnormal kinematics but also frequently results in major degenerative changes in the knee (p. 43).

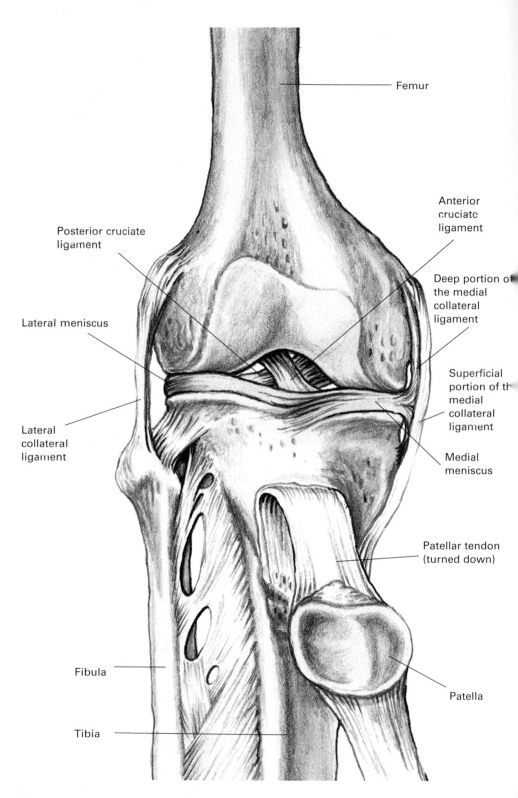

Figure 11.6 Anatomic diagram of the anterior right knee joint.

272

Anatomy

The human ACL is a complex structure at every level. The ligament is designed to act as a stabilizer while allowing normal joint motion throughout the functional range of motion. The ACL is a band of regularly oriented connective tissue that connects the femur and tibia (Figures 11.6 and 11.7). It has an average weight of 20 g (0.7 oz) and an average length of 35 mm (1.4 in). It is narrow in the middle, fanning out inferiorly and to a lesser extent superiorly. The ACL attaches to the posterior aspect of the medial surface of the lateral femoral condyle. The femoral attachment is in the form of a circle. Distally the ACL is attached to a fossa in front and lateral to the area in the middle of the knee, the anterior tibial spine. The tibial attachment is somewhat broader than the femoral attachment.

The ACL consists of an anteromedial band which is taut with the knee in flexion and relaxed when the knee is in extension and a posterolateral bundle which is tight in extension and relaxed in flexion. An intermediate band may be identifiable, which is tight through the whole range of motion from extension to flexion.

The ACL is an intra-articular ligament surrounded by synovium. It is well vascularized, and contains nerve endings which may have a proprioceptive function.

Biomechanics and function

The ACL is the second strongest ligament in the knee with a maximum load of around 500 lb (2200 N). At extreme extension, the anteromedial band is slack and the posterolateral band is tight; with increasing flexion, there is tightening of the anteromedial band and increased laxity in the posterolateral band.

The ACL prevents the anterior movement of the tibia in relation to the femur. The ligament takes up 75% of the anterior force in full extension, 87% at 30° of flexion, and 85% at 90° of flexion. Other restraining factors are the iliotibial band, the medial and lateral capsule, and the medial and lateral collateral ligaments. In ACL-deficient (malfunctioning) knees, the medial extra-articular structures resist anterior (forward) translation and valgus (to the outside) rotation at all flexion angles, while the lateral collateral ligament and the posterolateral structures resist anterior translation in extension only. The medial meniscus also resists anterior translation at all flexion angles. The ACL is the main stabilizer for anterior translation of the tibia in relation to the femur. Together with the PCL, the ACL resists and limits hyperextension (overstraightening), hyperflexion (overbending), and internal rotation (see Figure 11.7).

Mechanism of injury

Isolated injuries of the ACL can occur with a twisting impact, either in internal rotation and hyperextension, or in external rotation and valgus. In alpine skiing there are two typical injury mechanisms: the boot-induced ACL mechanism and the 'phantom foot' mechanism (pp. 77, 78).

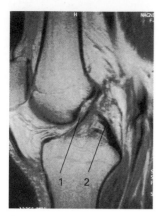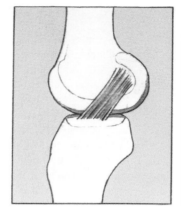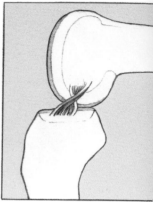

Figure 11.7 (**Left**) MRI of normal ACL (1) and PCL (2). (**Middle**) ACL in extension. (**Right**) ACL in flexion.

Combination injuries to the ACL, MCL, and the capsule can a[l] occur when the impact to the knee is from the lateral side; this forc[e] the knee into valgus and external rotation (Figure 11.8). The same inju[ry] could be caused by an impact to the medial side of the foot. A comb[i] nation injury of the ACL, the lateral collateral ligament (LCL), and t[he] posterolateral capsule can occur when an impact on the knee from t[he] medial side (or on the foot from the lateral side) forces the knee in[to] varus and internal rotation. Combination injuries with the PCL can [be] the result of any lateral or medial impact to the knee, as well as hyp[er] extension and hyperflexion injuries. These are usually high-ener[gy] injuries with dislocation or near-dislocation of the knee.

Bone avulsion injuries of the ACL can occur, especially in hyper[ex] tension and hyperflexion injuries in growing individuals. Avulsion of t[he] tibial insertion is not uncommon in young athletes.

Symptoms and diagnosis

Several clinical signs and tests indicate an ACL injury.

- A careful history is important. An ACL injury should always [be] suspected if there is a history of any kind of rotation or flexion inju[ry,] direct trauma, or rapid deceleration.
- The patient may have sudden pain or hear a 'pop'.
- The knee may give way. After the initial trauma, the athlete can oft[en] walk off the field; however, this should not fool the examiner.
- The patient may with time develop a recurrent 'giving way' probl[em] (the patient feels about to fall because of instability). This oft[en] indicates a serious ACL injury requiring surgery.
- Swelling may develop within a few hours, causing discomfort and pa[in.] The swelling is always a result of hemarthrosis (blood in the kne[e.] Any patient with traumatic hemarthrosis should be suspected of hav[ing] an ACL injury, the cause of hemarthrosis in 70% of cases.
- Sometimes a doctor can aspirate fluid, and if blood is present, an A[CL] injury is most likely. Aspiration of the blood also gives pain relief.
- The active and passive ranges of motion are limited. The athlete of[ten] has a motion deficit, especially if a couple of days have passed si[nce] the trauma.

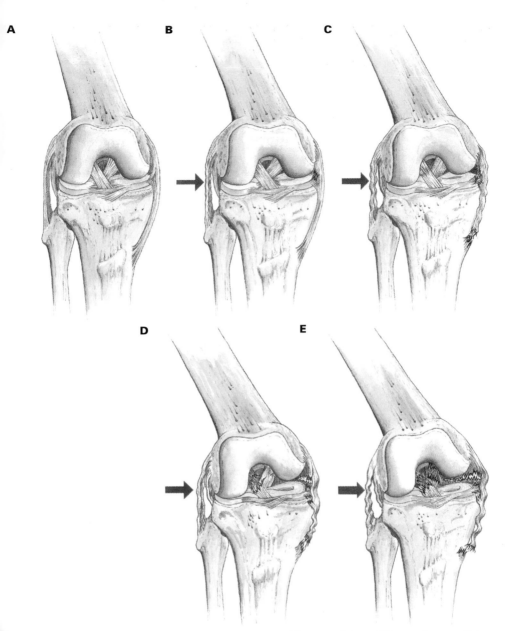

Figure 11.8 (**A**) Normal knee; (**B**) deep medial collateral ligament injury; (**C**) complete medial lateral ligament injury; (**D**) with ACL injury; (**E**) with PCL injury.

- An anterior drawer test with the knee in 20–30° of flexion and the tibia in neutral rotation (*Lachman's test*, Figure 11.9) is positive. The test is performed by pulling the tibia forward in relation to the femur. A positive Lachman's test is diagnostic for an ACL tear.
- An *anterior drawer test* in 70–90° of flexion, with the knee in neutral or internal rotation, is positive (Figure 11.10). This test is, however, not as reliable as the Lachman test, because the hamstrings and the medial posterior horn of the meniscus can resist this drawer.

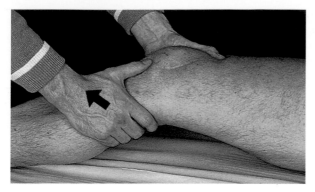

Figure 11.9 Lachman's test.

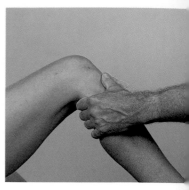

Figure 11.10 Anterior drawer test

- The *pivot shift examination*, or 'rotatory drawer test', may be positi (Figure 11.11). This test is difficult to perform, especially in acu injury. A positive pivot shift may be an indication for surgery in acti individuals since it indicates chronic ACL injury.
- Valgus and varus (side) stability of the knee at 20–30° of flexion a extension should be assessed to exclude injuries to the MCL and LC (see p. 283).
- The patellofemoral joint should also be examined.
- An X-ray examination is needed to exclude any bony injury.
- MRI is used by many; however, it is rarely needed as the diagno can be made from the history and clinical findings. On the other har MRI can help diagnose combination injuries and osseous (bony) lesio (Figure 11.12).
- Arthroscopy (Figure 11.13) will give the definite diagnosis, especia when combined with probing of the ACL. Diagnostic arthroscopy however, usually unnecessary as the diagnosis can be secured at t time of treatment.

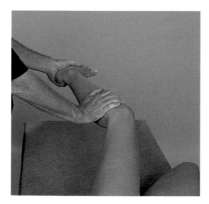

Figure 11.11 Pivot shift examination.

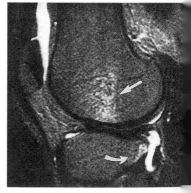

Figure 11.12 MRI of knee show bone bruise lesion (arrow) after A injury.

No single treatment protocol is applicable to all patients: treatment must be appropriate to the acuteness of the injury, the presence or absence of other lesions involving in the knee, the age and level of activity of the patient, the degree of instability, the type of injury to the ACL, and the ability of the patient to comply with a therapeutic program. The factors that decide the treatment are:

- The patient's age: there is no definitive limitation in age, however, since people are increasingly active on either side of the main spectrum. Patients 50–60 years old may be treated operatively if they are very active and the knee is very unstable.
- The activity level is probably the major factor in deciding whether to operate. Surgery is likely to be most beneficial in a very active patient, and these patients are often more willing to participate in an intensive rehabilitation program. Less active people who are not performing cutting or pivoting activities or can accept modifying their activities can often manage well and do not need surgery.
- Combined injuries are also an important factor in decision-making. Most people believe that injuries to other major ligaments increase the likelihood that nonoperative treatment of the ACL will lead to functional instability, but this is still controversial. Tears of the ACL often have an associated injury to one or both menisci. When a reparable meniscus lesion is observed in association with a complete tear of the ACL, reconstruction of the ACL at the same time as the meniscal repair is generally recommended. A meniscal tear often recurs if the ligament has not been repaired. However, in a patient with a chronic ACL tear, no history of pivot shift episodes, and an irreparable meniscus, the torn part of the meniscus can be removed from the knee with a reasonable chance that the symptoms will be eliminated.
- Degree of instability: whether patients who have generalized ligamentous laxity have more instability symptoms after ACL injury than those with normal laxity is controversial.
- Recurrent 'giving way' and positive pivot shift: athletes who have a torn ACL with abnormal anterior translation of the tibia on the femur compared with the other leg, but who have a negative or only a slightly positive pivot shift sign, have been shown to have fewer problems after nonoperative management than patients who have a more dramatic pivot shift result. Patients with a history of 'giving way' and a positive pivot shift usually need surgery.
- Patient compliance: a patient who undergoes ACL surgery must be able and willing to participate in a prolonged postoperative rehabilitation program. A patient who is compliant with the rehabilitation in the initial phase after the trauma is likely to be compliant with rehabilitation after surgery.

All these considerations mean that patients should be evaluated individually and candidates for surgery should be carefully selected.

Candidates for nonoperative treatment include very young and very old patients. Patients who are not very active and do not participate in activities that involve cutting and pivoting movements, can also manage

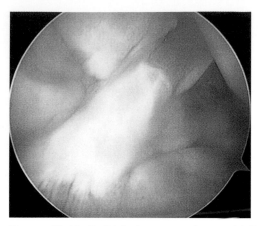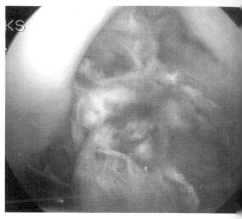

Figure 11.13 (Left) Arthroscopy of normal ACL. **(Right)** Arthroscopy of ruptured ACL.

without surgery. Sometimes patients choose to see what the outcome nonoperative management will be. If problems of 'giving way', pain, swelling develop, surgery can be carried out at a later date. This opti should be explained to the patient. A 'wait and see', nonoperati approach is not without risks, however, since further 'giving wa episodes can increase the damage to the knee, articular cartilage, a meniscus. Nonoperative treatment includes the following.

– Acute management of the injury with swelling and pain contr bracing, a gradual increase in range-of-motion exercises, ice, and an inflammatory medication. Rehabilitation of the muscles should advanced as rapidly as tolerated. Any immobilization splints need for the first day or two should be removed as soon as possible.

– Functional exercises should start as early as possible, to include act ities such as cycling, swimming, and straightforward jogging wh possible. These activities can start as soon as there is full range motion and there is no effusion in the joint. High-risk activities w cutting or pivoting should be avoided for 6–12 weeks after an AC tear.

– A brace may be used if the athlete returns to sports involving cutti or pivoting. Bracing may give the patient confidence and may prev hyperextension. It may also protect the tibia from forward translati in relation to the femur at low levels of load. The effectiveness functional braces has, however, not been completely establish Bracing should mainly be reserved for athletes who have occasio pivot shift and 'giving way' episodes.

– There may be a need for minimal operative intervention when sm meniscal tears are present, the stump of the torn ACL is imping in the joint, there is a catching or locking sensation or recurr effusions, or if there is unremitting pain and discomfort in the kn In such cases an MRI scan can be helpful preoperatively to ass these structures.

Patients who are treated without surgery should be advised about risks of this approach. They should be careful with their activities, avoid cutting and pivoting. If there are signs of 'giving way' episodes, knee buckling, or recurrent pain or swelling, there may be a need for surgery.

perative
eatment

Indications for surgery are most commonly activity-related, which means that very active persons have the greatest need for surgery. Knees that have marked instability, give recurrent effusion and pain, have large meniscal injuries that can be repaired, or have other articular cartilage injuries, should usually be treated operatively. The patient must also be compliant with the rehabilitation program.

Following acute trauma it is now considered advisable to delay surgery until the knee has settled down and the swelling and pain have resolved. The optimal time for the procedure is about 2–8 weeks after injury, although further delay does not significantly affect the results although the chances of a successful end result may decrease slightly.

Patients must be fully informed about the operation. They should be told that:
- the normal anatomic details of the ACL cannot be fully reproduced by any of the techniques now popular;
- the normal biomechanical behavior of the ACL cannot be totally reproduced by surgery;
- results are reasonably good, with a subjective success rate of 85–95%;
- not everyone can return to full activity.

The operation should be carried out by a surgeon experienced in this procedure in order to minimize the risks. The rehabilitation is cumbersome and requires an extremely compliant patient.

rgical
:hnique

- The surgical procedure should follow anatomical principles and allow early motion of the joint.
- Attention should be focused on the isometric placement, correct tensioning, and good fixation of the graft.

The graft selection is important. Most surgeons use the patient's own tissues, either from the patellar tendon or the hamstring tendons, for the reconstruction; both are very good grafts. Occasionally, especially in re-operations, allografts (tissue from cadavers) can be used, but it should not be the first choice in athletes. Synthetic ligaments should be avoided because of their stiffness and historically poor outcomes.

The procedure can be carried out arthroscopically or with a semiopen technique. A common arthroscopic technique for ACL surgery (endoscopic technique) allows for intra-articular insertion of the femoral fixation screws (Figures 11.14 and 11.15). Another variation of the technique requires an additional small skin incision on the lateral side of the knee. This variant is technically easier and more reproducible.

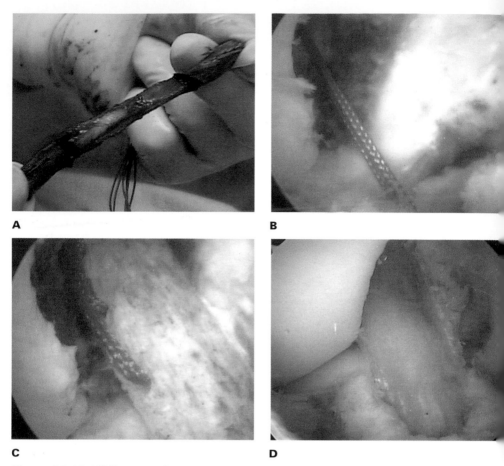

Figure 11.14 (**A**) Bone–patella tendon–bone graft used in arthroscopic ACL surgery. (**B**) (**C**) Bone plug is passed through tibial tunnel and joint to femoral tunnel. (**D**) New ACL graft in plac

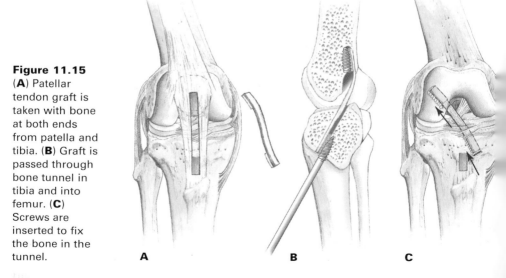

Figure 11.15 (**A**) Patellar tendon graft is taken with bone at both ends from patella and tibia. (**B**) Graft is passed through bone tunnel in tibia and into femur. (**C**) Screws are inserted to fix the bone in the tunnel.

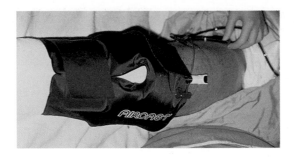

Figure 11.16
Cryo-cuff cold therapy
gives good pain relief.

Good pain control can now be achieved with injection of anesthetic and analgesic agents before, during, and after surgery, together with cryo-cuff cold therapy (Figure 11.16). This has resulted in many operations being performed on a day case (out-patient) basis. Some patients will, however, need to stay overnight.

Rehabilitation principles

Rehabilitation following ACL surgery starts with early range-of-motion exercises (p. 510; protocol on p. 518). Most commonly the surgeon allows 0–70° range of motion in the immediate postoperative period, but some allow full range of motion as tolerated. The most important aspect of the rehabilitation is to avoid muscle inhibition (inability to contract the muscle fully). Muscle inhibition is most often caused by pain and swelling, which may cause a vicious circle where wasting and weakness lead to further damage. Pain and swelling should therefore be treated first with compression and cold. Early motion can also be helpful in reducing the swelling.

- The most important muscles involved in rehabilitation are the quadriceps and hamstring muscles. The hamstring muscles work as an agonist to the ACL and should be exercised early. However, the muscle volume will not increase until the pain and swelling have been treated.
- A brace can be used during the rehabilitation phase to provide some protection. However, its stabilizing effect is limited, especially in high-speed activities. There is little evidence that bracing can provide adequate stress-shielding for reconstructed ligaments; however, braces do have some protective effect during normal daily activities. Many patients like them and feel they provide some stability; this also is of importance.
- The patient can return to increasing activity. Cycling has been shown to be a safe activity for ACL rehabilitation; patients can start as soon as the range of motion has reached 100°, usually 3–4 weeks after an ACL reconstruction. Straightforward jogging is often possible after 2 months, but activities that include cutting and pivoting should be avoided until the athlete has regained at least 85% of the strength in the thigh muscles as compared with the normal side. Such activities may be possible 4–6 months after surgery. The successful return to sports must, however, be customized to the individual and there can be no routine approach to this.

Results and prognosis

- The results of ACL reconstructive surgery are good: active people can return to the preoperative level in their sport after an acute ACL injury in around 80–90% of cases, and in about 70–80% of chronic cases.

– The management of chronic injuries follows the same surgical principle as acute injuries. The procedure is often a little more extensive, wit excision of more bone ('notchplasty') to give room for the ligament. There is often more articular cartilage damage and meniscal injury. Th prognosis is, therefore, not as good as for an acute injury, but the resul are still acceptable. Whether the surgery in the long run will prevel major degenerative disease is still unknown, but it seems that surgery least stops further major deterioration of the joint. The patients mo commonly experience good results from surgery and are very grateful.

The management of ACL injuries remains complicated and is not an exact science. The treatment should be customized to the individual.

Bibliography
Johnson RJ, Beynnon BD, Nichols CE, Renström PR (1992) Curre concepts review: the treatment of injuries of the ACL. *Journal of Bo and Joint Surgery* 74A:150–151.

Medial collateral ligament injuries

The MCL is the most commonly injured ligament in the knee. T incidence is probably higher than reported, because many minor MC injuries are never seen by physicians. The treatment of these injuries h changed; in the 1970s surgical treatment was common, but today mc MCL injuries are treated conservatively, with early rehabilitation.

Anatomy

Medial knee stability is primarily given by the medial static and dynan stabilizers extending from the midline anteriorly to the midline poste orly of the knee. The static structures are the superficial MCL, the pos rior oblique ligament, and the middle third of the capsule ligament (Figure 11.6). Dynamic stability is provided by the per anserinus tendo especially the semimembranosus tendon.

The three units of the MCL are the superficial MCL, the deep MC and the posterior oblique ligament. These structures do not wc independently, but as an integrated unit to resist abnormal loads.

The superficial MCL is on an average 4.4 in (11 cm) long and 0.2 (0.5 cm) wide. It originates from the medial femoral condyle just anter to the tubercle going distally to insert 2–3 in (5–7 cm) below the jo line on the anteromedial tibia just under the pes anserinus insertion. T anterior fibers tense throughout flexion and the posterior fibers slack in flexion. The MCL is tight in external rotation.

The middle third of the deep MCL is a short structure—abc 0.8–1.2 in (2–3 cm) long—which is attached to the meniscus underly the MCL. The deep and superficial layers are often integrated proxima

This ligament is relatively slack to allow knee motion, but short enough to hold the meniscus firmly along its periphery. The deep portion can be ruptured both proximally and distally to the meniscal attachment regardless of the location of the tear of the superficial MCL.

The posterior oblique ligament is a thickened capsular ligament originating just posterior to the superficial MCL at the condyle inserting just below the joint line. It is attached to the posterior horn of the medial meniscus. This structure is important in maintaining medial stability. The posterior oblique ligament becomes slack in flexion.

Biomechanical studies show that the MCL's main function is to resist valgus (outward side motion of the leg) and external rotation forces of the tibia in relation to the femur. The superficial MCL has been found to be responsible for 57% of medial stability at 5° of knee flexion and up to 78% at 25° of flexion. The deep MCL accounted for 8% at 5° and 4% at 25° and the posterior oblique accounted for 18% and 4% respectively.

Symptoms and diagnosis

- The history of injury can include noncontact valgus trauma, as well as external rotation injury in skiing. A major MCL injury may be caused by a lateral blow to the lower thigh or upper leg in soccer or American football.
- Pain occurs at the time of injury. Absence of severe pain does not exclude a severe injury; minor injuries may be more painful than more severe injuries.
- The ability to walk can be impaired after an MCL injury: 50% of athletes with severe (grade III) injuries cannot walk unaided by external support after the injury.
- Swelling of the joint is unusual; it indicates a more severe injury in the joint itself.
- Tenderness is usually present over the site of injury. The most common location for tenderness is the medial femoral condyle.
- Testing the laxity with valgus stress tests is important (Figure 11.17). The grading is as follows:
  • grade 0—normal, i.e. no joint opening;
  • grade I—0.2 in (1–4 mm) joint opening;
  • grade II—0.2–0.4 in (5–10 mm) joint opening;
  • grade III—0.4–0.6 in (10–15 mm) joint opening.

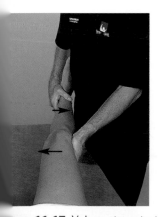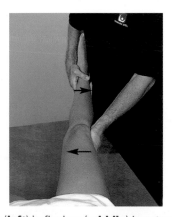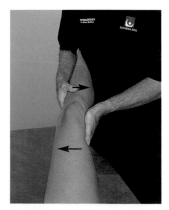

Figure 11.17 Valgus stress test: (**left**) in flexion; (**middle**) in extension; (**right**) alternative method.

- Grade I and II injuries have well-defined end points, but a grade III tear occurs only with the soft, mushy end point with valgus stress testing. It should be pointed out that even with a complete medial injury, there will be no valgus instability with the knee in full extension if the posterior cruciate ligament and the posterior capsule are intact. The medial instability should be primarily tested at 30° of knee flexion but include testing in extension.
- Lachman's test for ACL stability should be carried out when gross medial instability is present. A grade III MCL injury is associated with an ACL injury in 95% of cases.
- Anteroposterior, lateral, and patellofemoral X-rays are required for all patients with knee injuries. Fractures should be excluded. In doubtful cases, MRI may be used to identify the exact location of the MCL injury as well as associated meniscus and cruciate damage (Figure 11.18).

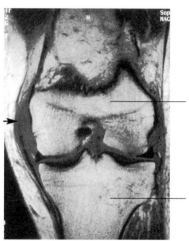

Figure 11.18 MRI showing complete tear of MCL (arrow). 1, Tibia; 2, femur.

Treatment

- Correct diagnosis is the basis for successful treatment. Acute grade I and II isolated MCL injuries are all treated conservatively with quick rehabilitation.
- For grade I and II injuries, weightbearing and early motion can start as early as possible (p. 514). A brace can be beneficial.
- If by the end of the first week there is satisfactory progress with full extension, no effusion, and decreased tenderness, the athlete will do well and may return to full activity (including contact sports) within 3–8 weeks.
- The treatment of grade III injuries depends on the associated injuries. Many believe that a significant anteromedial tibial subluxation (a major medial instability) cannot exist without a cruciate tear. The consensus is that in a combined MCL and ACL injury an intra-articular cruciate reconstruction should be carried out, with repair of the medial structures. The rehabilitation of these severe combined injuries is the same as for isolated ACL injuries. Early motion is important; surgery of the MCL structures can make the knee stiff.

In principle, MCL injuries are treated conservatively if isolated or sometimes surgically if combined with cruciate injuries.

Complications of MCL injuries are rare. Some residual pain may occur over the proximal origin. Stiffness used to be a problem, but is now less frequent because of earlier motion. Chronic instability can still be a problem if the MCL structures are not healed or repaired well. Occasionally, a secondary medial reconstruction may be needed. The importance of intensive rehabilitation of these injuries cannot be stressed enough. Early motion, weight-bearing and muscle exercises should be started as early as possible.

Return to sports is permitted as soon as the athlete is comfortable with it. In a grade I sprain this may be within 1–2 weeks. Grade II sprains need a little longer, but sport can be allowed when there is no pain or valgus stress, or only slight tenderness—about 2–4 weeks. Grade III injuries are the problem: athletes need acceptable stability with a valgus stress test and 80% strength on strength testing. Functional activities can be well tolerated. Sometimes these athletes need a brace.

Combined ACL–MCL injuries

Combined injuries of the ACL and MCL are quite common, especially in skiing. The general principle of this injury is to first treat the MCL injury with a functional rehabilitation program: this generally involves using a functional brace for complete MCL tears for about 4–6 weeks. After this the ACL tear can be addressed, usually by surgical reconstruction in active individuals. This allows optimal treatment of both injuries since it is best to wait a few weeks after an ACL tear to avoid excess stiffness of the knee, which can occur after early surgery. There is, however, some controversy about treatment of complete MCL tears that have also torn the capsule of the knee and the two ends of the MCL are far apart; in such cases, the MCL may not heal well without surgery to reapproximate the ends. An MRI scan can assess this. Any operation on the MCL should be performed within 2 weeks of injury and the ACL can be reconstructed at the same time.

Posterior cruciate ligament injuries

PCL tears of the knee are not very common; they constitute only 5–10% of all major knee ligament tears.

Anatomy

The PCL has an average width of 0.5 in (13 mm) and length of 1.5 in (38 mm). It is fan-shaped, being narrowest in the midportion and fanning out superiorly and, to a lesser extent, inferiorly. The PCL originates on the posterior surface of the tibia and passes superiorly and anteriomedially to insert on the lateral wall of the medial femoral condyle. The PCL consists of a larger anterior band which is taut in flexion and relaxed in extension, and a smaller posterior band which is taut in extension and relaxed in flexion (Figure 11.19). In 70–100% of knees there is either an

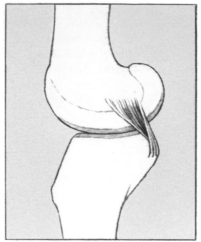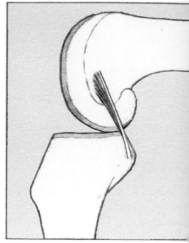

Figure 11.19 PCL (**left**) in extension and (**right**) in flexion.

anterior or a posterior meniscofemoral ligament (passing from the meni
cus to the femur). The posterior meniscofemoral ligament is called t
ligament of Wrisberg and is more frequently present than the ligame
of Humphrey, which is the anterior meniscofemoral ligament. It shou
be pointed out that the PCL is an intra-articular ligament (inside t
joint), but has an extra-articular (outside the joint) distal insertion.

Biomechanics and function

The PCL is stronger than the ACL. The PCL is relatively taut
extreme extension, but it becomes more slack when the knee is flexe
being most relaxed at about 30° of flexion. With increasing knee ang
the PCL begins to tighten again, being maximally taut in full flexic
The PCL provides 95% of the strength to prevent the poster
movement of the tibia in relation to the femur. Secondary stabilizers
the posterior lateral capsule, popliteus muscle and tendon, MC
posteromedial capsule, LCL, and midmedial capsule. The propos
functions of the PCL are to resist posterior drawer forces, to resist hyp
extension, to limit internal rotation, to limit hyperflexion, and to preve
varus and valgus.

Mechanism of injury

A posteriorly directed force on the upper front of a flexed knee, such
a dashboard injury in a motor vehicle accident, is the most common ca
of a PCL injury. In soccer, a player may receive a blow to the ante
proximal surface of the tibia while attempting to slide-tackle
opponent, and thereby force the tibia posteriorly to cause a PCL t
(Figure 11.20). The PCL may also tear from a fall on a flexed knee wl
the foot is in plantar flexion (Figure 11.21). An isolated PCL tear n
also occur when the athlete's knee is forced to hyperflex while the f

286

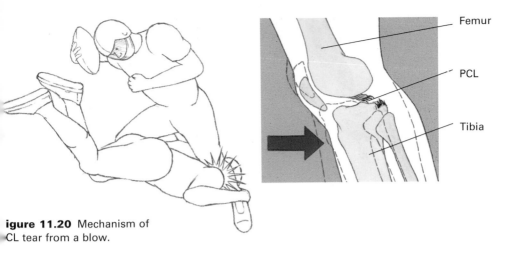

Figure 11.20 Mechanism of PCL tear from a blow.

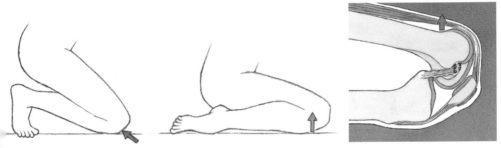

Figure 11.21 Mechanism of PCL tear from a fall.

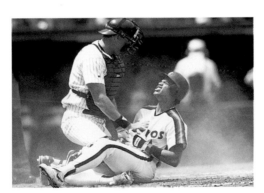

Figure 11.22 Sudden forces acting on the knee may cause a PCL injury (by courtesy of All Sport: photographer, Stephen Dunn).

is in dorsiflexion. Another mechanism of an acute PCL injury is a sudden, unexpected hyperextension of the knee (Figure 11.22).

Injuries to the PCL are often avulsions and disruptions of the tibial insertion, which have been said to occur most typically in dashboard and hyperextension injuries. An avulsion from the tibial attachment is more frequent in growing individuals than in adults.

Diagnosis

In athletes with an acute isolated PCL injury, there is only a mild hemarthrosis. Typically there is an increase in pain with flexion beyond 90°. Generally, the swelling and the pain are less than in ACL injuries.

287

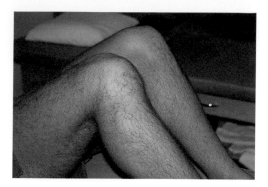

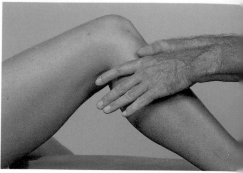

Figure 11.23 Posterior sag sign.   **Figure 11.24** Posterior drawer test.

In patients with symptomatic chronic PCL deficiency, there is often patellofemoral pain and recurrent instability to support the diagnosis.

There are several tests that indicate a PCL injury.

- The *posterior sag sign* is a straight posterior increased displacement of the tibia when the knee is flexed 70–90° (Figure 11.23).
- The *posterior drawer test* is a classic test revealing straight posterior translation of the tibial plateau in relation to femur with the knee flexed to 90° (Figure 11.24). The tibia should be in neutral rotation during the test. there is 0.12–0.4 in (3–10 mm) of increased excursion this usually indicate a partial PCL tear. If there is more than 10 mm (0.4 in) increased posterior drawer, there is a complete PCL tear and the indication for surgery increases. A posterior drawer test is sensitive in chronic PCL deficiency but in acute cases, false negative findings are not uncommon. The posterior drawer test has been shown to be positive in 31–76% of cases in which serious disruption of the PCL was verified. The structures of the posterior lateral corner may provide an important secondary restraint, which may block the posterior drawer test to give false negative results.
- In the *quadriceps active test*, the patient is supine and the knees are flexed to 90° (Figures 11.25). In this position, the tibia translate posteriorly if there is PCL insufficiency.
- Pathological hyperextension of the knee is not uncommon, but can be a nonspecific finding in chronic PCL injuries. This test is usually easy to perform without pain in chronic PCL-deficient knees, but in acute injuries may be hindered by pain.

Imaging can support the diagnosis:
- Plain X-rays will exclude major fractures and bony avulsions.
- Magnetic resonance imaging is a useful diagnostic tool, but it is expensive. MRI may miss a tear if there is only ligament elongation without a failure in ligament continuity. An MRI scan is indicated for the diagnosis of PCL injuries if the clinical impression is uncertain, planning revision surgery for postoperative complaints, and for research (Figure 11.26).

The diagnosis can be verified by:
- examination under anesthesia; this may be general, epidural, spinal, local. When the patient is relaxed, the diagnosis is usually clear;

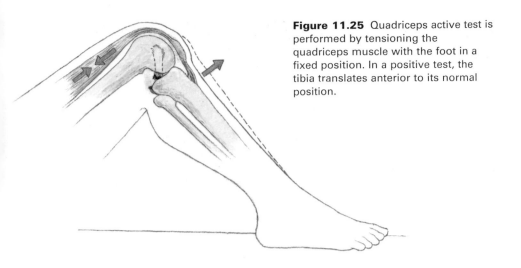

Figure 11.25 Quadriceps active test is performed by tensioning the quadriceps muscle with the foot in a fixed position. In a positive test, the tibia translates anterior to its normal position.

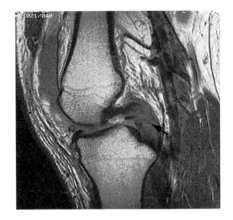

Figure 11.26 MRI of PCL tear (arrow).

– arthroscopy. This will give a definitive answer about the injury, especially when probing is included. This is important, since in some cases there is no detectable failure in ligament continuity, but the ligament is elongated.

Natural history

The natural history of PCL injuries is not yet clearly understood. Some reports showed that nonoperatively treated isolated injuries resulted in 80% satisfaction and return to sport. Other studies found that 90% complained of pain with activities, and 50% had difficulties walking 6 years after injury. Long-term reports with over 15 years' follow-up indicate osteoarthritis (see p. 00) in 80%. This outcome may be activity related. There is patellofemoral osteoarthritis in 62% of cases after 15 years. Poor outcome is correlated with chondromalacia, meniscus injury, quadriceps hypotrophy and degenerative changes in the knee. The proposed natural history in PCL-deficient knees is as follows:

– functional adaptations: 3–18 months;
– functional tolerance with some osteoarthritis development: 15–20 years;
– osteoarthritic deterioration of the knee after 25 years.

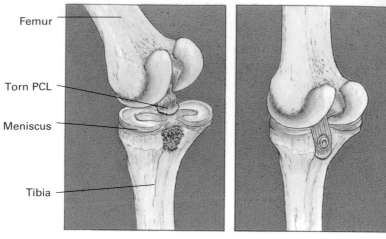

Figure 11.27 (**Left**) PCL injury, (**right**) reattached with screws.

Treatment

PCL injuries with bony avulsion

In dislocated PCL bone avulsions, open reduction and internal fixatic is the method of choice. Excellent results can be achieved after reattacl ment with sutures through drill holes or by fixation with screws (Figur 11.27). Early controlled mobilization in a knee brace is usually possibl

Isolated intrasubstance tears

Nonoperative treatment with aggressive rehabilitation is often used f isolated PCL injuries, especially if the posterior translation is less th 0.4 in (10 mm). Conservative treatment includes a brace or splint f comfort for up to 2 weeks, and then early functional rehabilitatio Quadriceps strengthening is important and can compensate for function PCL disability. Studies indicate that injured knees of conservative treated athletes may remain posteriorly more lax than the uninjured kn but the great majority of athletes seem to be functionally stable and a often asymptomatic. Return to full activity following an isolated PC injury is possible within 2–8 weeks of injury. The short-term outcome usually acceptable if a strong quadriceps function can be maintained. the posterior translation is not prevented with quadriceps activity, the l outcome may be medial compartment and patellofemoral osteoarthritis

Surgical treatment of acute PCL injuries is controversial. If the post rior translation on a drawer test is more than 0.4 in (10 mm), surge should be considered because it is then likely that secondary stabilize also have been injured. The indication for surgery is increased if the PC tear is combined with other ligamentous injuries. The surgical techniq is the same as for chronic PCL instability.

Chronic PCL instability

If the athlete in spite of vigorous muscle rehabilitation has functio symptoms of 'giving way' or discomfort, or more than 0.4 in (10 m posterior laxity on the posterior drawer test, surgery should be seriou considered. Many surgical techniques have been described. The major have failed fully to prevent some remaining objective clinical poster instability, with some patients having a persistent posterior drawer or sag compared with the normal contralateral knee.

The most commonly used grafts for PCL reconstruction are:
1. the patellar or quadriceps tendon from the injured knee;
2. an allograft (graft from a cadaver); today, Achilles tendon allograft is mostly used;
3. augmentation of the existing PCL with the hamstring tendons.

An arthroscopically assisted technique is most commonly used; this is technically demanding and great attention to detail is necessary.

Early motion is usually allowed after PCL surgery, but is usually limited to 0–60° during the first few weeks. Partial weightbearing is usually recommended for 8–10 days and thereafter as tolerated. Isometric quadriceps exercises are started within the first few days, followed by straight-leg raising as soon as possible. Hamstring muscles should be activated later. Functional activities should start as soon as possible. However, there is controversy over the best postoperative rehabilitation protocol.

Depending on the sport, 75–85% of patients can return to activity in 4–8 months after surgery.

Lateral cruciate ligament injury and posterior lateral instability

The LCL is the primary restraint to varus stress of the knee (when the distal lower leg is pressed inward). It is most commonly injured in combination with one of the cruciate ligaments. The mechanism of injury is usually hyperextension in combination with a varus loading of the knee. An injury to the posterolateral complex can produce severe functional instability and disability, and is a major problem in sports medicine.

The posterior lateral complex consists of the biceps tendon, the tendon of the lateral head of the gastrocnemius muscle, the arcuate ligament, the LCL, and the popliteus muscle–tendon unit. Depending on the tissues involved, the physical examination and the treatment will vary.

agnosis and
atment

LCL insufficiency

Diagnosis of LCL insufficiency is made by eliciting varus instability during an applied varus stress on the tibia with the knee flexed at 30° (Figure 11.26). 0.2 in (5 mm) of laxity indicates LCL insufficiency. Varus opening of 0.2–0.4 in (5–10 mm) indicates combined LCL and popliteus injury, and more than 0.4 in (10 mm) indicates an LCL, popliteus, and ACL or PCL injury. In these cases there is also instability in the extended knee.

Serious LCL insufficiency may be treated by surgical advancement of the existing ligament and/or augmentation of the ligament with, for example, the biceps tendon, a hamstring tendon, or an allograft.

Popliteal tendon injury

If there is symptomatic posterior lateral instability with a varus (side) opening of more than 0.2–0.4 in (5–10 mm), or if there is a 10–15° increase

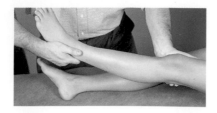

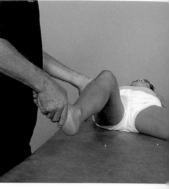

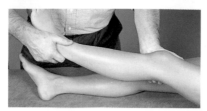

Figure 11.29 Reverse pivot shif

in external rotation of the lower leg when measured at 30° of knee flexio
a popliteal tendon injury should be suspected (Figure 11.28).

Posterolateral instability and PCL injury

The posterolateral drawer test assesses external rotatory instability. T
reverse pivot shift can also detect posterolateral instability (Figure 11.29
The lateral tibial plateau is subluxed posteriorly by placing the joint
flexion and by holding the foot in external rotation. When the knee
extended with pressure on the lateral aspect of the tibia, a shift, whi
relocates the joint, occurs at about 30° of flexion. A reverse pivot shi
however, can occur in 35% of normal knees. When diagnosing the
injuries, it is important to observe the gait for increased external rotati
of the foot, painful heel strike, or the presence of a varus thrust (i.e. t
injured knee is moved outward in a sudden jerking motion when the l
is weightbearing).

Athletes who have acute posterolateral rotatory instability need urge
surgical repair. The peroneal nerve needs to be evaluated during t
procedure. Postoperatively the patient is fitted with a brace allowi
motion of 0–60° and restricted to partial weightbearing for 1–2 weel
Thereafter, range of motion and weightbearing can increase as tolerate

The greatest attention should be paid to injury of the posterolate
corner of the knee, as this is perhaps the most disabling of all ligame
injuries to the knee. Many questions remain unanswered concerning PC
and posterolateral corner injuries. It is unclear what functional mecha
ical characteristics of the posterolateral structures makes this injury m
disabling than other combined or isolated knee ligament injuries.

Combined ACL–LCL injuries

Injuries to the LCL and posterolateral corner (Figure 11.30) are prol
bly the most disabling of all three ligament injuries (this is even m
true of combined injuries). If such injuries are recognized late they
extremely difficult to treat and have high failure rates; the best option
to repair them within the first 2 weeks. In combined ACL–LCL injuri
the ACL should be treated at the same time, usually by reconstructic

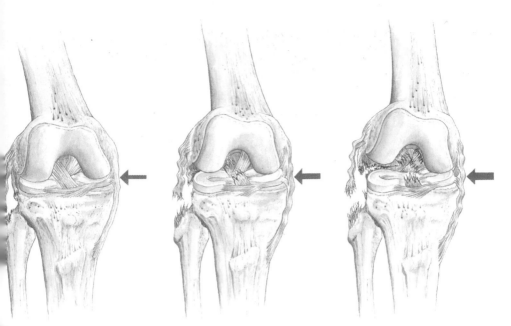

gure 11.30 The stages in development of injury caused by impact against the inner side of e knee joint. (**Left**) LCL ruptures on moderate impact. (**Middle**) With a more violent impact, L also ruptures. (**Right**) In an extremely violent impact, PCL also ruptures.

Knee dislocation

Dislocation of the femorotibial joint requires major trauma. Most of these injuries are due to motor vehicle accidents, but occasionally they do occur in sports. Additional injuries to the blood vessels around the knee occur about 30% of the time, and injuries to the nerves are common. Because of the possible loss of blood supply to the lower leg it is important to reduce the dislocation immediately; this is one of the few true orthopedic emergencies. Following reduction, the arteries of the leg must be evaluated by arteriogram where possible. Close observation of Doppler blood pressure measurements has been advocated as an alternative. Knee dislocation almost always requires hospitalization for observation. If the artery is injured and is impairing the blood supply to the lower leg, immediate surgery is required to repair or bypass the injured area. Knee dislocation will tear several ligaments: which ligaments are torn will depend on the direction of the dislocation. Often both ACL and PCL are torn in combination with lateral (or medial) ligament and capsular structures. Operative repair and reconstruction of the injured ligaments is becoming more common, although some have reported satisfactory results with nonoperative treatment using a brace for 6-8 weeks. If operative treatment is elected, ideally it should be performed within the first 2 weeks when at least the collateral and capsular ligaments should be repaired. The ACL and PCL can be reconstructed later. If the patient's condition delays the procedure, reconstruction can be done later but the results are not as good. Knee dislocation is a devastating injury and most athletes will have difficulty returning to their previous level of activity. Return to sport may be possible within 9-12 months.

Meniscus injuries

Injuries to the knee joint cause more problems for athletes than injuries to any other joint. The most common knee injuries are lesions of the medial and lateral menisci. The sports with the highest prevalence of meniscal injuries are soccer, football, basketball, and baseball, i.e. sports with rotational and 'cutting' motion. The incidence of meniscal injury that results in meniscectomy is 61 per 100 000 population. Treatment of meniscal lesions with arthroscopy has become the most common orthopedic surgical procedure, and in many orthopedic centers constitute 10–15% of all surgery.

In the past, the meniscus was thought to be an expendable structure. Such thinking prompted many surgeons to remove it completely when it was damaged; meniscectomy was considered a relatively benign procedure, allowing the athlete to return quickly to sport, and the results were good in short-term studies. Several authors suggested that the excised meniscus was replaced by a functional fibrocartilaginous structure, but this has not been verified.

The meniscus has now been shown to serve a significant function, and poor functional results and degenerative changes in the knee joint after meniscectomy have been reported. Progressive articular cartilage damage was observed on the weightbearing areas of the medial condyles after medial meniscectomy. Long-term follow-up studies of patients after meniscectomy showed degenerative changes in 20–80% and unsatisfactory results in 32–50%.

Since the 1980s knowledge of the biomechanical function of the knee has increased. The consensus of recent research is that the meniscus plays an important role in the function of the knee joint, emphasizing loadbearing function and its stabilizing character during flexion–extension and rotation.

Gross anatomy

The medial and lateral menisci are C-shaped wedges of fibrocartilage located between the condyles of the femur and tibia. The medial meniscus is somewhat more C-shaped than the more circular lateral meniscus because the posterior and anterior horns of the lateral meniscus attached to the nonarticular area of the tibia plateau, whereas those of the medial meniscus are clear of the plateau anteriorly and posteriorly (Figure 11.31). The meniscus has a thick convex periphery and a thin concave central marginal edge. The anterior and posterior halves of the medial meniscus differ in width: the anterior portion is much narrower than the posterior portion. There are, however, variations, and occasionally there may be little difference in width between the two halves. A narrow meniscus is less likely to be injured than a broad one.

The medial meniscus is approximately 1.4 in (3.5 cm) in length. The anterior horn of the medial meniscus is attached to the anterior surface of the tibia well off the tibial plateau. The anterior fibers of the anterior cruciate

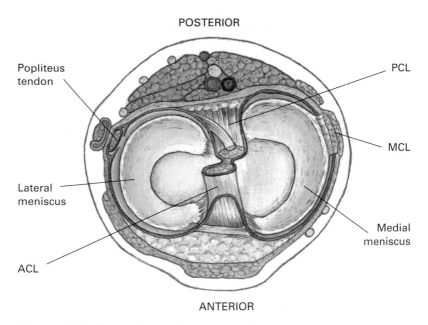

POSTERIOR

Popliteus
tendon

PCL

MCL

Lateral
meniscus

Medial
meniscus

ACL

ANTERIOR

Figure 11.31 The medial and lateral menisci.

ate attachment merge with the transverse ligament, which connects the anterior horns of the medial and lateral menisci. The posterior horn of the medial meniscus is firmly attached to the posterior aspect of the tibia just anterior to the insertion of the PCL. The medial meniscus is continuously attached along its periphery to the joint capsule. At its midpoint, the meniscus is firmly attached to the femur and tibia through a condensation in the joint capsule known as the deep medial ligament. The medial meniscus has no direct attachment to any muscle, but indirect capsule connections to the semimembranosus may provide some retraction of the posterior horn.

The lateral meniscus is almost circular and covers a larger portion of the tibial articular surface than the medial meniscus. The lateral meniscus is consistent in width throughout its course. The anterior horn of the lateral meniscus blends into the attachment of the anterior cruciate ligament, whereas the posterior horn attaches just behind the intercondylar eminence, often blending into the posterior aspect of the ACL (Figure 11.32). There is no attachment of the lateral meniscus to the LCL. Its peripheral attachment is interrupted posterior to where the popliteal tendon passes. The capsular components attach the lateral meniscus to the tibia less firmly than the medial meniscus. The lateral meniscus is more mobile than the medial meniscus, and has a range of movement that may be as great as 10 mm (0.4 in) in an anteroposterior direction. This mobility is explained by the close proximity of the attachments of the anterior and posterior horns and the lack of attachment to the capsular ligament posterolaterally. The firm attachment of the arcuate ligament to the lateral meniscus and the attachment of the popliteus muscle to both the arcuate ligament and meniscus ensure the dynamic retraction of the posterior segment of the meniscus during internal rotation of the tibia on the femur as the knee begins to flex from its fully extended position.

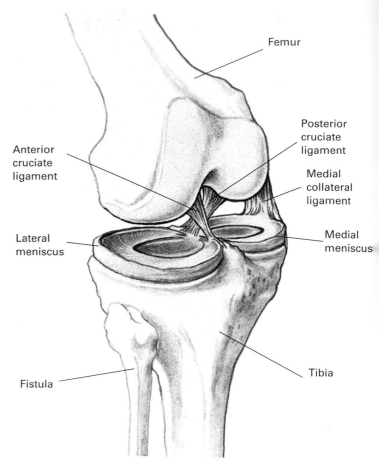

Figure 11.32 Anatomic diagram of the anterior relationship between menisci, cruciate ligaments and MCL.

Structure, circulation, and neuroanatomy

Collagen fibers within the menisci are primarily oriented in a circumf
ential fashion, thus resisting the loads applied to them by the femur.
this manner they are suitably aligned to resist elongation, much as ho
prevent expansion of a barrel.

The vascular supply of the menisci originates predominately from
inferior and superior lateral and medial genicular arteries. In ad
menisci, the degree of peripheral vascular penetration is 10–30% of
width of the medial meniscus and 10–25% of the width of the late
meniscus. With age, there is a decline in meniscus vascularity which m
be associated with weightbearing. Cells within the central and in
regions of the menisci are dependent on diffusion of synovial fluid
their nutrition.

In human menisci, the meniscal horns are significantly more innerva
than the meniscal bodies. The central thirds are totally devoid of inn
vation. The nerve endings in the menisci have sensory function; they m
therefore, provide some proprioceptive function relating to joint positi

Meniscal functions

The meniscus has an important role as a protective load-sharing structure. It transmits 30–70% of the load applied across the joint. The meniscus can resist large compressive loads. Because of its wedge shape, its circumferentially oriented collagen fibers and the firm attachment of the anterior and posterior horns allow the weightbearing meniscus to elongate as the femur presses down on the tibia. The posterior horns carry a greater proportion of the load than the anterior segments, and the distribution of the load depends on the amount of knee flexion. At least 50% of the compressive load at the knee joint is transmitted through the menisci in extension, with 85% being transmitted in 90° of flexion. The ability of the joint to transmit load is significantly reduced by the removal of all or part of the meniscus. Meniscectomy profoundly alters the manner in which loadbearing occurs at the knee joint. Medial meniscectomy reduces the contact area by 50–70%, the greater reduction occurring at greater loads. Removal of part of the meniscus reduces the weight-transmitting function less than removing the entire structure, so long as the circumferential continuity of the meniscus is intact. The joint space narrowing, osteophyte formation, and flattening of the femoral condyles frequently observed following meniscectomy probably result from the loss of this function.

Menisci and subchondral bone assist cartilage in absorbing shock. The meniscus absorbs energy by undergoing elongation when a load is borne by the knee joint. As the joint compresses, the wedge-shaped meniscus extrudes peripherally and its circumferentially oriented collagen fibers elongate. Thus, the meniscus absorbs energy and reduces the shock that the underlying cartilage and subchondral bone would otherwise endure. The menisci absorb the greatest amount of energy at relatively low loading rates, but even at more rapid rates the shock absorption characteristics probably still contribute significantly. The shock absorption capacity of the normal knee is reduced 20% by meniscectomy.

Menisci have a role to play in stress reduction. Stress (load per unit area) across the knee joint was experimentally found to increase approximately 3 times in dogs and 2.5 times in human cadavers after removal of both menisci.

Another important function of the menisci is to increase joint congruity by filling in the space between the tibia and the femur where they are not in contact.

The menisci have an important stabilizing function within the knee joint as they serve to maintain proper positioning of the femur relative to the tibia. The menisci increase stability by deepening the articular surfaces of the tibial plateau and filling the dead space that would otherwise exist at the periphery of the condyle. This also prevents the intrusion of the capsule and synovial membrane between the adjacent articular surfaces. The close relationship of the meniscal attachment to the cruciate ligaments and to the capsular structures also supports the stabilizing role of the menisci. The menisci apparently play an important part in preventing an increase in anterior laxity when cruciate function has been lost. Tears of the medial meniscus frequently develop after an apparently isolated disruption of the ACL. The firm fixation of the medial menis-

cus to the tibial plateau allows it to restrain anterior translation effectively, whereas the less rigidly fixed lateral meniscus is unable to do s
One would, therefore, expect the frequency of delayed tears of the medi
meniscus following ACL injury to exceed those of the lateral meniscu

The role of the meniscus in the dynamic stability of the knee joint
suggested by the close relationship of the quadriceps, popliteus, ar
semimembranosus tendons to the menisci. Contraction of the quadricep
will thus actively pull both menisci forward as the knee extends.

The menisci also limit extremes in flexion and extension. Before fu
extension of the knee is attained, there is an 18° external rotation of th
tibia with respect to the femur. There is a spiral or a helicoid motion
the tibiofemoral joint, which occurs from 30° or 15° of flexion to fu
extension of the knee. This action, the 'screw-home motion', is due
the existence of a larger area of bearing surface on the medial condy
than on the lateral. During the 'screw-home' motion, the menisci a
forced far forward by the impinging femoral condyles. The anterior hor
of the menisci then act as a block to further extension. The greater t
hyperextension, the more tightly the anterior segments of the menisci a
held. In full flexion, the posterior horns are driven far posteriorly a
assist in blocking any further flexion as long as the ligaments and caps
lar structures are intact.

The menisci may contribute to joint lubrication by spreading a film
nutrient synovial fluid over the articular surfaces. The menisci probab
assist in lubrication by reducing the space available within which flu
can pool.

Finally, during weightbearing the menisci serve to compress t
nourishing synovial fluid into the articular cartilage.

Biomechanics of meniscus injury

Meniscus injuries commonly occur in contact sports; often in combin
tion with ligament injuries, particularly when the medial meniscus
involved. This is partly because the medial meniscus is attached to
medial collateral ligament, and partly because tackles are often direc
towards the lateral side of the knee, causing external rotation of the ti
Injury to the medial meniscus is about 5 times more common than inji
to the lateral meniscus. Meniscal injuries are frequently caused by a tw
ing impact to the knee. In cases of external rotation of the foot and lo
leg in relation to the femur, the medial meniscus is most vulnerable, wh
in internal rotation of the foot and lower leg the lateral meniscus is m
easily injured (Figure 11.33). Meniscus injuries can also occur as a re
of hyperextension and hyperflexion of the knee. In elderly individual
meniscus injury can occur during a normal body movement such as d
knee bends, because of decreased strength due to degenerative change

When meniscus injuries have been caused by trauma, the ruptures
vertically through the meniscal tissue; in elderly people, horizontal ruptu
are more common (Figure 11.34). Every suspected or confirmed menis
injury should be subjected to a stability test by a doctor to exclude ligam
deficiency.

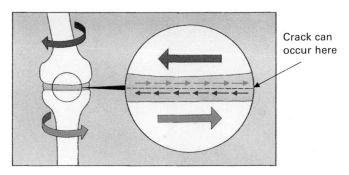

Figure 11.33 The mechanism involved in a horizontal tear within a meniscus.

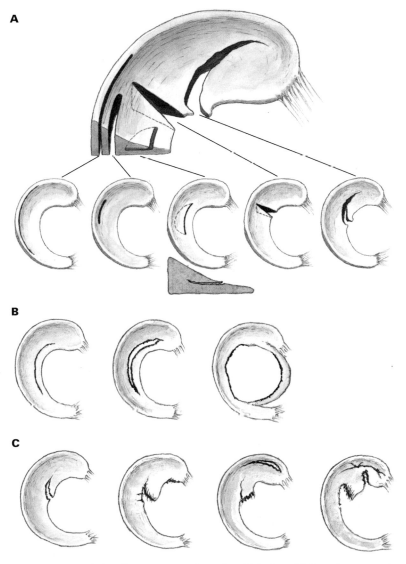

Figure 11.34 (**A**) Different types of meniscal injuries. (**B**) Development of meniscus bucket handle tear. (**C**) Development of meniscus flap tear.

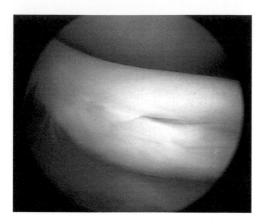

Figure 11.35 Arthroscopic view of 'bucket handle' tear of meniscus.

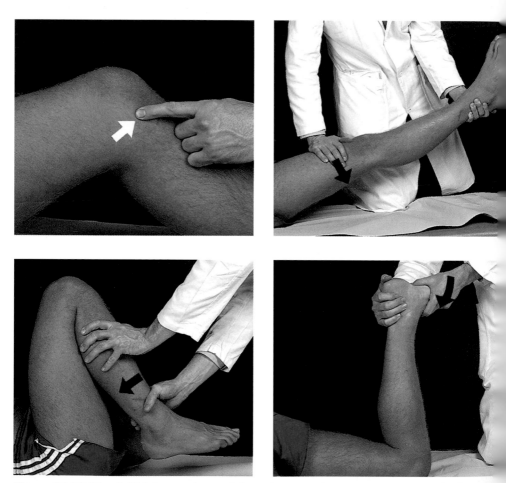

Figure 11.36 (Top left) Injury to the medial meniscus: tenderness can occur over the inner synovial cavity (see arrow). (**Top right**) Injury to the lateral meniscus: pain can occur if the kne joint is over-extended. (**Bottom left**) Injury to the medial or lateral meniscus: pain can occur the knee joint during vigorous flexion of the joint. (**Bottom right**) Injury to the medial menisc pain can occur when foot and lower leg are rotated externally with knee bent at 90°. Injury to external meniscus: pain can occur when foot and lower leg are rotated internally with knee be at 90°.

Medial meniscus injury

- Pain on the medial (inner) side of the knee joint occurs during and after exertion.
- 'Locking' happens when the torn part of the meniscus is lodged in the joint, forming a 'bucket handle' (Figure 11.35), blocking mobility so that full extension or flexion is impossible. The joint can lock momentarily of its own accord in certain positions.
- Pain in the area of the medial joint line occurs during hyperextension and hyperflexion and also on turning the foot and lower leg outward when the knee joint is flexed.
- Sometimes there is an effusion of fluid in the joint, especially after exertion.

The diagnosis of an internal meniscus injury is considered to be fairly certain if three or more of the following findings are present (Figure 11.36):
- tenderness at one point over the medial joint line;
- pain in the area of the medial joint line during hyperextension of the knee joint;
- pain in the area of the medial joint line during hyperflexion of the knee joint;
- pain during external rotation of the foot and the lower leg when the knee is flexed at different angles around 70–90°;
- weakened or hypotrophied quadriceps muscle.

An MRI scan will verify the diagnosis (Figure 11.37). Arthroscopy of the joint is the most certain way of confirming a diagnosis of meniscus injury (Figure 11.38).

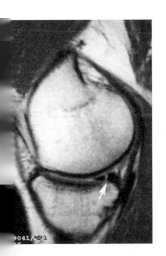
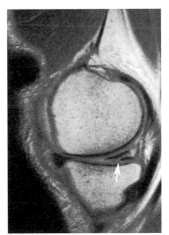
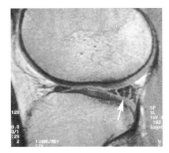

Figure 11.37 MRI of meniscal tears (arrows). (**A**) Vertical tear; (**B**) horizontal tear; (**C**) degenerative tear.

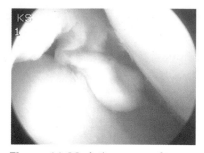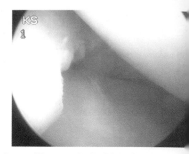

Figure 11.38 Arthroscopy of torn meniscus (flap tear): (**left**) before and (**right**) after treatment.

Lateral meniscus injury

– Pain in the lateral aspect of the joint occurs in connection with exertion of the knee joint. In many cases the pain appears consistently after specific amount of exertion.
– 'Locking' occurs (see above).
– Pain in the area of the lateral joint line occurs on hyperextension and hyperflexion of the knee and also on internal rotation of the foot and the lower leg in relation to the femur when the knee joint is flexed to 70-90.
– Sometimes there is an effusion of fluid in the joint.

The diagnosis of a lateral meniscus injury is considered to be fairly certain if three or more of the following findings are present:
– tenderness at one point over the lateral joint line;
– pain in the area of the lateral joint line during hyperextension of the knee joint;
– pain in the area of the lateral joint line during hyperflexion of the knee joint;
– pain during internal rotation of the foot and the lower leg when the knee is flexed at different angles;
– weakened or hypotrophied quadriceps muscle.

An MRI scan or arthroscopy confirms the diagnosis.

Treatment

The *athlete* should carry out static quadriceps muscle exercises. It important that anyone waiting for knee surgery should exercise the thigh muscles daily. This prevents unnecessary weakening of the muscles, and enables rehabilitation to be shortened considerably.
The *doctor* may:
– operate during arthroscopy by removing or suturing back the damaged part of the meniscus. In cases of acute locking the injury should operated on within a few days. The damaged part of the meniscus held with forceps and is cut loose with small scalpels or scissors inserted into the joint under arthroscopic observation;
– prescribe training of the quadriceps and hamstring muscles (pp. 5 509; protocol on p. 516). The training is started as soon as possible after surgery. Crutches can be used for 1–2 days so that the injured leg relieved of some weight. Weightbearing of the knee joint to the pain threshold is allowed as tolerated.

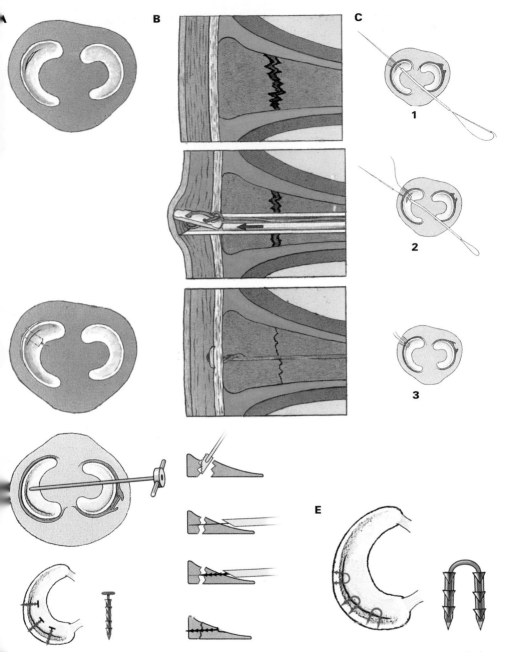

Figure 11.39 (**A**) Untreated meniscal tear. (**B**) T-fix technique. (**C1–3**) Cross-sectional surgical repair ('inside out') of torn meniscus. (**D**) Repair with resorbable meniscal arrow. (**E**) Repair with resorbable meniscal staple.

It is well established that retention of as much of a stable, well-balanced meniscus as possible is important to protect the articular carti-lage from further stress and degeneration. The amount of degenerative change in the joint is directly proportional to the amount of meniscus removed. The tibiofemoral contact stresses increase in proportion to the amount of meniscus excised and the extent to which the meniscal structure is disrupted. Even damaged menisci can transmit loads as long as a portion of the circumferential continuity remains intact. Following partial meniscectomy, a significant load is borne by an intact peripheral rim. There is no abnormally high pressure at the cut edge of the remaining meniscus. Leaving a peripheral rim of the meniscus intact in an uncomplicated bucket-handle tear gave good results.

There is a renewed interest in surgical repair of the torn meniscus and clinically good results have been reported (Figure 11.39). It is better to create a stable degenerative meniscus out of an unstable degenerative meniscus than to perform a partial meniscectomy. Nonoperative treatment of meniscal tears is possible in stable, vertical, longitudinal, rather small tears which tend to occur in the peripheral vascular portions of the menisci.

Healing and complications

An athlete who has been operated on for a meniscus injury should not return to ordinary training until almost full mobility and strength of the knee joint have been regained. This usually takes 2–6 weeks after transarthroscopic surgery, depending on the size and location of the tear. When there is a large posterior horn tear, return to sport can take longer, up to 12-16 weeks. Return to sport after a repair usually takes 4 months because of the healing process (rehabilitation protocol on p. 517).

Even after return to sporting activity the athlete should continue training the quadriceps and hamstrings muscles.

The menisci should be preserved whenever possible. Only when their ability to function is destroyed and they produce localized pain, locking, and recurrent effusion should all or part of their substance be removed. Partial meniscectomy and retention of a well-balanced intact peripheral rim is sound biomechanically and results in a better long-term result than total meniscectomy. Partial arthroscopic meniscectomy not only has the biomechanical advantage of reducing the increase of stress, but also has a lower operative morbidity and fewer effects on postoperative stability, and results in fewer degenerative changes in the articular cartilage. Meniscus repair should save as much meniscal tissue as possible. Meniscal transplantation from deceased donors (allograft) is emerging as a possibility but is still experimental.

Discoid meniscus

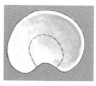

Figure 11.40
Discoid meniscus.

A discoid meniscus is a thickened, enlarged abnormal meniscus covering most of the surface of the tibial condyle; it may be complete, covering the entire articular surface of the tibial condyle, or incomplete, partially covering the surface, and may vary in thickness (Figure 11.40). The entire posterior portion of the meniscus may be hypermobile. Discoid menisci usually occur on the lateral meniscus. Their incidence varies, but is reported to be 1.4–16.6%.

The diagnosis of discoid meniscus can sometimes be made from the history. The athlete may describe a large snap during flexion or extension of the knee, which can be heard on examination. There may be a 'catching' or 'giving way' feeling. This history may be present in children as well as adolescents. The diagnosis is verified by arthroscopy or MRI.

Treatment

The treatment varies. An intact discoid meniscus that is an incidental finding needs no specific treatment. It is not known how many cases of untreated discoid meniscus will eventually develop tears. Treatment must be individual. If there is a tear in the discoid meniscus that produces pain or snapping in the knee, or if there is a hypermobile medial segment, the best treatment is subtotal arthroscopic meniscectomy (removal of part of the meniscus). If the discoid meniscus is unstable, repair or removal of the meniscus may be needed. Return to sports is usually the same as after conventional meniscus surgery.

Bibliography

DeHaven KE (1981) Peripheral meniscus repair. An alternative to meniscectomy. *Orthopedic Transactions* 5: 399–400.

Henning CE, Lynch MA (1985) Current concepts of meniscal function and pathology. *Clinical Sports Medicine* 4: 360–365.

Johnson RJ, Kettlekamp DB, Clark W et al. (1974) Factors affecting late results after meniscectomy. *Journal of Bone and Joint Surgery* 56A: 719–729.

Articular cartilage injuries

Injuries to the articular cartilage (chondral) surfaces can affect the joint surfaces of the femur, the tibia, and the patella. Such injuries are often disregarded as they can be difficult to identify (see p. 17). They may result from direct impact against the knee joint, but can also occur in association with meniscal and ligament injuries. Indeed, any condition that leads to excessive repetitive forces can cause cartilage damage, in the form of small or large cracks and defects on the joint surfaces and continued degeneration. The result can be premature osteoarthritis.

**Symptoms
and diagnosis**

- Swelling occurs in the knee joint with recurrent effusions.
- Pain is felt during and after weightbearing activities.
- 'Locking' or 'catching' mimics meniscal injury.
- Crepitations are heard on weightbearing activities.
- Loose bodies may be felt.
- The injury can be diagnosed by arthroscopy (Figure 11.41) and sometimes by MRI.

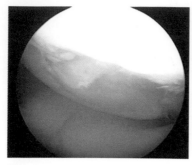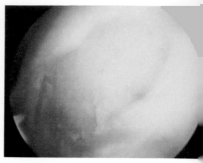

Figure 11.41 Arthroscopy of articular cartilage injury (**left**) on medial femoral condyle and (**right**) on patella.

Treatment

The *athlete* should:
- avoid symptomatic activity;
- train the thigh musculature;
- use a knee support or a heat retainer;

The *doctor* may:
- recommend a change to a sport that makes fewer demands on the knee joints;
- surgically remove the damaged cartilage, which is gradually replaced by less elastic fibrocartilage; where there is disabling knee pain or swelling from isolated articular cartilage injuries, the doctor may operate using one of the newer techniques described below.

Alternative surgical treatments

Several new techniques have been developed to treat small, isolated articular cartilage defects. Although they are still under evaluation, early results are promising.

With abrasion, picking, or drilling of the defect, the defect is abraded to encourage cells to infiltrate the area from the underlying bone, forming new cartilage to fill the defect. No long-term results or comparative studies are available.

Tissue engineering methods are described on pp. 21, 22. None of the methods has consistently been shown to form new normal cartilage, and isolated articular cartilage defects continue to be a difficult problem in orthopedics.

Osteochondritis dissecans

Osteochondritis dissecans, the detachment of fragments of bone and cartilage into the knee joint, often afflicts young people aged 12–16 years permanently affecting the articular surface of the femur. The location of the injury is often obvious (Figure 11.42). The condition causes the

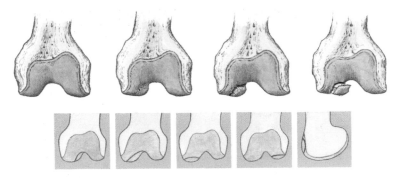

Figure 11.42 Common locations affected by osteochondritis dissecans.

Figure 11.43
(A) MRI of osteochondritis dissecans on the femoral condyle: lateral view. (B) X-ray showing lateral femoral condyle osteochonditis dissecans.

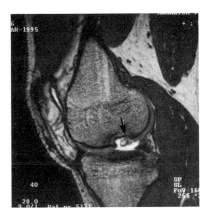

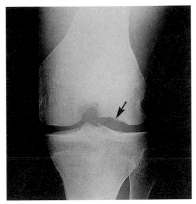

cartilage and bone to disintegrate in an area which may be as large as a hazelnut (Figure 11.42). Gradually the whole of the altered area or parts of it can break away from the underlying bone and give rise to loose bodies in the joint. The result is locking and recurrent effusions.

Symptoms and diagnosis

See page 24.

Treatment

See page 24.

Healing

The affected athlete may return to sporting activity after the ligament has healed, which may take 3–6 months after the operation, but only after having consulted a doctor. Before returning, the athlete should have built up muscular strength and mobility by training.

Plica syndrome

Synovial plica syndrome is not very common, but may occasionally cause pain in the knee. A plica is a normal synovial septum (thickened knee capsular fold) which sometimes can become inflamed and thereby cause

pain. Plicae are present in the knee in 20–60% of the population. Th
plica traversing the area proximal to the patella is the suprapatellar plica
The area distal to the patella is filled with the infrapatellar plica, whic
connects the fat pad to the superior part of the notch. The most involve
plica is the medial patellar plica, which runs from the medial side of th
suprapatellar area to the anterior fat pad. There is also occasionally
lateral patellar plica.

Symptoms and diagnosis
- Pain is felt with activities such as running, skiing, and cycling.
- Sometimes the athlete may complain of clicking and catching, whic
  can imitate locking of the knee. This is often experienced durin
  flexion and when the inflamed plica runs over the epicondyle.
- The plica can sometimes be palpated as a thick band on the edge
  the articular surface.

Treatment
- Conservative treatment is rest, avoiding pain-causing situations an
  gradually increasing activities. Painful activities should be avoided.
- Anti-inflammatory medication may be prescribed.
- Arthroscopy may confirm the diagnosis (Figure 11.44). Resection
  the plica is effective in 70–90% of the athletes.
- Return to sports is possible within 2 weeks.

Knee extension mechanism injuries

The knee extension mechanism includes the quadriceps muscle–tendo
the patellar bone, the patellar tendon, and its insertion into the tibi
Injuries can occur in all these structures.

Quadriceps tendon injuries

The distal quadriceps tendon attaches to the patella and its adjacent s
tissue structures (the retinaculum). It is important for the extensor mech
nism. This tendon is extremely strong and only ruptures in rare situ
tions, mostly in older athletes, such as golf players falling on slippery gra
slopes, or weightlifters lifting excessive loads. It can also be an overu
injury in weightlifters doing repeated knee bending work (Figure 11.4

Rupture

The typical history of a rupture of the quadriceps tendon includes
sudden pop when increased stress is applied to the extensor mechanis
When there is a complete rupture, the disability will be immediate a
the athlete cannot support the body weight on the injured side. There
often a gross displacement of the patella distally. These injuries are oft
complete, and therefore pain is not prominent.

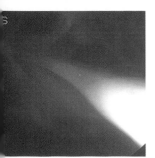

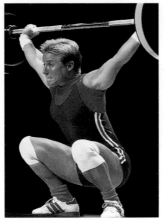

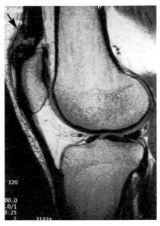

gure 11.44 Synovial plica
the knee, as seen with the
throscope.

Figure 11.45 Repeated knee
bending can cause problems
for weightlifters (by courtesy
of All Sport: photographer,
Jim De Frisco).

Figure 11.46 MRI of almost
complete quadriceps tendon
tear (arrow).

mptoms **d diagnosis**	– Tenderness and swelling occur where the muscle merges into the tendon above the patella or where the tendon inserts into the patella. – A gap can be felt where the rupture has occurred. – The injured person cannot actively extend the knee. – MRI will confirm the diagnosis (Figure 11.46).
eatment	The *doctor* may: – treat with bandaging and gradually increasing strength and mobility training; – refrain from operating in cases of a partial rupture as the injury usually does not lead to any noticeably impaired function in the long run; – X-ray the joint to show the pathological position of the patella; – operate in cases of major ruptures in athletes or active persons when the tendon is avulsed from the patella; – operate on old injuries of this type.

Early mobilization is important, but return to sports is not possible before
4–6 months.

Overuse injuries

Chronic overuse injuries to the distal quadriceps tendon area are not very
common; they are most likely to occur in weightlifters. Problems can also be
seen in basketball or team handball players who jump frequently. They
complain of pain when they push off for the jump, or on rising from squatting or kneeling positions (Figure 11.47). There is localized tenderness over
the proximal area of the patella where the quadriceps tendon inserts.
Sometimes there is discomfort when contracting the quadriceps, especially
against resistance or when the extended knee is lifted against resistance. The

309

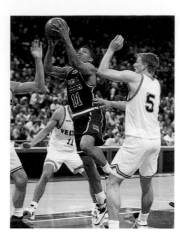

Figure 11.47 Chronic overuse injuries of the distal quadriceps tendon may present in basketball players (by courtesy of All Sport: photographer, Doug Pensinger.)

treatment of these overuse injuries are according to the principles on p. 4
The prognosis is often reasonably good and gradual return to sports m;
follow a rehabilitation period including stretching and strengthening exercise

Patellofemoral pain syndrome

Patellofemoral disorders are a common problem in all age groups. T
cause of this pain is complex and not well known. It is therefore impo
tant to make a precise diagnosis, otherwise the treatment will not
successful.

Functional anatomy

Normally the patella has a wedge shape, with a medial and a lateral fa
and a central crest. The patella has the thickest cartilage of any joi
The patella slides on extension and flexion in the intercondylar sul
(on the central distal part of the femur, called the trochlea), which crea
the geometric stability of the joint.

Etiology

Damage to the articular surface of the patella usually occurs in indiv
uals aged 10–25 years, and is associated with pain, especially on walk;
up and down hills and stairs and when squatting.

It is common for pain to occur in the knee when walking up and do
hills. Compared with the normal flexion of the joint on flat ground, k;
flexion increases considerably during these activities, increasing comp
sion between the patella and the femur. Walking *uphill* causes less pain t

walking *downhill*, because during ascent the knee joint is flexed at an angle of about 50° under load, while on descent it is flexed at an angle of about 80° under load. The body does not lean forward when walking downhill, so knee flexion is controlled by the quadriceps muscles alone, increasing the compression forces between the patella and the femur.

The cause of anterior knee pain may not always be found (*idiopathic pain*). Possible causes are trauma, malalignment or instability.

Idiopathic anterior knee pain

Anterior knee pain is often present in growing individuals and often there is no cause to be found (idiopathic). Before the pain is labeled as idiopathic, other pathological causes must be excluded, such as bursitis, fat pad syndrome, plica syndrome, and meniscus problems. The reason for the pain is unknown. The articular cartilage itself lacks a nerve supply and is not painful. Lesions of the articular cartilage can, however, irritate the synovia lining the joint. This is usually the primary source of pain in the patellofemoral joint. The synovium can be stretched. The load transfer to subchondral bone can be altered because of biomechanical failure of the articular cartilage. This bone can thicken and thereby contribute to pain. The extensor mechanism can also be responsible for the pain.

Trauma

Many athletes with patellar knee pain have a history of direct trauma to the patella joint. This can damage the subchondral bone, as well as the articular cartilage, and cause pain. The patella can dislocate (completely out of joint) and subluxate (partially out of joint) laterally. This injury is combined with tearing of the medial retinaculum and the vastus medialis muscle. Osteochondral (bone and cartilage) fractures of the lateral femoral condyle or of the patella can also occur. Predisposing factors include high-riding patella (patella alta), hypermobile patella, generalized ligament laxity, increased Q angle (see below) and changes in the relationship between the femur and tibia, hypotrophy of the muscles, valgus deformity of the knee, and abnormal shape of the patella and the patella groove. Dislocation may recur in 15–45% because of these predisposing factors.

Malalignment/instability of the extensor mechanism

Instability is believed to be a frequent cause of patellofemoral pain. Patellofemoral disorders are very common in the general population, and symptoms related to the extensor mechanism of the knee are the most common complaint in sports-related injuries. About 30% of all overuse injuries are related to the knee and 35% involve the extensor mechanism. In activities, involving strenuous use of the legs, such as running, jumping, gymnastics, or ballet dancing, the incidence can be as high as 75%.

Patella instability and malalignment are important background factors for patellofemoral disorders. The *passive stability* of the patellofemoral joint

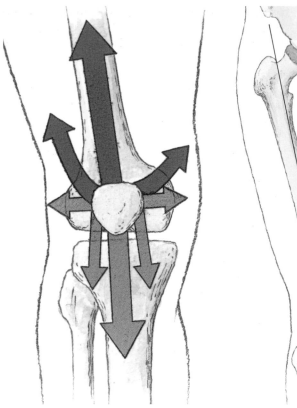

Figure 11.48 Forces acting on the patella: red, active stabilizers; green, passive stabilizers.

Figure 11.49 The quadriceps angle (Q angle).

is dependent on the geometry of the articular surfaces of the trochlea and the patella. The anatomy of the intercondylar sulcus, especially in the proximal part of the articular surface of the trochlea, is important for the stability of the patella, when the joint is close to extension. Other passive structures stabilizing the patellofemoral joint are the lateral and medial transverse and longitudinal retinacula, active during flexion and extension both in weightbearing and non-weightbearing movements (Figure 11.48).

The lateral and medial transverse retinacula run from the medial and lateral epicondyle of the femur and insert on the medial and lateral aspect of the proximal patella. The medial and lateral longitudinal retinacula are tendinous connections between the vastus medialis obliquus and the vastus lateralis muscles and insert on the medial and lateral aspect of the proximal tibia. The longitudinal retinacula act both as passive and active stabilizers over the vastus medialis obliquus and the vastus lateralis muscles.

The patellar ligament has also both passive and active functions. It acts as a ligament in stabilizing the patella for proximal traction, and acts as a tendon via the patella to the quadriceps muscle.

The *active stability* of the patella is controlled by the quadriceps muscles: the vastus medialis obliquus exerts medial traction, the vastus lateralis lateral traction, and the rectus femoris and the vastus intermedius medius axial traction on the patella.

The quadriceps angle (Q angle) is the angle formed between the lines through the longitudinal axis of the rectus femoris muscle and through the patellar ligament (Figure 11.49). These lines meet in the center of the patella. An increased Q angle will during quadriceps contraction cause lateral tracking of the patella.

Even minor abnormalities in the passive and active stability of the patella may give rise to patellofemoral symptoms and patellar instability.

Patella instability due to patellofemoral dysplasia (underdevelopment of the patellofemoral joint) seems to be an important contributing factor for patellofemoral pain. Patellofemoral dysplasia may be a genetic or developmental abnormality.

For normal development of this joint, the trochlea needs the stimulation of the patella to create an intercondylar sulcus and a congruent joint. Without such stimulation, the trochlea may develop only a shallow sulcus, or it could be flat or even convex, especially in the proximal part of the femoral trochlea. The patella then often has a flat surface, or loses its wedge shape with a dominating lateral facet.

Dysplasia (developmental abnormality) of the patellofemoral joint and the femoral trochlea, may be associated with patella alta, an increased Q angle, or genu valgum (lower leg directed outwards). Tibial and femoral torsion (rotation) has also been implicated. The lack of geometric stability along with an increased Q angle will create patellar instability and could be increased by muscular imbalance especially due to weakness of the vastus medialis obliquus.

Grading of patellar instability

Grade I/*Patellar lateral tracking*: owing to an increased Q angle, the patella will move laterally before moving proximally on quadriceps contraction, which will give a lateral patellar compression syndrome with a small area of contact with increased rest on the articular surfaces of the patella and the trochlea (Figure 11.50). The patella will not dislocate but will track laterally on quadriceps contraction on an extended knee. There is a negative apprehension test (p. 316).

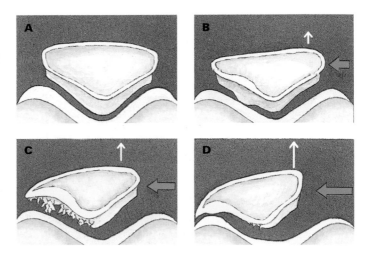

Figure 11.50 Patellar tracking. (**A**) Normal. (**B**) Lateral tracking causing some damage on the lateral angle. (**C**) Subluxation and some lateral tilt, causing further damage. (**D**) Subluxation and severe lateral tilt.

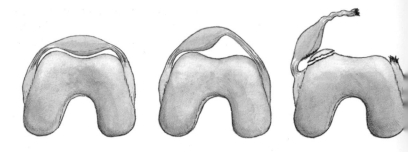

Figure 11.51 Patellar dislocation causing osteochondral (bone–cartilage) o chondral (cartilage only) injury. Simultaneous or alternative injury can occu on the patellar cartilage surface.

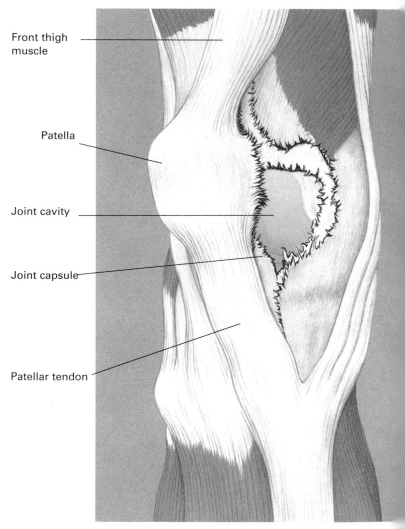

Front thigh
muscle

Patella

Joint cavity

Joint capsule

Patellar tendon

Figure 11.52 Lateral dislocation of the patella. Note the extensive injury soft tissues with rupture in and around the knee capsule.

Grade II/*Patellar subluxation*: subluxation of the patella could either be a straight lateral subluxation or a tilt of the patella. Both conditions could be defined as subluxations with only a part of the articular surfaces in contact. The diagnosis is confirmed by CT scan.

- (A) *Patellar lateral tilt* is observed in chronic knee pain. Shortening and thickening of the lateral retinaculum and capsule occur, and as a result, the lateral facet is forced into the femoral trochlea during knee flexion, causing a lateral compression and a tilt. Over time, however, the patellar lateral tilt will cause cartilage damage. The diagnosis is confirmed by X-rays or CT scans.
- (B) *Patellar lateral subluxation* includes a straight subluxation of the patella elicited by quadriceps contraction on an extended knee. Recurrent subluxation of the patella will with time cause articular cartilage damage to both the patella and the trochlea. Sometimes there is a combination of patellar lateral subluxation and patellar tilt, which will increase the instability. The diagnosis is confirmed by CT scan during quadriceps relaxation and contraction.

Grade III/*Patellar dislocation*: this is a severe condition with frequent recurrence (Figures 11.51 and 11.52). 'Giving way' symptoms due to instability and progressive articular cartilage damage will occur over time. It is a severe dysfunction of the joint and should be corrected early. On quadriceps contraction there could be a subluxation or even dislocation on testing and there is a positive apprehension test. Patellar dislocation in a normal knee can be traumatic (p. 314), caused by a fall on or an acute blow to the patella with a lateral dislocation and articular cartilage damage. It can also occur in an athlete with patellofemoral dysplasia and an increased Q angle. In such cases surgical repair of the medial retinaculum is an opportunity to correct the other defects.

Symptoms and diagnosis

- Widespread anterior pain occurs in the knee joint and behind the patella during exertion or load such as sitting with a bent knee.
- The pain problems are accentuated in walking and running, and on hills and stairs, especially during descent.
- Pain and stiffness can be felt when rising from a sitting to a standing position, typically after watching a film or movie (the 'movie sign').
- Pain problems are often made worse by squatting.
- Pain occurs with isometric contractions of the quadriceps under resistance at $0°$ and $20°$.
- Local tenderness may be present on the medial or lateral patellar facets around the patella and on compression of the patella.
- Crepitation or creaking during flexion and extension of the knee may be experienced behind the patella, indicating chondromalacia (p. 318).
- Sometimes a slight swelling in the knee joint is noticeable.
- The Q angle should be measured: at $30°$ of flexion, the angle is normally less than $10°$ in men and less than $15°$ in women, and at $90°$ of flexion it is less than $8°$.
- Malalignment of the lower limb including increased pronation of the foot, malrotation of the tibia or the femur (femoral anteversion), genu valgum (increased angle between the tibia and femur), and tight lateral retinaculum may be significant factors, which also increase the Q angle and may cause recurrent dislocation of the patella (Figure 11.53).

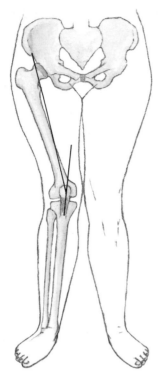

Figure 11.53 Malalignment of the lower limb.

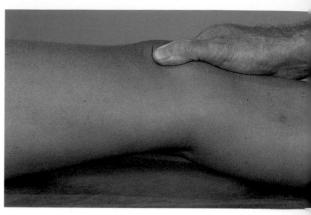

Figure 11.54 Apprehension test showing lateral patella provocation.

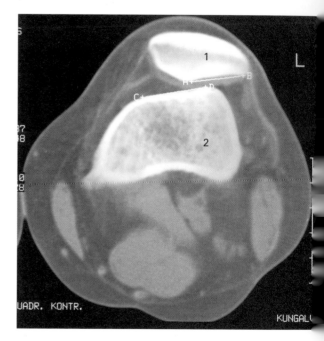

Figure 11.55 CT of patellofemoral joint during quadriceps contraction, showing cross-sections of the patella (1, subluxed laterally) and the distal femur (2, note the flat surface).

- Active and passive tracking of the patella should be evaluated.
- The *apprehension test* is positive. This test is performed with the kn in 0° of flexion. The examiner fixes the patella laterally with the har When the athlete bends the knee, the patella tries to sublux a thereby causes pain (Figure 11.54).
- The *passive patella tilt test* evaluates the tension of the lateral retin ulum structures.
- Plain X-rays of the knee should be taken. The patella in relation the joint line can be evaluated by lateral plain views. The Merch infrapatellar view can be valuable, i.e. X-rays of the patella with knee flexed at 40°.
- A CT scan is effective in evaluating different malalignment patte as well as assessing bone lesions and patellofemoral relationsh

(Figure 11.55). The CT scan is also valuable for diagnosis of recurrent patellar subluxation in adolescents. An MRI scan is less valuable, as it is difficult to perform if the knee is flexed more than 30°; however, it is useful for evaluating the articular cartilage surface.
- A bone scan can be used in cases with prolonged symptoms and anterior knee pain. The diagnosis is confirmed by increased uptake of nuclide (radioactive agent) by both patella and femur, and indicates a poor prognosis.
- Arthroscopy can evaluate the extent of the patella articular damage and confirm the clinical and radiographic alignment and establish whether synovitis is present (Figure 11.56).

The *athlete* should:
- rest from painful activities;
- in the acute phase, apply ice;
- use a brace with a notch and support for the patella; sometimes taping can be helpful;
- exercise the quadriceps and hamstring muscles, especially the vastus medialis, by a specific exercise protocol (p. 515). Stretching is important. The effect of this type of training may, however, take time.

The *doctor* may:
- explain the cause of the pain and involve parents if necessary. This should be done at the first visit to the clinic;
- carry out the tests necessary to secure a correct diagnosis;
- prescribe active rest, avoidance of pain-causing situations, and physical therapy. The athlete often needs to be educated by a knowledgeable physical therapist and by the physician. The athlete must really understand the nature of the injury in order to accept it, and must realize that with a conservative exercise program, 80% of athletes with idiopathic patellofemoral pain usually improve over a period of 6 months. It should be stressed that this injury will take time to heal;
- prescribe anti-inflammatory medication in the acute stage. Even if there are no major objective symptoms the goal of the treatment is to regain homeostasis (metabolic equilibrium). This is the key to success;
- sometimes perform arthroscopy to confirm the diagnosis and assess the articular cartilage of the patella;
- operate in cases of prolonged symptoms. There are more than a hundred surgical procedures for the treatment of patellofemoral disorders, addressing the different malalignments. Surgery can also include treatment of the articular cartilage lesions (p. 17). Below are specific treatment possibilities.

Treatment of patellar lateral tracking
The athlete should rest from painful activities and protect the knee; a brace with lateral support or taping is used for stabilizing the patella. Eccentric strength training, specifically of the vastus medialis obliquus muscles, is important.

The *doctor* may:
- prescribe avoidance of painful activities, and physiotherapy focusing on exercises of vastus medialis obliquus;

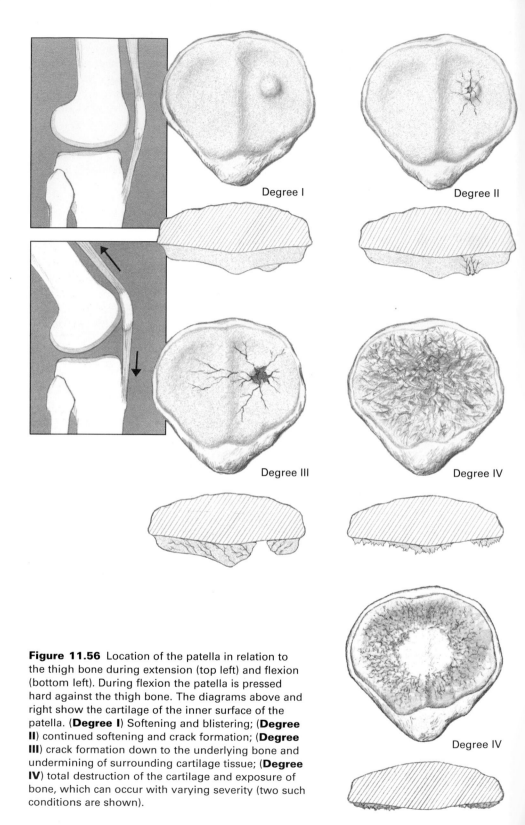

Figure 11.56 Location of the patella in relation to the thigh bone during extension (top left) and flexion (bottom left). During flexion the patella is pressed hard against the thigh bone. The diagrams above and right show the cartilage of the inner surface of the patella. (**Degree I**) Softening and blistering; (**Degree II**) continued softening and crack formation; (**Degree III**) crack formation down to the underlying bone and undermining of surrounding cartilage tissue; (**Degree IV**) total destruction of the cartilage and exposure of bone, which can occur with varying severity (two such conditions are shown).

Degree I

Degree II

Degree III

Degree IV

Degree IV

- prescribe anti-inflammatory medication;
- carry out arthroscopy and surgically release tight lateral structures. When articular damage exists with flaps, or softening with mechanical locking or catching, gentle debridement of the damaged area may be helpful. If other background factors are present, such as increased Q angle and patellofemoral dysplasia, further realignment procedures may be necessary.

Patellofemoral symptoms caused by patellar lateral tracking where no articular cartilage damage is present may have a good prognosis with conservative treatment.

Treatment of patellar lateral tilt

If there is no articular cartilage damage, the prognosis could be good with conservative treatment such as stabilizing braces and vastus medialis obliquus strengthening, but in the long term surgery may be needed. In chronic cases there may be a tight, thickened retinaculum and capsule. If a tight lateral retinaculum only is present, the treatment could be lateral release, followed by strengthening of the vastus medialis obliquus. If other contributory factors are present, further realignment procedures may be necessary.

Treatment of patellar lateral subluxation

Patients should be treated early, initially by using conservative methods such as with stabilizing braces, taping, vastus medialis obliquus strengthening exercises, and a change of activities. If conservative treatment fails, stabilizing procedures of the patella should be performed, with correction of all contributory factors.

Treatment of patellar dislocation

The diagnosis is confirmed with CT scan with or without quadriceps contraction. Exercises and braces should be tried. Surgical treatment should be performed if conservative treatment fails, especially if there is a loose bone fragment. The prognosis may be good if there is no articular cartilage damage in the patellofemoral joint. For treatment of articular cartilage surface injury, see p. 17.

ealing and :turn to ports

Problems caused by patellofemoral disorders can disappear spontaneously, especially in young athletes. Athletes must therefore be prepared to change their training habits to avoid running up and down hills and to avoid activities that trigger the pain. Surgery should be avoided or postponed if possible.

Patellofemoral pain syndrome is one of the most difficult syndromes to manage in sports, because of the long period of rehabilitation and the need for great patience on the part of the athlete. Education of the athlete about this injury is of the utmost importance.

Bibliography

Fulkerson JP, Hungerford DS (1990) *Disorders of the Patellofemoral Joint* 3rd edn. Baltimore: Williams & Wilkins.

Papagelopoulos PJ, Sim FH (1997) Patellofemoral pain syndrome diagnosis and management. *Review of Orthopaedics* 20(2): 148–157.

Fractures of the patella

The patella can be cracked by transverse or longitudinal fractures or shattered by stellate fractures. The injury often occurs as a result of fall on the knee. When the fragments are displaced, surgery is required followed by use of a brace for about 4 weeks. When there is no displacement a plaster cast will usually suffice. A longitudinal patellar fracture often requires no more than bandaging if there is no displacement. The patient should subsequently be instructed in isometric thigh muscle training. Healing time is usually 6–8 weeks, depending on the fracture type.

Patellar tendon rupture

The patellar tendon is very strong (almost the strongest soft tissue in the whole body); it originates from the patella and inserts in the tibial tuberosity (the prominence on the anterior proximal part of the tibia). This tendon is essential for the knee extensor mechanism, i.e. it is impossible to extend the knee unless this tendon is intact.

Ruptures of the tendon can be complete or partial. A complete patellar tendon rupture is not very common as the tendon is so strong. Biomechanical studies have shown that a patellar tendon rupture may occur during weightlifting when the patellar tendon tension at the time of failure was equal to approximately 17.5 times the lifter's body weight. A risk factor for patellar tendon rupture is previous steroid injections.

Symptoms and diagnosis

At the time of injury the athlete experiences a sudden 'pop' with intense pain, typically when pushing-off or landing after a jump. The disability will be immediate and the athlete cannot support weight on the injured side. The patella will be proximally displaced and there will be a palpable cleft over the rupture site. There will be tenderness over that area and some swelling, but usually little pain. An X-ray will show a patella bone that is proximally retracted.

Treatment

A complete patellar tendon rupture, which may be proximal or distal, is treated surgically. Usually it is enough to suture the tendon back to bone but occasionally it has to be reinforced by addition of tissue such as, e.g. the hamstring tendon. Rehabilitation is slow, with a gradual increase in range of motion and thereafter strengthening. Return to sports may be possible after 6–8 months. Cycling and sports such as golf may be possible before that.

Jumper's knee (patellar tendon overuse injury, patellar tendinosis)

Patellar tendon overuse injuries are common because the patellar tendon is essential in almost all sporting activities. Injuries may be associated with the high demands on the extensor mechanism, and also with the load on the patellar tendon in explosive jumping and running, which may result in partial tears or chronic overload of the tendon. Injury becomes more likely if there are degenerative changes in the tendon (p. 43).

The mechanism behind this injury is debated. There may be an impingement between the distal pole of the patella and the tendon itself during flexion as an additional cause of this injury. Most injuries, especially partial tears, are located in the proximal posterior aspect of the tendon, indicating that the impingement may well be the main reason for these injuries (Figure 11.57).

Symptoms and diagnosis

- Pain at the inferior pole of the patella is common, especially during activity, typically jumping in volleyball, basketball, and team handball.
- There is tenderness at the inferior pole of the patella at the attachment of the patellar tendon. This tenderness is often very focal and distinct, indicating a partial tear or tendinosis. The tenderness can be more pronounced when palpating by pressing on the proximal pole of the patella with the knee fully extended.
- Thickening of the proximal patellar tendon may be present.
- Hypotrophy of the muscles is often associated with this injury, as well as tightness of the quadriceps.

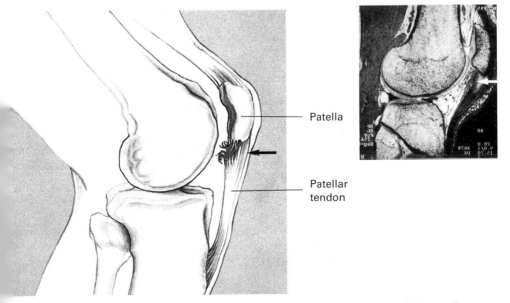

Patella

Patellar tendon

Figure 11.57 'Jumper's knee' – a partial rupture of the top posterior portion of the patellar tendon (arrow). (**Inset**) MRI of partial patellar tendon tendinosis (arrow).

- An MRI or ultrasound scan will verify the injury: MRI in particular can show the area of degeneration (tendinosis) or the indications of chronic partial tear (see Figure 11.57).

Treatment

The *athlete* can:
- avoid painful situations;
- exercise the extensor mechanism muscles by strengthening and stretching;
- be encouraged to cycle.

The *doctor* can:
- prescribe anti-inflammatory medication (which has limited effects);
- correct malalignments;
- send a patient to physical therapy, as these injuries often need expert help. Patient education is very important;
- recommend strength training including eccentric action, which gradually increased according to the principles on p. 510; rehabilitation activities are presented on p. 510;
- prescribe therapeutic modalities such as phonophoresis (p. 99) and iontophoresis (p. 100) or ultrasound alone;
- prescribe an infrapatellar strap that encircles the area of the patellar tendon and compresses it. This may alter the mechanical stress within the tendon in a similar way to the straps used in tennis elbow (p. 166). 77% of patients using such a strap experienced enough relief from pain to resume 'normal' activity. These results are, however, controversial. The treatment should be individualized, as these straps have a variable effect. The same can be said of patellofemoral taping techniques.

Steroid injections should be avoided. Injection into a patellar tendon will increase the risk for patellar tendon rupture.

If conservative therapy is not enough, surgical treatment with removal of the pathological area is indicated. Sometimes the tip of the distal pole of the patella should be partially removed with the aid of an arthroscope. The rehabilitation will take time and will require patience from the athlete. Return to activity depends on the sport, but it is usually possible to resume strenuous sports within 4–8 months, depending on the character of the injury.

A well prescribed exercise program stimulates healing of tendinosis.

Traction tendinitis

Sinding–Larsen–Johansson disease

Sinding–Larsen–Johansson disease is a traction tendinitis of the distal pole of the patella, caused by microtrauma. It is seen in growing individuals; who have pain at the inferior pole of the patella in association with running and jumping. Typical clinical signs are point tenderness at the inferior pole of the patella, swelling, limitation of motion, and a protective limp. Radiography may show fragmentation or ossification of the distal pole of the patella where the tendon inserts.

The treatment consists of alleviation of symptoms, as the syndrome is self-limiting. Resolution may occur within 12 months. During this time there should be restriction of activities. Strength training and stretching are components of rehabilitation. Education of the athlete is important. When the athlete is fully grown, there are usually no residual problems.

It should be remembered that the differential diagnosis could be stress fracture of the patella.

Osgood–Schlatter disease

Traction tendinitis of the distal patellar tendon, known as Osgood–Schlatter disease, is common in adolescent athletes and is seen in 13% of cases of knee pain in a typical sports medicine center (Figure 11.58). These adolescents have often undergone rapid growth and are involved in sports requiring tensile quadriceps contraction, such as jumping and running.

In Osgood–Schlatter disease the tibial attachment of the patellar tendon becomes a seat of inflammation and degradation of bone (traction apophysitis of the tibial tuberosity). The pole of the patellar tendon causes detachment of small cartilage fragments from the tibial tuberosity. The cause of this injury is unclear; possibly it is traction microtrauma. Very active boys between 10–16 are primarily affected, and the symptoms disappear when the athlete is fully grown.

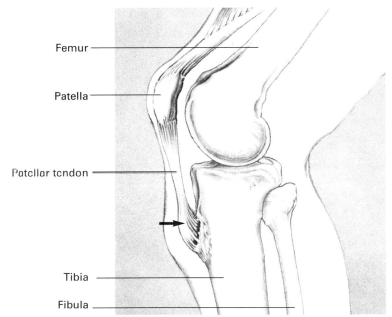

Femur

Patella

Patellar tendon

Tibia

Fibula

Figure 11.58 Osgood–Schlatter's disease: the bone is inflamed and broken up at the attachment of the patellar tendon to the fibula (arrow).

Symptoms and diagnosis	– Pain is felt at the attachment of the tendon to the tibia during and after physical activity.

<table>
<tr><td>Symptoms
and diagnosis</td><td>

– Pain is felt at the attachment of the tendon to the tibia during and after physical activity.
– Pain can be triggered by contraction of the quadriceps against resistance.
– Localized tenderness and soft tissue swelling of the attachment of the patellar tendon to the tibia.
– The skin may be hot and red, with a prominence at the affected area.
– Tightness of the muscles is often present.
– An X-ray examination may show fragmentation of the bone; soft tissue swelling and thickening of the distal portion of the patellar tendon may also be seen.

</td></tr>
</table>

Symptoms and diagnosis

– Pain is felt at the attachment of the tendon to the tibia during and after physical activity.
– Pain can be triggered by contraction of the quadriceps against resistance.
– Localized tenderness and soft tissue swelling of the attachment of the patellar tendon to the tibia.
– The skin may be hot and red, with a prominence at the affected area.
– Tightness of the muscles is often present.
– An X-ray examination may show fragmentation of the bone; soft tissue swelling and thickening of the distal portion of the patellar tendon may also be seen.

Treatment

The *athlete* can:
– avoid painful situations: the athlete need not stop being active, but should be careful to avoid jumping and running, and anything else causing pain;
– apply ice to the area after activity, and sometimes heat before activity;
– carefully exercise the quadriceps muscles.

The *doctor* may:
– educate the athlete and the parents about the condition. Inform the patient that this injury is self-limiting provided activities are restricted and pain-causing situations avoided;
– apply a brace or a cast for 2 weeks if the athlete is uncooperative the pain is severe;
– prescribe an infrapatellar strap or knee sleeve to help participation sports;
– refer to physical therapy—this can be helpful as part of the education process;
– rarely, operate to remove small bone fragments, if the pain remains.

Healing and complications

Osgood–Schlatter disease heals spontaneously and problems seldom occur after the athlete's legs are fully developed at 17–18 years of age. Problems in older athletes may be caused by loose bodies formed at the site of the insertion of the patellar tendon or even at the bursa beneath the patellar tendon. These can be removed surgically with good results.

Bursitis

The knee is surrounded by several bursae. The principles of bursitis are discussed on p. 52.

Prepatellar bursitis

The prepatellar bursa is located anterior and distal to the patella. location makes it vulnerable to traumatic bursitis (Figure 11.59). Te

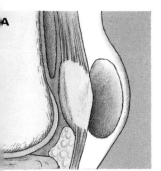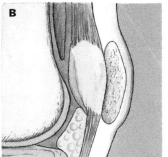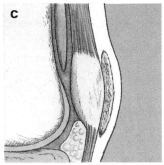

gure 11.59 (**A**) Acute bleeding in anterior patellar bursa. (**B**) Untreated bleeding, adhesions d loose bodies. (**C**) Residual condition with adhesions, scar tissue and loose bodies.

handball players, American football players, soccer players, wrestlers, and gymnasts are at increased risk. One study reported that 9.5% of wrestlers had prepatellar bursitis over a 6-year period.

Acute traumatic bursitis is caused by a single direct blow to the area resulting in hemorrhagic bursitis. Diagnosis and treatment are described on p. 52. Healing may take a week. Return to sport is possible as soon as the symptoms have disappeared, the swelling and inflammation have subsided, and there is a more or less normal range of motion. Protective padding is important to prevent recurrence.

Recurrent bursitis can result from recurrent trauma. This chronic situation is more difficult to treat. Aspiration is usually necessary and then cortisone can be injected into the area. A compression bandage is helpful. Immobilization for a short period may be necessary. Sometimes surgical excision of the bursa is indicated when there are multiple recurrences, or the inflamed bursa extends beyond the patella. Return to sport after surgery is possible within 2–3 weeks.

Septic (infected) bursitis requires aggressive medical treatment as detailed on p. 52.

Infrapatellar bursitis

A small bursa is located under the distal part of the patellar tendon and the proximal anterior part of the tibia. Pain in this area can be a residual problem after Osgood–Schlatter disease. Bursitis may be combined with the presence of a small bone fragment. The symptoms are pain in this area, localized tenderness, and sometimes problems with extending the knee against resistance. Treatment is conservative; occasionally surgery is needed.

Pes anserinus bursitis

The pes anserinus is the tendinous insertion of the hamstring muscles (sartorius, gracilis, and semitendinosus) on the anterior medial aspect of the proximal tibia. There is a bursa between the aponeurosis of these tendons and the medial collateral ligament approximately 2.4 in (6 cm below the medial joint line. This bursa may be inflamed by overus friction. Occasionally there may be a direct contusion. As the diagnos of this injury is not easy, it is probably commoner than is recognized.

Symptoms are localized pain during activity. Physical examinatio shows localized tenderness, swelling, and sometimes crepitus.

Treatment is conservative, including anti-inflammatory medication an restricted activity. Occasionally corticosteroid injection and ultrasoun treatment have been successful. If conservative therapy does not hel surgery to remove the bursa will usually give good results.

Baker's cyst (popliteal bursitis)

A distended bursa in the hollow behind the knee (the popliteal space) a relatively uncommon condition which manifests itself as a swelling the posterior joint capsule of the knee joint (Figure 11.60). The bursa sometimes connected with the joint, and when an irritant condition present with an effusion in the joint, synovial fluid may be pressed o into the bursa so that it becomes distended.

Symptoms and diagnosis

– A sensation of pressure mainly affecting the popliteal space is exper enced, especially on bending. This feeling may also be transmitted the calf muscles.
– It is difficult to bend and straighten the knee joint completely.
– Aching and tenderness are felt after exertion of the knee joint.
– The distended bursa appears as a rounded, fluctuant swelling, usual the size of a golf ball but sometimes as big as a tennis ball, when t knee joint is held in extension.
– Ultrasonography or MRI of the knee (see Figure 11.60) can show t elements of the bursa.
– Arthroscopy may reveal the cause of the effusion in the knee joint.

Figure 11.60
Baker's cyst.
(**Right**) MRI of multilobular Baker's cyst (white areas).

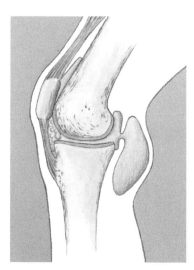
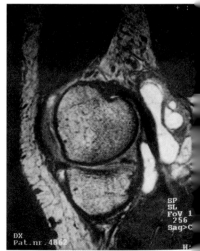

The *athlete* should rest; the symptoms may then disappear.
The *doctor* may:
- treat any cause of the effusion in the knee joint;
- remove the bursa surgically if it is causing problems.

The injured athlete can return to sporting activity 4–8 weeks after surgery. Baker's cyst often disappears spontaneously in children.

Runner's knee (iliotibial band friction syndrome)

This painful condition is localized on the lateral side of the knee joint. It is particularly common in athletes who run downhill for prolonged periods. The iliotibial tract originates from the tensor fasciae latae, and passes the greater trochanter and runs distally on the lateral side of the leg. It inserts into the lateral tibial condyle. When the knee is in extension, the iliotibial band lies anterior to the lateral epicondyle of the femur. When the athlete flexes the knee, the iliotibial band passes over the condyle at 30° of flexion, increasing friction. Inflammation of the iliotibial band occurs over the prominent epicondyle secondary to this friction. There may be associated bursitis. After 30° of flexion the iliotibial band is posterior to the epicondyle (Figure 11.61). Excessive foot pronation, genu varum, rotation of the tibia, and excessive tightness of the iliotibial band have been associated with the injury. This injury is also seen in athletes who run on cambered roads, resulting in a leg-length discrepancy.

- Pain localized to the lateral side of the knee may limit activity. It may radiate proximally or distally. This pain may start after the athlete has run a certain distance and then increase so that further running becomes impossible. After resting the pain may disappear, but it recurs if running is resumed.
- Running downhill or climbing stairs may aggravate the symptoms, as these activities cause excessive friction of the iliotibial band on the lateral condyle.
- Localized tenderness on the lateral condyle is felt approximately 1.2 in (3 cm) proximal to the lateral joint line (Figure 11.62).
- A compression test (*Noble's test*) can reproduce the typical pain. With the patient supine, the examiner's thumb is placed over the condyle and active extension/flexion is performed. Pain results with a maximum of 30° of flexion.
- *Ober's test* evaluates the iliotibial band tightness. The unaffected hip and knee are flexed. The involved knee is flexed to 90° and the same side hip is abducted and hyperextended. The tight iliotibial band will prevent the extremity from dropping below the horizontal plane.

- Athletic activity should be modified to avoid pain-causing situations and running downhill or on the side of the road.

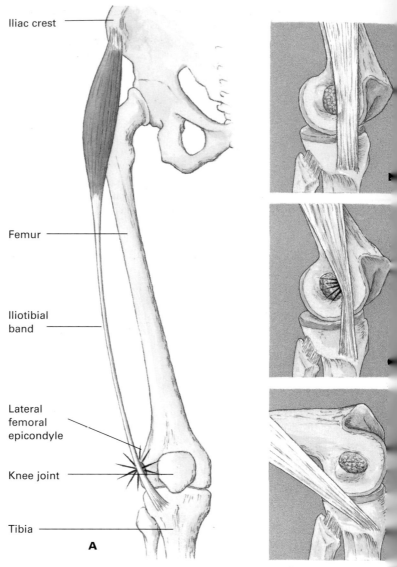

Iliac crest

Femur

Iliotibial
band

Lateral
femoral
epicondyle

Knee joint

Tibia

A

Figure 11.61 (**A**) Iliotibial band friction; anterior view. (**B**) Knee extended
(illotibial band anterior of epicondyle). (**C**) Knee bent 30° (iliotibial band ru
over epicondyle). (**D**) Knee flexed more than 30° (illotibial band behind
epicondyle).

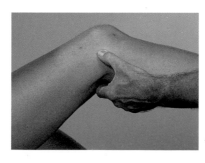

Figure 11.62 Palpation tendern
over the lateral epicondyle.

- When training resumes, alteration of the training program may be helpful.
- Apply heat before activities.
- Ice can be applied immediately after activity.
- Practice static stretching (p. 508) of the tissues on the lateral aspect of the thigh.

The *doctor* may:
- prescribe anti-inflammatory medication;
- prescribe a period of rest;
- prescribe a lateral wedge orthosis, which may be help an athlete with a tight iliotibial band;
- administer a local steroid injection;
- operate if conservative therapy fails. A small incision can be made from posterior in the iliotibial band over the lateral condyle with knees at 30° of flexion. Return to sports may be possible within 3–4 weeks.

Bibliography

Noble CA (1980) Iliotibial band friction syndrome in runners. *American Journal of Sports Medicine* 8: 232–234.

Popliteal tendon overuse injury

Overuse injuries to the popliteal tendon are uncommon. They cause pain on the lateral side of the knee joint. The popliteal tendon has its wide origin on the posterior aspect of the tibia above the insertion of the soleus muscle; it courses supralaterally and anteriorly and runs beneath the lateral collateral ligament to insert in front of it on the femur. The major function of the popliteal tendon is to initiate and maintain internal rotation of the tibia on the femur and to assist the posterior cruciate ligament in its actions. This injury usually occurs in runners and can also occur in people involved in downhill walking such as backpackers.

The pathological basis of this injury is usually peritendonitis or tendinosis. Ruptures are rare, and occur mostly with major trauma.

nptoms
l diagnosis

- Pain is located at the lateral femoral condyle. It usually occurs during weightbearing with knee flexion at 15–30°.
- The onset of pain is often insidious and there is no history of acute injury. The pain occurs when walking or running downhill or downstairs.
- Local tenderness is noted on palpation over the tendon attachment and lateral aspect of the femur just anterior to the LCL insertion. This tenderness is most apparent if the injured person sits, holding the knee joint of the injured leg at an angle of 90° with the foot placed on the healthy knee.
- Pain can occur while rotating the lower leg inwards.
- Before the diagnosis is made, the doctor should check that there is no injury to the lateral meniscus.
- The physical examination may often be normal. The patient should therefore be examined immediately after running.

Treatment

The *athlete* should:
– avoid pain-causing situations: it is often possible to continue runnin on even surfaces, cycling, or crosscountry skiing;
– apply local heat before activities and ice after activities.
The *doctor* may:
– prescribe anti-inflammatory medication;
– in persistent cases, administer a local injection of steroids around t tendon, followed by restriction of activities for 1–2 weeks;
– send the patient to a physical therapist for education and treatment
– encourage stretching;
– operate in cases of prolonged and severe problems.

Injury to the distal bicep femoris muscle–tendon at the knee

The symptoms and treatment for this injury are the same as describ on p. 263 for the thigh.

Bibliography
Brittberg M, Lindahl A, Nilsson A, et al (1994) Treatment of deep car lage defects in the knee with autologous chondrocyte transplantatic *New England Journal of Medicine* 331:889–895.
Minas T, Peterson L (1997) Chondrocyte transplantation. *Operat Techniques in Orthopaedics* 7/4:323–333.
Peterson L (1996) Articular cartilage injuries treated with autolog chondrocyte transplantation in the human knee. *Acta Orthopaed Belgica* 62/1:196–200.

12 Lower leg

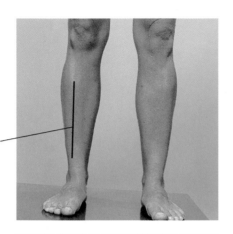

Figure 12.1 Anteromedial aspect of lower leg and location of associated injuries.

;ute and ronic anterior mpartment ndrome 336, 337); ialis anterior ndrome (338)

Figure 12.2 Anterolateral and anteromedial aspects of lower leg and associated injuries.

leus rupture 345)

sterior deep npartment drome (342); dial tibial ess syndrome 9)

tal tibial stress ctures (341)

ntaris longus ry (360)

Common peroneal nerve injury (p. 346)

Proximal tibial stress fractures (341)

Lateral compartment syndrome (346)

Central and anterior tibial stress fractures (341)

Fibula stress fractures (341); muscle hernia (346); superficial peroneal nerve entrapment (347)

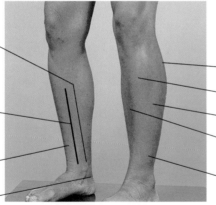

Figure 12.3 Posterior aspect of lower leg and location of associated injuries.

nis leg 344)

rtionitis of illes tendon)

Posterior superficial compartment syndrome (p. 343)

Achilles tendon partial and complete rupture (350, 352); Achilles tendinosis (354); Achilles peritenonitis (355)

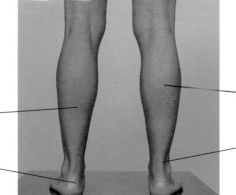

Common peroneal nerve injury (p. 346)

Achilles tendon partial and complete rupture (pp. 350, 352); Achilles tendinosis (354); Achilles peritenonitis (355)

Fibula stress fracture (341)

Achilles bursitis (357)

Functional anatomy

The musculature of the lower leg is enclosed in four tight, inflexible compartments by fascias of connective tissue which are anchored to the tibia and fibula. A cross-section through the lower leg about 4 in (10 cm) below the knee shows that the four compartments are clearly defined. In front, between the tibia and the fibula, there is an anterior compartment which contains the toe extensors, the tibialis anterior muscle, and the blood vessels and nerves that supply the anterior aspect of the lower leg and foot. At the back, the lower leg is divided into two compartments, one deep and one superficial. The deep one, which is located between the tibia and the fibula and behind the tight connective tissue band (interosseous membrane) that connects the two, contains the long flexors (flexor digitorum longus and flexor hallucis longus) and tibialis posterior muscle. Nerves and blood vessels pass to the back of the lower leg and the sole of the foot through this deep compartment. The posterior superficial muscle compartment at the back contains the broad deep calf muscle (the soleus) and the superficial calf muscle (the gastrocnemius). On the lateral aspect of the leg, around the fibula, is a lateral compartment which encloses the peroneus longus, the peroneus brevis and the peroneal nerve.

Fractures

Fractures of the lower leg occur most frequently in alpine skiers but also in crosscountry skiers, riders and participants in contact sports such as American football, soccer, rugby, and ice hockey (Figure 12.5).

In alpine skiing, the injury occurs most frequently in young skiers and there is no difference in incidence by sex. Snow conditions are an important consideration in tibial fractures: on icy or hard-packed surfaces the incidence of tibial fractures is much lower than on powder snow. A contributory factor may be the failure of the ski binding to release

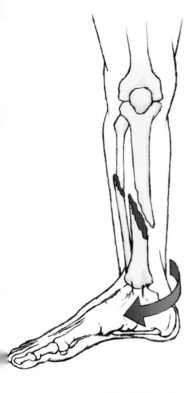

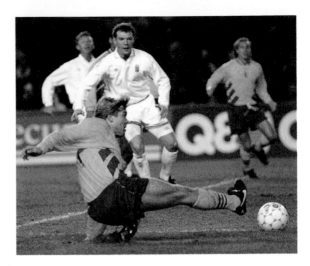

Figure 12.5 (**Left**) Lower leg fracture. (**Right**) During a cutting maneuver the foot was caught and twisted against the ground. A distal lower leg fracture and syndesmosis rupture occurred. Surgery was necessary (by courtesy of Fotograf Roland Rygin).

88). Tibial fractures are relatively unusual in crosscountry skiing but they do occur. Soccer fractures can occur when the lower leg is kicked by an opponent while the foot is loaded. Rugby tackles or an opponent tripping over an outstretched leg may also cause fractures. Lower leg fractures are not uncommon in motor sports.

Fractures of the tibia and fibula

The tibia and fibula may fracture simultaneously or separately. As a rule the injury is more serious if both bones are affected, particularly if the broken ends penetrate the skin causing a compound fracture. The different types of fracture can be seen on p. 6.

Symptoms
and diagnosis

- Intense, instantaneous pain is felt in the injured area.
- Tenderness and swelling occur over the fracture.
- The athlete is unable to use the injured leg.
- The normal contour and alignment of the lower leg may be altered by displacement of the fractured bones.

Treatment

When treating fractures it is important to remember that the soft tissues around the injury are also damaged. Guidelines for acute treatment can be found in Chapter 5. The injured athlete should not be given anything to eat and drink before transportation to hospital in case general anesthesia is required.

The *doctor* may:
- examine the injured area and nerve function and circulation distal t
  the injury;
- X-ray the injury;
- realign the bones if necessary and put the leg in a walking boot,
  brace, or a plaster cast, which for the first 4–8 weeks should includ
  the foot, the lower leg, and sometimes the thigh up to the groin. Th
  treatment usually lasts for 8–12 weeks or sometimes longer;
- operate if necessary. The bone ends can be fixed with a steel rod or
  plate and screws. After surgery, external support may be applied fc
  4–12 weeks, but motion of the knee and ankle should be allowed :
  soon as possible;
- realign the bones and use an external fixation instrument. This allow
  early range-of-motion training. Acute compartment rupture may occ
  and should be treated along with the fracture (see below).

Healing and complications

After the period of protection, mobility and strength are improved k
continued training. A return to competitive sports is usually not poss
ble for at least 6 months after the injury. In cases of tibial fractures the
can be complications such as delayed union or nonhealing pseudarthr
sis formation. This condition is difficult to treat and may require surger

Fractures of the fibula

When the fibula alone is fractured, a simultaneous injury often occurs
the syndesmosis, the strong ligaments that unite the fibula and the til
at the ankle joint. It is therefore important that the ankle joint
examined for stability by a doctor and X-rayed.

Symptoms and diagnosis

- Pain and tenderness are felt over the fracture.
- Pain occurs when the leg is under load.
- When the syndesmosis (p. 372) is damaged the ankle joint sho
  swelling, tenderness and instability, when tested with external rotatic
- An X-ray of the lower leg and the ankle joint confirms the diagnos

Treatment

An isolated fracture of the fibula without displacement often requi
only rest and no immobility treatment, but when the syndesmosis
severely injured surgical repair of the ligaments may be necessary.

Healing

The healing time is 4–6 weeks, depending on the extent of the fractu
If an injury of the syndesmosis is present the deltoid ligament can
ruptured (p. 371).

Compartment syndrome

Compartment syndromes are painful conditions caused by increas
pressure inside the different muscle compartments. They may be ac
or chronic (Figure 12.6).

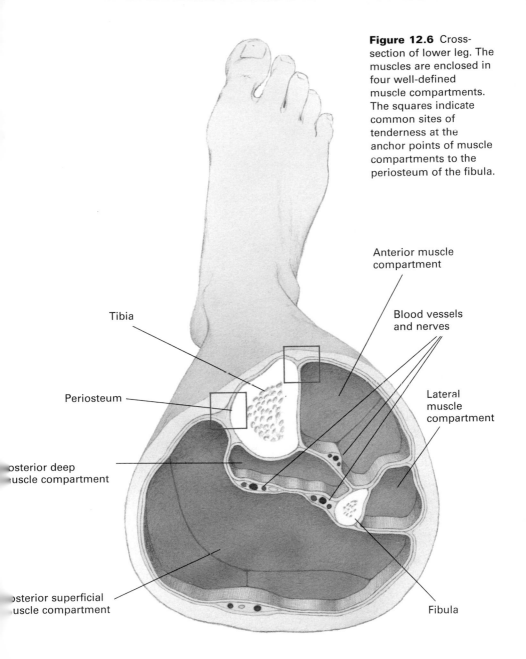

Figure 12.6 Cross-section of lower leg. The muscles are enclosed in four well-defined muscle compartments. The squares indicate common sites of tenderness at the anchor points of muscle compartments to the periosteum of the fibula.

Anterior muscle compartment

Tibia

Blood vessels and nerves

Periosteum

Lateral muscle compartment

Posterior deep muscle compartment

Posterior superficial muscle compartment

Fibula

Acute compartment syndrome can arise as a result of:
- external impact which causes a fracture and/or soft tissue injury with bleeding inside a compartment;
- muscle rupture with bleeding inside a compartment;
- overuse, e.g. from running on a hard surface without adequate preparation or time for adjustment.

Chronic compartment syndrome can result from muscular hypertrophy (an increase in muscle volume) following prolonged training. The increase in volume causes the musculature to expand more than is allowed for by the surrounding fascia, since these tight membranes are

335

not particularly elastic. When the muscles are at rest there is no problem, but during muscular work thousands of small blood vessels dilate in order to increase the blood flow, thereby increasing the intracompartmental pressure. The blood flow may be obstructed by excessive pressure, depriving the muscle of oxygen, and leading to formation of lactic acid. This changes the cell environment, and fluid begins to leak from the capillaries, causing swelling (edema) within the muscle and further increasing the pressure in the muscle compartment, impairing the blood flow even more. This vicious cycle continues unless exercise ceases. Muscular contraction within the compartments can also exert traction on the periosteum, causing it to become inflamed (periostitis).

Compartment syndromes can occur at the front, at the back, and on each side of the lower leg.

Anterior lower leg pain

Anterior lower leg pain is caused by chronic compartment syndromes of the anterior (10–20%) and lateral (1–2%) muscle compartments, peroneal nerve syndromes (20%), muscle hernia (5%) or medial tibial stress syndromes (50%).

Acute anterior compartment syndrome

Acute anterior compartment syndrome can occur as a result of direct impact, such as a kick or a blow, to the tibialis anterior muscle. This is however, uncommon, as the muscle lies well protected laterally to the tibia. Acute bleeding in the anterior compartment of the lower leg can lead to greatly increased pressure which in turn impairs the blood flow of the vessels that pass through the muscle compartment. Of most importance is the artery supplying the anterior part of the dorsum of the foot which can become completely blocked, causing an acute condition which requires surgery.

Acute anterior compartment syndrome can also be caused by overuse triggered by the athlete training or competing too intensively, perhaps on a hard surface and without proper preparation.

Symptoms and diagnosis
- A characteristic symptom is acute pain which gradually increases until it becomes impossible to continue running.
- Weakness can occur when the foot is dorsiflexed (bent upwards).
- A sensation of numbness extending down into the foot may be felt.
- Local swelling and tenderness can be present over the tibialis anterior muscle.
- Pain can be triggered when the foot or toes are passively plantar flexed (bent downwards).

The *athlete* should:
- rest actively;
- cool the injured area.

The *doctor* may:
- prescribe diuretics;
- prescribe anti-inflammatory medication;
- check the effectiveness of the treatment by measuring the pressure in the muscle compartment;
- operate to divide the fascia if the pressure in the muscle compartment is too high and does not diminish. Treatment should be started early, because the increased pressure can cause permanent damage to muscle and other soft tissues in the muscle compartment.

Chronic anterior compartment syndrome

Chronic anterior compartment syndrome mainly affects athletes who run long distances, or compete in specialized sports such as walking. These athletes have increased the volume of their lower leg muscles (by up to 20%) by extensive training, and the muscles have thus become larger than the surrounding fascias will allow. During exertion, as first the venous blood supply and then the arterial flow become obstructed, the pain due to lack of oxygen and increased pressure gradually worsens until the athlete can no longer continue training, either because of the pain itself or because of weakness of muscular function.

- Pain increases under load and finally makes continued muscle work impossible.
- The pain disappears after a short rest but recurs when activity is resumed.
- Local swelling and tenderness over the muscle belly on the antero-lateral side of the tibia is often present (Figure 12.7).
- Pain and muscle weakness occur on dorsiflexing the foot after provocation by muscle work.
- Passive plantar toe flexion may provoke pain.
- A sensation of numbness in the space between the big toe and the second toe, weakness in the foot, and marked difficulty in dorsiflexing the foot are experienced.
- The pressure in the muscle compartment can be measured at rest and during muscle work. Increased pressure is present in cases of chronic anterior compartment syndrome.

The *athlete* should:
- rest until pain has resolved;
- stretch the involved compartment;
- apply local heat and use a heat retainer;
- analyze running surfaces, running technique, training, type of shoes, and so on.

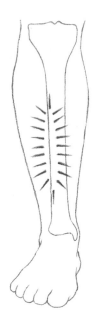

Figure 12.7
Area affected by chronic anterior compartment syndrome.

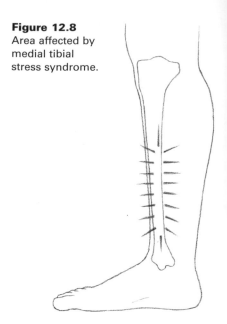

Figure 12.8
Area affected by medial tibial stress syndrome.

The *doctor* may:
- analyze anatomical background factors;
- treat the injured athlete with diuretics and anti-inflammatory medication
- perform compartment pressure measurements (pressure of more tha 35 mmHg after effort suggests the diagnosis);
- operate to divide the fascia and give the enlarged muscle more spac (there are good results after surgery in over 90% of cases).

Tibialis anterior syndrome

An acute inflammation of the tendon sheath of the tibialis anterior musc may arise from overuse of the ankle joint, e.g. in jumping and runnin (especially on a hard surface), in racket sports, and so on. Dorsiflexic of the ankle joint precipitates the problem. It can also be caused increased pressure from shoes or skates that are laced too tightly.

Symptoms and diagnosis
- Local pain is felt on dorsiflexing the ankle joint.
- Crepitus (creaking) occurs over the tendon on moving the ankle joir
- Temperature increase, skin redness and swelling may be present ov the lower anterior part of the tibia.
- Tenderness over the tendon and its sheath is felt on direct pressure ov the lateral side of the tibia and also when the foot is bent up and dow If the hand is placed over the tendon, crepitus sometimes can be fel

Treatment
The *athlete* should:
- rest actively;
- apply cooling both in the acute stage and later, when it may be alte nated with heat treatment;
- have proper footwear and equipment;
- unload the anterior area of the shoe or skate.

338

The *doctor* may:
- prescribe anti-inflammatory medication;
- prescribe crutches for 2–3 days to take the weight off the leg. Brace treatment is rarely needed in acute injury, but may be helpful in cases of prolonged symptoms.

Medial lower leg pain

Pain on the medial side of the lower leg can arise from medial tibial stress syndrome, a stress fracture of the tibia or from posterior deep muscle compartment syndrome.

Medial tibial stress syndrome

Medial tibial stress syndrome (periostitis of the medial margin of the tibia or 'shin splints') is a common complaint in athletes, especially those who change from one playing surface to another in spring and autumn, change their type of shoes, alter their techniques, or subject themselves to intensive training on hard tracks, streets, or floors. This syndrome can be triggered by running and other sports with elements of jumping, the main cause of the pain being repeated landing and take-off from the surface. Runners who run with forefoot strides or with externally rotated feet ('Charlie Chaplin runners') or who use spiked shoes can suffer from these complaints. Increased pronation can be a contributory cause.

Symptoms and diagnosis
- There is diffuse longitudinal tenderness over the distal medial margin of the tibia which can be intense. It can be local but also spreads diffusely longitudinally. The tenderness is usually pronounced over the lower half of the bone.
- A certain degree of diffuse swelling can be felt and seen.
- The pain ceases at rest but returns on renewed activity. The injured athlete can enter the pain cycle.
- Pain is triggered when the toes or ankle joint are bent in plantar flexion.
- Local tenderness occurs usually in the lower half of the tibia (Figure 12.8). A certain degree of irregularity can sometimes be felt along its edge.
- An X-ray examination is needed when symptoms are prolonged, to exclude a stress fracture. Otherwise findings are normal, although there may be hypertrophy of the posterior cortex of the tibia.
- There is normal pressure in the compartment.
- A triple-phase bone scan may help to distinguish this syndrome from a tibial stress fracture. There is a moderate increase of activity along the posteromedial border of the tibia on the delayed images.
- Magnetic resonance imaging can be of value to show bone edema, indicating that this condition may be a stress reaction of bone and a precursor to a stress fracture.

Preventive measures
Every change of surface should be made gradually while the intensity of training is adjusted accordingly.

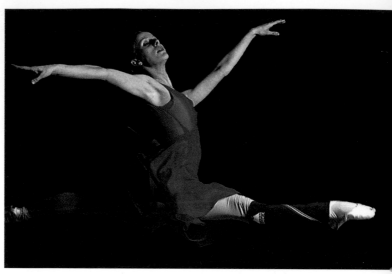

Figure 12.9 It can be of value to use a heat retainer to prevent or treat injuries during activities involving hard and repeated loading.

- Correct clothing and equipment should be used. Shoes should b chosen to suit the surface: shoes with cleats should be avoided whe training on unyielding hard surfaces such as asphalt. Orthotic treat ment may be required.
- The technique should be adjusted to the surface.
- Careful warm-up is essential.

Treatment

The *athlete*:
- should interrupt training and competition and rest as early as poss ble. The sooner training is given up, the more rapidly the injury wi heal. A chronic condition can then be avoided. Pain is a warning th should signal rest;
- should not start training again until there is no pain under load ar the tenderness over the tibia is gone;
- maintain physical fitness by cycling or swimming. If cycling, the ped should be held under the heel rather than the front of the foot;
- can apply local heat and use a heat retainer (Figure 12.9). Sometim alternating heat and cooling can be of value;
- should see a doctor if the complaint persists.

The *doctor* may:
- prescribe anti-inflammatory medication;
- measure the pressure in the posterior deep muscle compartme during provocation in cases of persistent complaints to exclude de posterior compartment syndrome;
- analyze malalignment as a cause: examine the anatomy of the low extremity and the foot, particularly with regard to pronation and a hi longitudinal arch, or genu valgum (foot orthoses can be effective in to 30% of patients);
- operate to divide the periosteum from the medial margin of the tib

Return to sport is possible within 2–4 months in most cases. It requires gradual increase of activity, education of athlete and coaches about the chronicity of this injury, and skilful teamwork. The prognosis is usually good, but the cause of the injury must be identified, whether it is a training error or a biomechanical deviation.

Medial tibial stress syndrome can occur as an isolated condition but can also be a symptom of a chronic posterior deep compartment syndrome. If conservative treatment fails to relieve pain due to loading within 2 weeks, then a stress fracture should be suspected and excluded by X-ray or bone scan.

Lower leg fractures

Both tibia and fibula can be the site of stress fractures (p. 8), often after prolonged and repeated running. Skeletal asymmetry, leg-length discrepancy, variations in gait, poor running conditions, hard or cambered surfaces, or prior injury can predispose to injury. Stress fractures are more common in women.

pes

1 *Fibula stress fractures:* these are usually located 2–3 in (5–7 cm) from the tip of the medial malleolus. They are typical injuries of long-distance runners.
2 *Proximal and distal tibia stress fractures:* these are most common in the proximal area and are usually located posteromedially. This part of the tibia is a compression site and these fractures develop slowly. They allow remodeling and hypotrophy and often heal well in 4–8 weeks. They are seen mostly in runners.
3 *Central and anterior tibial stress fractures:* these are located in the anterior aspect of the tibia, which is called the tension side. They heal very poorly and must be treated with special attention. They typically have an opening of the anterior side called the 'dreaded line' (see Figure 12.10). They are seen in sports that include jumping, such as volleyball or team handball.

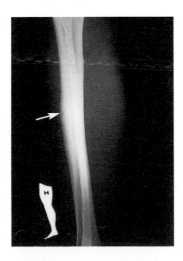

Figure 12.10 The 'dreaded line' (arrow) is a chronic stress fracture of the anterior middle portion of the tibia.

Symptoms and diagnosis	– These are typical of stress fractures (see p. 8).
	– It is possible to differentiate a stress fracture from medial tibial stress syndrome by a triple-phase bone scan. In medial tibial stress syndrome the scan is only positive on the delayed phase and covers a long segment, while in stress fractures the scan is positive on all phases and has a focal location.
	– MRI can verify the stress fracture. Bone edema (swelling) can be seen as a reaction to the stress fracture.
Treatment	– Rest and avoidance of abuse from painful activities.
	– Crutches may sometimes be needed in the early phase if there is pain on weightbearing.
	– Conservative treatment of these stress fractures can be combined with electrical stimulation.

For anterior tibial stress fracture of the central tibia a more aggressive approach has been advocated, since these fractures may take a long time to heal. Among the different surgical alternatives are:
– shock wave therapy: in some hands this has given good results, but the treatment, despite promising results, should still be considered experimental;
– early surgery with excision of the excessive sclerotic (hard) bone the delayed union, combined with drilling;
– early surgery with intramedullary (marrow canal) nailing, which has allowed return to sports in a few months.

Since stress fractures (especially those of the anterior central tibia) have a tendency to heal poorly, an early consultation with an orthopedic sports medicine specialist is recommended.

The anterior tibial stress fracture located on the central tibia should be treated with special care.

Posterior deep compartment syndrome

The *acute posterior deep compartment syndrome* can result from external impact or acute overuse of the muscles, e.g. during running and jumping (especially when taking-off). Such an injury may affect all the muscles simultaneously, or one (e.g. tibialis posterior, flexor hallucis longus, flexor digitorum longus) in isolation. It can be difficult—sometimes impossible—to decide which muscles have been affected, but clues can be found if each muscle group is tested individually:
– plantar-flexing the big toe against resistance triggers pain, the flexor hallucis longus muscle tendon is involved;

- if plantar-flexing the whole of the foot inward against resistance triggers pain, the tibialis posterior muscle is primarily involved;
- if plantar-flexing all the toes against resistance triggers pain, the long toe flexors are involved.

In *chronic posterior deep compartment syndrome*, increased pressure during activity in the muscle compartment, in addition to the increased muscle contraction, can cause increased pressure on the vessels and nerves in the compartment, as well as traction on the fascial attachment to the periosteum on the inside edge of the tibia. The result may be pain and inflammation of the periosteum (periostitis).

Symptoms and diagnosis

The examination should if needed be performed after provocation.
- Pain occurs on kicking or pushing-off from the ground and also on heel-raising. The pain starts insidiously and gradually intensifies until physical activity is rendered impossible.
- A sensation of numbness in the foot and weakness on taking-off are felt.
- The symptoms abate after rest but recur when there is renewed exertion.

Treatment

The treatment is the same as for chronic anterior compartment syndrome (p. 337).

Table 12.1 offers a differential diagnosis between the causes of medial tibial pain.

Table 12.1

Sign	Medial tibial syndrome	Stress fracture	Compartment syndrome
Pain during activity	500 m	Immediate	3 km
Need to stop	No	Yes	Yes
Pain after activity	Yes	No	No

Posterior lower leg pain

Posterior superficial compartment syndrome

Posterior superficial compartment syndrome is an uncommon condition affecting the muscle compartment containing the broad, deep calf muscle (the soleus) and the superficial calf muscle (the gastrocnemius). Symptoms, diagnosis, and treatment are in principle the same as for anterior compartment syndrome (p. 337).

'Tennis leg' (rupture of the gastrocnemius muscle)

Ruptures of the calf musculature usually occur at the point where t'
Achilles tendon merges with the inner belly of the calf muscle (Figu
12.11). The injury occurs most frequently in tennis, badminton, squa
volleyball, basketball, and team handball, and also in the jumping spor

Symptoms and diagnosis

- There is a sudden pain in the calf which may feel like a blow on t
  leg from behind.
- There is difficulty in contracting the calf muscle and walking on tipt
- Local tenderness occurs over the injured area.
- Effusion of blood in the region of the rupture.
- A gap can be felt in the muscle–tendon junction over the injured ar
- In middle-aged and elderly individuals a muscle–tendon juncti
  injury may be misinterpreted as thrombosis.

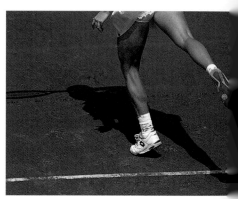

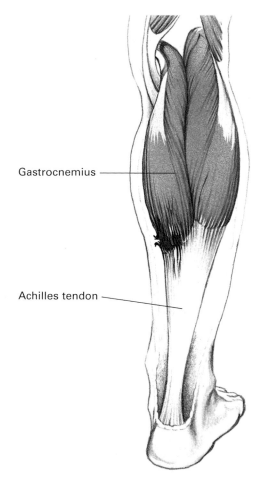

Gastrocnemius

Achilles tendon

Figure 12.11 (**Left**) Rupture of the inner belly of the gastrocnemius muscle at the merger of muscle and tendon – 'tennis leg' (**Above**) Ruptures of muscles and tendons common in dynamic sports with rapid movements (by courtesy of All Sport: photographer, Pascal Rondeau).

Treatment	The *athlete* should:
	– treat the injury immediately by cooling, apply a compression bandage, and elevate the leg;
	– avoid any 'pushing-off' activity;
	– use crutches.

The *doctor* may:
- in cases of minor ruptures and in elderly patients, prescribe a support bandage and early introduction of mobility and progressive strength training;
- advise the athlete to wear a walking boot to keep the ankle stiff and prevent 'pushing-off' activity;
- occasionally operate when the injury and the hematoma are extensive in an active athlete.

Healing and complications

Muscle rehabilitation should start within 3–5 days and increase progressively (p. 337). The injured athlete can return to training 2–6 weeks after a minor rupture. After surgery, rehabilitation will demand another 6–10 weeks.

An untreated muscle rupture leads to scarring which carries with it the risk of repeated discomfort if the muscle is overexerted.

Rupture of the soleus muscle

On vigorous take-offs or jump-ups the soleus muscle deep in the calf can be overloaded and rupture. Such ruptures are uncommon, and are usually only partial.

Symptoms and diagnosis

- Pain is located deep in the calf and recurs on repeated loading.
- Pain is triggered when the foot is plantar-flexed against resistance and also on attempting to walk on tiptoe.
- Bleeding most often makes itself felt only some 24 hours after the injury. Bruising becomes visible on the inner side of the proximal and middle parts of the shin.
- Deep local tenderness is felt over the rupture, often along the soleus at the tibial margin.
- In cases of long-term problems MRI may be helpful.

Treatment

The *athlete* should:
- immediately treat the injury by cooling, apply a compression bandage, and elevate the leg;
- start motion and strengthening gradually after 3–5 days.

The *doctor* may:
- prescribe further strength and mobility training;
- prescribe anti-inflammatory medication if the leg is painful.

If the bleeding accompanying the muscle rupture is extensive, acutely increased pressure can occur in the posterior superficial muscle compartment (see p. 343).

345

The injured athlete should not return to regular training until there i
no further pain during movements under load, which usually takes 2—
weeks.

Lateral lower leg pain

In the lateral side of the lower leg, pain can occur in the fibula as a resu
of stress fractures (p. 341) and also in the lateral muscle compartment a
a result of acute or chronic lateral compartment syndrome.

Lateral compartment syndrome

Acute lateral compartment syndrome can result from external impact (
sudden overuse of the muscles. Symptoms, diagnosis and treatment a
in principle the same as for cases of acute anterior compartme
syndrome (p. 336).

Chronic pressure increase in the lateral muscle compartment occu
mainly in runners and is often associated with deficient ligaments on th
lateral aspect of the ankle joint. The muscle group of the lateral compar
ment acts to stabilize the lateral side of the ankle joint and can be overloade
in cases of instability of the joint. Symptoms, diagnosis and treatment a
the same as for chronic anterior compartment syndrome (p. 337).

Muscle hernia

A muscle hernia is a defect in the muscle fascia. It exists in 40%
athletes with chronic compartment syndrome, compared with 5%
normal athletes. The muscle can herniate through this fascia defect. T
hernia is characterized by localized muscle swelling. Pain and swelli
increase with exercise. There are negative findings on X-ray and bo
scan. Occasionally, pressure studies may be abnormal if there is an assoc
ated compartment syndrome.

As there may be increased intracompartmental pressure after fasc
closure, the most common treatment is completion of the herniation wi
complete fasciotomy. Occasionally, the fascia can be closed with t
addition of transplanted fascial material.

Injury to the common peroneal nerve

Injuries to the peroneal nerve in its course down the lateral aspect of
upper part of the fibula can occur as a result of impact—a blow, kick

fall—or as a result of external pressure in the form of a tape or plaster cast. This pressure is most common when the nerve goes around the proximal 0.8 in (2 cm) of the fibula.

Symptoms and diagnosis

- The pressure on the nerve causes paralysis creating a weakness in dorsiflexion of the ankle joint and eversion (pronation) of the foot. The result can be a 'drop foot'.
- The skin in the area may lose some sensitivity.
- An EMG test may be used to analyze the injury.

Treatment

Treatment includes:
- strength and mobility training;
- taking the pressure off the injured area;
- a bandage or an extension orthosis to keep the foot in its normal position, if necessary;
- electrical stimulation by a physiotherapist to reduce muscle wasting in cases of paralysis;
- anti-inflammatory medication if needed.

Healing

The function of the ankle joint usually returns after a period that varies from a few days to several months. The function usually returns if the nerve is damaged only by pressure.

Entrapment of the superficial peroneal nerve

The superficial peroneal nerve pierces the deep fascia 4 in (10 cm) proximal to the lateral malleolus of the ankle. It is the most common nerve compression in the lower leg. The symptoms are vaguely localized pain at the lateral ankle and these may be foot pain. This pain is usually associated with exercise. There is a positive Tinel sign (tapping on the nerve gives discomfort) and a positive nerve conduction velocity test. Treatment is by surgical decompression and fasciotomy.

Lower leg neurological pain

In elderly athletes there can be neurological pain in the lower leg, which may have the following causes:
1. Neuropathy or 'nerve pain', is not uncommon in middle-aged women with diabetes. The symptoms with pain are worse at night or at rest. This problem is best treated by the doctor who regulates the diabetes. Sometimes orthoses are valuable.
2. Neuroradiculopathy (nerve pain radiation), which often is associated with back pain, causes sensory pain spread according to the nerve distribution. There can be some muscle weakness present. The treatment is rest or occasional surgery.

c

3. Spinal stenosis (a narrow spinal canal) can also give problems. These patients often can exercise without pain with flexed spine and knee and continue cycling and stairclimbing, but have pain with other activities. Associated back pain with exercise and spinal imaging will give the diagnosis.

Vascular pain in the lower legs

Elderly people may have problems with their circulation. *Arterial insufficiency* is characterized by claudication, which is pain in the legs with any activity. These patients should go through a vascular evaluation. *Venous insufficiency* is seen in older age groups. These elderly athletes may have distal pretibial bone pain, tenderness, and swelling, which increases as the day progresses. Vascular examination is often normal in these patients, who should be evaluated by a doctor. An *exertional deep vein thrombosis* (blood clot) is very rare in active individuals. It is characterized by constant pain localized to the posterior compartment. The pain is not associated with exercise.

Achilles tendon injuries

The principles of tendon injuries are discussed on p. 42. The main role of the Achilles tendon is as part of the muscle–tendon unit generating forceful plantar flexion activities. The Achilles tendon is part of the soleus and gastrocnemius–soleus complex. The gastrocnemius component of the tendon is longer (4.4–10.4 in, 11–26 cm) than the soleus component (1.2–4.4 in, 3–11 cm). The soleus component occupies the medial portion of the tendon at the level of its insertion and the gastrocnemius occupies the lateral aspect at this level. There is a spiral orientation of the most distal 0.8–2 in (2–5 cm) of the tendon, which may contribute to injuries. The Achilles tendon extremely strong.

Etiology

Achilles tendon injuries may have many causes, both intrinsic (related the body) and extrinsic.

Extrinsic factors

Probably the most common extrinsic factors are a sudden change in activity, excessive training, sudden change in training surface characteristics, or suboptimal footwear. Most Achilles tendon ruptures or injuries occur in transition from inactivity to activity. This is especially true in formerly active athletes: after a period of limited sporting activity, typically when marriage and careers take priority, many athletes resume strenuous exercise at the age of 35–45 years. A sudden change in activities, e.g. from crosscountry skiing or running to tennis, is also a factor. Excessive training, especially by middle-aged athletes, may cause Achilles tendon damage.

Particular movements in sports such as the tennis serve or high-jump push-off, may cause Achilles tendon injuries. The tennis serve action includes a heavy push-off followed by lower leg rotation which increases the load in the Achilles tendon and calf muscles. This motion may cause 'tennis leg' which is a partial tear of the muscle–tendon junction of the Achilles tendon and gastrocnemius (p. 344). A sudden change in direction which includes a sudden deceleration and then a major push-off which forces the foot and the lower leg into major rotation may also damage the Achilles tendon. This is the most likely cause for complete Achilles tendon tears in the middle-aged tennis player.

The sport surfaces may vary considerably. Unforgiving surfaces such as asphalt or concrete often have high friction and are fatiguing for the legs; this kind of surface will often produce an overuse syndrome in the Achilles tendon. More forgiving surfaces such as clay are less likely to result in tendon problems, as the deceleration load is decreased by gliding on the surface.

Shoes are an important support for the Achilles tendon. Modern jogging and tennis shoes have a high heel counter which supports Achilles tendon rotation, and may thereby protect the tendon from damage.

Intrinsic factors

Common intrinsic factors are malalignment, excessive pronation, gastrocnemius–soleus stiffness, muscle imbalance, and age.

Functional hyperpronation can be physiologic, but can also be excessive, caused by malalignments such as tibia varus (inward direction of lower leg) or forefoot varus. A forefoot varus (inward direction of forefoot) of more than 7° has been found in roughly half the runners with Achilles tendon problems. It is therefore felt that it may be a common cause of functional hyperpronation in the running population. Pronation is discussed on p. 397.

The biomechanical evidence for increased localized stress of the Achilles tendon with hyperpronation is lacking. Pronation of 10° increases the strain on the medial side by 20% compared with the neutral position. The increase of the load on the medial side may be explained by the fact that the subtalar joint axis around which the majority of the pronation occurs lies to the lateral side of the Achilles tendon insertion. The medial side is therefore eccentric to the axis. Thus, as the foot pronates, the fibers on the medial aspect will be expected to rotate further away from the region, increasing the relative tension and stress.

The tendons begin to show degenerative changes (p. 43) at the early age of 25–30 years. The changes bring about weakness in the tendons but to some extent they can be prevented or at least delayed by regular physical activity.

Injuries to the Achilles tendon can be divided into complete Achilles tendon tears, partial Achilles tendon tears, tendinosis, peritenonitis with or without tendinosis, and insertionitis. Injuries may also occur around the Achilles tendon, such as Achilles bursitis.

Complete rupture of the Achilles tendon

A rupture of the Achilles tendon is one of the most common tendon injuries in sport, affecting 1 in every 10 000 inhabitants per year, with an incidence increasing with age (Figure 12.12). The ratio of men to women affected is 6:1 and the average age of sufferer 35–40 years. The tear can be complete or partial. The injury mainly afflicts participants in football, team handball, volleyball, basketball, tennis, squash, and especially badminton, and also athletes such as runners and jumpers. Complete rupture of the Achilles tendon usually occurs in degenerate tendons that are subjected to increased load.

Symptoms and diagnosis

- Intense pain is felt over the ruptured area of the Achilles tendon the time of injury. The injured person will often state that 'something hit me from behind' at the moment the pain began. There is not much pain, however, after the acute phase, and the athlete experiences improvement of the condition. Attention must be focused on the functional impairment.
- The injured athlete cannot walk normally on the foot or on tiptoe, and cannot 'push off' on that leg.
- Increasing swelling is caused by bleeding, which can gradually cause bruising over the lower part of the leg and the foot.
- Localized tenderness is felt over the ruptured area, which is often located about 2–8 cm (0.8–3.2 in) above the calcaneus, while the athlete is lying prone.
- A gap can be seen or felt in the tendon.
- The ability to bend the foot downwards (plantar flexion) is impaired.
- *Thompson's test* gives a positive result. For this test the injured athlete lies face down with the knee of the injured leg slightly bent. When the examiner compresses the calf muscle of the injured leg with one hand, the foot is bent downwards (plantar flexed) if the Achilles tendon is intact, but remains in its initial position if the tendon is torn.
- An MRI or ultrasound scan will verify the tear (see Figure 12.12), but is not needed if surgical treatment is planned. If conservative treatment is planned, it is sometimes necessary to exclude a 'mop tear' (see below), which can best be done by MRI or ultrasound. A mop tear may give poor results if treated conservatively.
- It should be pointed out that the diagnosis of a complete Achilles tendon rupture is usually straightforward, but is missed in 20% cases by the first examining doctor.

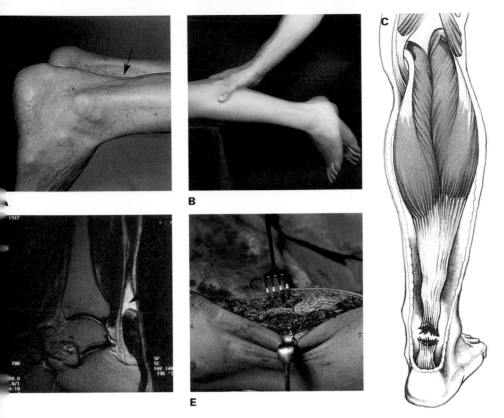

Figure 12.12 Achilles tendon rupture. (**A**) A gap (arrow) is seen in the tendon. (**B**) Thompsen's st. (**C**) Anatomic drawing. (**D**) MRI scan indicating ruptured tendon (arrow). (**E**) Rupture seen during surgery.

Treatment

The *doctor* can treat the injury with a cast with the foot in physiologic plantar flexion to bring the torn ends in contact. The case should then be worn for 8–10 weeks and gradually moved into the neutral position. There are indications that this can be done after 4 weeks, but the scientific support for this is not yet clear. Conservative treatment with a cast may be successful if the treatment starts within 48 hours of injury. One problem with conservative treatment is that there is more risk of a second rupture than with surgical treatment. This could be because the tendon tears are 'mop tears', in which the distal fragment of the tendon is folded down, making repositioning of the tendon ends impossible. Mop tears occur in 20% of cases. If the rupture gap is less than 0.08 in (2 mm) on ultrasound scan, the patient may be treated conservatively with success.

Alternatively, the doctor can operate to suture the ends of the tendon together, whether in an open or closed operation, with or without mini-incisions. This creates tension in the tendon, which encourages the proper orientation of its constituent collagen fibers, which is necessary to regain good strength. This reduces the risk of re-rupture and allows an early return to sports. Furthermore, surgical treatment allows early motion, which is the key to rehabilitation and regaining strength. Motion should start after the first week with plantar flexion of 0–20°. The patient wears a walking boot and can start weightbearing as tolerated, usually

351

after 2 weeks. After 6 weeks the patient can start using jogging shoes and return to sport is usually possible within 3–4 months (rehabilitation protocol on p. 523).

| Healing and complications | There is an increased risk for re-rupture with conservative treatment (10–15%). The treatment should therefore be carefully monitored by a trainer or physical therapist. Return to sports such as running and jumping is usually not possible until after 9–12 months. Healing with elongation may cause decreased strength in plantar flexion. |

Surgery with early functional mobilization and treatment allows an early return to sport. Return to sport at the same level as before a complete tear is 75% in top-level tennis players and 90% in recreational tennis players. These figures were much lower in a conservatively treated group. There are, however, complications to surgery such as delayed healing of the wound and infection. The re-rupture rate in the operative group is less than 2%.

Partial rupture of the Achilles tendon

A partial rupture of the Achilles tendon can occur in runners, jumpers and throwers and also in participants in racket sports, basketball, volley ball, and soccer (Figure 12.13). This injury can lead to scar formation which is liable to cause increased degenerative breakdown in the tendon and tendinosis (p. 43). This often becomes chronic and can cause prolonged problems.

Symptoms and diagnosis

- Some young patients experience a sudden onset of pain at the time of injury, but others may not notice pain at the actual moment of rupture, the pain becoming more evident after the completion of the activity.
- When the injury is in its acute stage, a defect can be felt in the tendon (sometimes no larger than the top of the little finger) over which there is extreme tenderness.
- When physical activity is resumed, the injured athlete feels an intense shooting, cutting, or stabbing pain.
- During the following training period the symptoms may disappear for a while after warm-up, but they return with even greater intensity when the training is over. The result can be that the injured person enters a vicious circle of pain in which the condition becomes progressively more painful and progressively more difficult to treat.
- Stiffness occurs in the morning and also before and after exertion.
- When the healing process has started, local swelling is often found over which a distinct tenderness is present when the area is pressed from the sides. The swelling is usually slight but can sometimes cause a change in the contour of the tendon.
- If the injured athlete is in severe pain, there is often tenderness when the swollen area is touched directly from behind.
- In cases of prolonged symptoms there is often a decrease in the strength and size (hypotrophy) of the calf muscle.

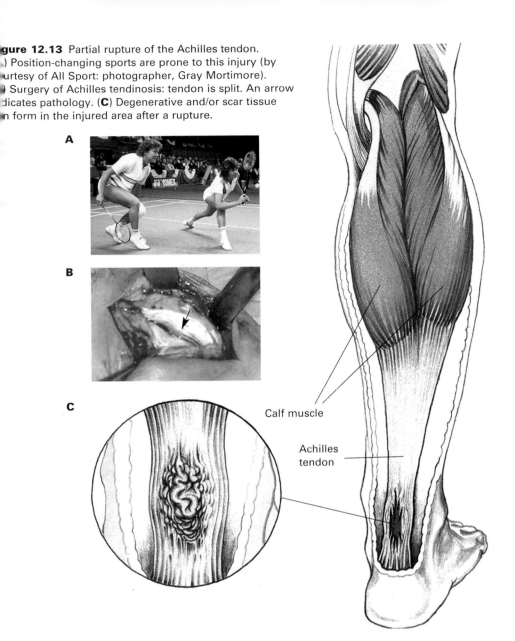

Figure 12.13 Partial rupture of the Achilles tendon.
(A) Position-changing sports are prone to this injury (by courtesy of All Sport: photographer, Gray Mortimore).
(B) Surgery of Achilles tendinosis: tendon is split. An arrow indicates pathology. (C) Degenerative and/or scar tissue can form in the injured area after a rupture.

A

B

C

Calf muscle

Achilles tendon

– An X-ray of the soft tissues is of value in showing local swelling of the ruptured area and swelling of the adjacent soft tissues.
– An MRI will provide a detailed assessment of the location of the tear, as well as the extent of the injury. Ultrasonography may support the diagnosis and permit evaluation of the size of the injury.

Treatment

The *athlete* should:
– rest and treat the injury with ice in the acute phase;
– use crutches if pain is severe;
– use shoes with 1 cm (0.5 in) heel wedges;
– consult a sport medicine specialist.

The *doctor* may:
- when the rupture is small and acute, apply a walking boot or a plaste cast for 4-6 weeks, holding the foot in slight plantar flexion; a walkin boot can also be tried for 3–4 weeks in chronic cases;
- prescribe an exercise program;
- in cases of prolonged chronic symptoms, operate to remove damage tissue.

Studies showed that 70% of athletes with verified and conservative treated chronic partial Achilles tendon ruptures still had major proble 10 years after the initial injury. Pain persisting for more than 6 mont in the distal part of the Achilles tendon is often resistant to conservati treatment. In such patients, surgery, which includes excision of the sc and granulation tissue in the tendon, is often necessary. The treatme after surgery is a plaster cast or a walking boot which is worn for 5 weeks. A careful progressive rehabilitation program with early moti within 1–2 weeks is necessary (p. 523) and should be carried out wi supervision..

Healing and
complications

After surgery the healing time is usually around 2 months. The rehab itation period is then 3–4 months before the athlete can resume full trai ing. The injured athlete should not count on resuming competition f at least 4–6 months. The average time is 6–8 months for serious chror injury. Surgery gives excellent to good results in most patients, with 80 returning to former levels of activity.

The problem with the rehabilitation after this injury is that the patie often feels cured and starts to use the tendon too much after 2–4 mont The healing of a chronic tendon condition always takes a long time.

Exercise promotes healing, but too much, too soon will result in pain, so it is necessary for the injured athlete to 'listen to the tendon'.

Achilles tendinosis

By the age of 25 years, the Achilles tendon begins to show signs of deg erative changes (p. 43); these may be aggravated by changes in traini (the 'principle of transition', p. 44), leading to tendinosis.

Symptoms
and diagnosis

- Stiffness occurs in the morning and often before and/or after activ
- A local swelling can often be palpated with distinct tenderness. T tenderness can be located on one side of the tendon.
- An MRI or ultrasound scan will provide details of the tendinosis a its extent in the tendon (Figure 12.14). An MRI scan can provid detailed evaluation of the tendon continuation but it is expensi Ultrasonography is less expensive and can therefore be used to foll the healing of the injury.

354

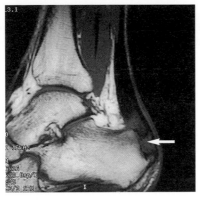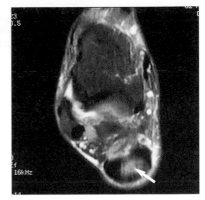

Figure 12.14 MRI of Achilles tendinosis (arrows).

The *athlete* should:
- avoid pain-causing situations and abuse of the tendon;
- keep active with nonpounding activities such as cycling and jogging in water;
- carry out stretching and eccentric strength exercises after instructions;
- follow the principles outlined on p. 45.

The *doctor* may:
- prescribe an exercise program which includes stretching and strength training. If the tendinosis is chronic, eccentric activities have been shown to give a good result; however, these should, be carried out after instruction and initially under supervision. Close cooperation with a physical therapist or trainer is often important;
- instruct the injured athlete how to 'listen to the tendon' so that optimal training is achieved;
- operate in cases of prolonged chronic symptoms where the conservative therapy has been tried for 6–12 months. Surgery often includes excision of the damaged tissue. The postoperative treatment is early motion after the wound has healed, with some protection from an orthosis. The postoperative program should be carried out under supervision.

The rehabilitation time varies from individual to individual. Often the athlete can quickly resume cycling and swimming. Running may begin after 3–6 months, depending on the seriousness of the injury. Surgery gives acceptable results in most patients, with 80% returning to former levels of activity.

Tendon overuse injuries constitute a real challenge and should be managed with great respect.

Achilles peritenonitis (tendon sheath inflammation)

There is rarely much inflammation present in the Achilles tendon. The surrounding tissues are more sensitive to an inflammatory reaction.

Acute inflammation

Acute inflammation of the Achilles tendon sheath (peritenonitis) oft
occurs in untrained individuals who start training too intensively, b
may also occur in well trained athletes who change surface, type of sh
or technique, or who train in cold weather. Running on a very se
surface (sand) and running uphill can trigger pain.

Symptoms and diagnosis
- Pain is felt on using the Achilles tendon.
- Diffuse swelling occurs around the tendon.
- There is intense, diffuse tenderness and impaired function.
- In cases of severe inflammation, skin redness appears over the tendc
- When the fingers are pressed on the tendon during ankle jo
  movement, a crepitus (creaking sensation) can be felt.

Preventive measures

Warm-up and stretching exercises are important. Well designed traini
and competition shoes of good quality should be used. A heel wedge
1 cm (0.5 in) will relieve tension in the Achilles tendon.

Treatment

The *athlete* should:
- rest; in the acute phase, crutches may be helpful;
- cool the injury with ice to reduce pain and swelling;
- use a 1 cm (0.5 in) heel wedge;
- apply local heat after the acute phase and use a heat retainer;
- consult a doctor if the complaint does not abate after a few days.

The *doctor* may:
- prescribe anti-inflammatory medication;
- apply a plaster cast in severe cases;
- prescribe a training program after the acute phase which sho
  include strength training and static stretching (p. 523). Eccen
  exercises which put high load on the tendon should become part
  the program when healing allows.

Healing

When treatment of acute inflammation of the Achilles tendon and
sheath has been started early, the prognosis is good and the injury he
in 1–2 weeks. The risk of recurrence is small if the athlete does not ret
to sporting activity too early. Acute inflammation of the Achi
peritenon can develop into a chronic condition which is very difficul
treat. It is therefore of the utmost importance that athletes should
when there are signs of Achilles peritenonitis.

Chronic inflammation

Chronic inflammation of the Achilles tendon sheath occurs in athl
(often elderly) who have been training intensively on a hard surface
a long time and who have ignored warning pains. These pains at
tend to disappear after the warm-up exercises before a training perioc
that the affected athlete can continue training. The symptoms ret
after training is over and gradually become more and more severe. Soo

or later continued running is impossible, and the athlete is trapped in the pain cycle.

- Pain, aching, and stiffness in the Achilles tendon occur before, during, and after exertion.
- There is diffuse swelling in the tendon.
- The tendon is diffusely tender on palpation.
- The athlete may suffer pain in the tendon when walking, especially uphill and upstairs.
- Athletes with this condition have in 50% of cases some kind of malalignment, such as increased pronation or forefoot varus.
- In cases of persistent Achilles tendon problems a combination injury with tendinosis should be suspected and investigated by a doctor.

The *athlete* should:
- avoid pain-causing situations;
- apply local heat and use a heat retainer;
- use shoes with 1 cm (0.5 in) heel wedge.
The *doctor* may:
- analyze the injured athlete's training considering especially the design of the shoes and the type of training surface;
- prescribe an exercise program with strength training and stretching (p. 523). The strength training should include eccentric exercises (p. 45);
- prescribe anti-inflammatory medication for a short time;
- prescribe ointments to stimulate blood flow and control the inflammation;
- apply a walking boot or a plaster cast for 3–6 weeks if there is severe pain or malfunction;
- operate in prolonged cases, releasing the tendon from the surrounding sheath scar tissue, which is then removed. Be aware that this injury can be combined with tendinosis.

Inflammation of the Achilles tendon sheath should be treated at an early stage.

Achilles bursitis

Bursitis over the calcaneus (heel bone) can occur in a superficial bursa located between the skin and the posterior surface of the Achilles tendon, which is vulnerable to pressure from shoes and often becomes inflamed. There is also a deeply located bursa (the retrocalcaneal bursa) between the Achilles tendon and the calcaneus, which can become inflamed if it is irritated either by external pressure or by a partial tendon rupture (Figure 12.15). If prolonged pressure against the tendon attachment, for example by repeated dorsiflexion, is the cause of the inflammation of the bursa, a bony prominence often appears on the posterior aspect of the calcaneus; this further increases the risk of the bursa being subjected to pressure or impingement between the bone and the tendon.

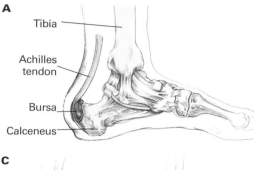

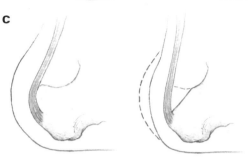

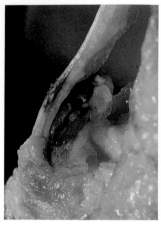

Figure 12.15 (A) Chronic bursitis at the attachment of the Achilles tendon to the posterior calcaneus. **(B)** Bursa (dyed blue to show location). **(C)** Enlarged posterior corner of calcaneus; and after removal.

Symptoms and diagnosis

– Redness and thickening of the skin may occur over the calcaneus the lateral side of the Achilles tendon attachment if the superfic bursa is involved.
– Pain can be experienced when running uphill or on soft surfaces.
– There are often symptoms such as tenderness and swelling which ma it difficult for the athlete to wear ordinary shoes.
– When the deep bursa is pressed from both sides anterior to the Achil tendon, a spongy resistance and pain can be felt as well as discomfo
– An MRI or ultrasound scan will confirm the diagnosis, but is seld indicated.

Treatment

The *athlete* should:
– relieve the calcaneus of pressure immediately symptoms begin, wearing shoes without backs such as sandals or clogs;
– relieve the area when the superficial bursa is inflamed with a fo rubber ring which is placed around the bony prominence if one formed;
– adjust the shoes, for example by raising the heel and softening counter in order to avoid pressure against the area;
– apply local heat.

The *doctor* may:
– prescribe anti-inflammatory medication;
– give ultrasound treatment;
– give a local steroid injection and prescribe rest;
– operate when the inflammation in the bursa has become chronic a a bony prominence has appeared. During the operation the bursa the prominence are removed.

Return to running is possible in 3–6 months depending on the type surgery.

Insertionitis (apophysitis calcanei)

Injury to the Achilles tendon apophysis insertion to the calcaneus occurs in both elderly and young athletes.

The elderly often have degenerative changes in the tendon which can form calcifications and cause tendinosis at the insertion site; these athletes have pain during running, and in chronic cases also after running. The distal tendon area is very stiff in the morning, and the athletes have difficulty starting activities. Treatment is conservative, but surgery may be needed if problems last for more than 9–12 months. The distal tendon may be the site of a partial tear of the tendon.

In active individuals aged 8–15 years the Achilles tendon attachment (apophysis) to the calcaneus can become the site of fragmentation (Figure 12.16), a condition which is probably caused by overloading and can be seen on X-ray examination (compare Osgood–Schlatter disease, p. 323).

Symptoms and diagnosis
- Pain in the calcaneus is felt when running and walking. The complaint often remains after exertion, when stiffness sets in and causes a limp.
- Some swelling and tenderness occur over the Achilles tendon attachment to the calcaneus.
- An X-ray confirms the diagnosis.

Treatment
The *athlete* should:
- rest from painful activities until the pain has gone (the symptoms, however, often return);
- use shoes with 1 cm (0.5 in) heel wedge which can alleviate the symptoms by relieving the Achilles tendon from tension.

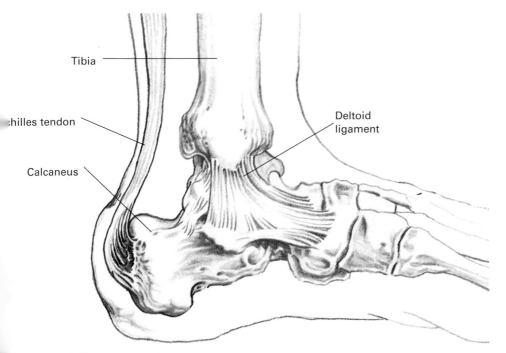

Tibia

Achilles tendon

Calcaneus

Deltoid ligament

Figure 12.16 Inflammation and breaking up of the Achilles tendon attachment to the calcaneus.

The *doctor* may:
- apply a walking boot or a plaster cast for about 3 weeks, which c give permanent pain relief;
- prescribe an orthotic device to unload the Achilles tendon (in t elderly) and plantar fascia;
- operate if major calcifications and tendon degeneration are present.

Healing

The condition resolves spontaneously in the younger athlete on reachi the age of 16–18 years when ossification of the skeleton is complete. the older athlete conservative treatment may be successful but may ta a long time.

Plantaris longus injury

The plantaris longus muscle has a long, thin tendon that inserts on t medial aspect of the calcaneus close to the Achilles tendon. It can injured with partial and total ruptures on explosive activities with pro tion involved. Only partial ruptures give remaining symptoms.

Symptoms and diagnosis
- Pain is felt on the medial aspect of the Achilles tendon when runni and jumping.
- Local tenderness occurs medial to the Achilles tendon inserti Sometimes there is swelling, and pain on plantar flexion.
- Ultrasonography or MRI may confirm the diagnosis.

Treatment

The *athlete* should:
- rest until the pain and tenderness is gone;
- use a heel wedge, and unload the tender area.

The *doctor* may:
- prescribe anti-inflammatory medication;
- excise the damaged tendon in chronic cases;
- allow use of a walking boot and early motion after surgery;
- allow gradual return to sports activities 1–3 months after surgery.

Bibliography
Kannus P, Jozsa L (1991) Histopathological changes preceeding spor neous ruptures of a tendon. *Journal of Bone and Joint Surg* 73A:1507–1525.
Leadbetter WB (1992) Cell matrix response in sports injury. *Clinic Sports Medicine* July: 533–579.

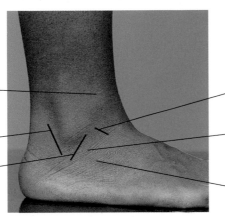

Figure 13.1 Lateral aspect of the ankle and location of associated injuries.

ndesmosis
ury (p. 372);
iofibular
nostosis (374)

roneal tendon
ury (386)

L tear (369)

ATFL tear (p. 366)

Subtalar sprain and instability (378)

Sinus tarsi syndrome (378)

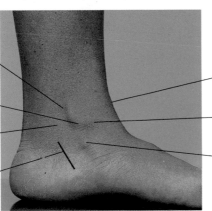

Figure 13.2 Medial aspect of the ankle and location of associated injuries.

sterior tibial
don injury
387)

ltoid ligament
r (371)

sterior
pingement
4)

xor hallucis
gus tendon
ury (389)

Anterior tibial tendon injury (p. 390)

Osteochondral lesion of the talus (379)

Posterior tibial tendon injury (387)

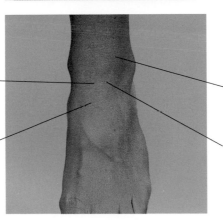

Figure 13.3 Anterior aspect of the ankle and location of associated injuries.

ne
pingement
382)

terior tibial
don injury
0)

Syndesmosis injury (p. 372); tibiofibular synostosis (374)

Soft tissue impingement (383)

The ankle joint is a remarkable example of the functional interpl[a]
between bones, joints, and ligamentous structures, with their protecti[ve]
action upon one another. The ankle joint is maintained by the wedg[e]
shaped talus and its sculptured fit between the tibia and fibula. In t[he]
neutral position of the ankle, there are strong osseous (bony) constraint[s]
With increasing plantar flexion, the osseous constraints decrease and t[he]
soft tissues and ligaments maintain the joint stability. It is in this positi[on]
that the ligamentous tissues are most susceptible to injury.

Fractures

The ankle joint is one of the areas that most frequently suffers fractur[es]
in sports. As the bones and surrounding ligaments cooperate to maint[ain]
stability in the ankle joint, combination injuries are common.

Mechanism of injury

The most common mechanism of injury is an *inward* turning of the s[ole]
of the foot and the front of the foot (supination–internal rotation). Depen[d]
ing on the force and degree of supination, different injuries can occur:
- tearing of the ligament between the talus and the fibula (the anter[ior]
  talofibular ligament);
- fracture of the fibula on a level with the joint line;
- fracture of the medial malleolus;
- dislocation of the talus.

Another common injury is an *outward* turning of the sole of the foot a[nd]
the front of the foot (pronation–external rotation). Again, differe[nt]
injuries occur depending on the force of pronation:
- tearing of the deltoid ligament or a fracture of the medial malleolu[s]
- tearing of the syndesmosis;
- fracture of the fibula above the level of the ankle joint;
- dislocation of the talus.

Other mechanisms of injury are also possible.

Symptoms   – Intense aching and pain are felt when the foot is under load.
and diagnosis   – Tenderness and considerable swelling occur.
- Sometimes there is visible displacement.
- An X-ray shows a skeletal injury.

Treatment   The *athlete* should:
- immediately cool the injury, apply a compression bandage, and elev[ate]
  the foot (see Chapter 5);
- consult a doctor.

The *doctor* may:
- apply an ankle brace, a walking boot, or a plaster cast for 4–8 week[s if]
  there is no major displacement and the ankle joint is assessed as sta[ble]

362

– operate in cases of a fracture with displacement or where there is instability of the ankle joint.

The recovery time is about as long as the immobility period, i.e. 4–8
weeks. The injured athlete can start range-of-motion and strength training exercises (p. 512) and proprioceptive training at an early stage,
depending on the type of fracture. An ankle joint fracture needs at least
2–3 months to heal to full stability, and the injured athlete should allow
a break from competition of at least 4 months. When training is resumed
a brace should be used.

After surgery during which the injured bone has been realigned to its
exact position, the prognosis is good. Slight displacement in the fracture
during healing, however, can result in wearing of the cartilage and
impaired future functioning owing to osteoarthrosis.

Ligament injuries

Ligament injuries of the ankle are among the most common sports injuries.
They occur in most ball sports, jumping sports, and so on (Figure 13.4).
There is approximately one sprain per 10 000 persons each day.

The soft tissue structure of the ankle is maintained by three groups of
ligaments functioning as static stabilizers: the lateral ligament, the deltoid
ligament and the syndesmosis complex.

The *lateral ligament* complex of the ankle is composed of three
ligaments: the anterior talofibular ligament (ATFL), the calcaneofibular
ligament (CFL), and the posterior talofibular ligament (PTFL). The
origin and insertion of these ligaments and their orientation at various

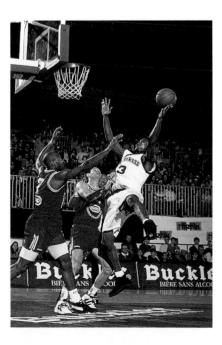

Figure 13.4 Participants in ball
sports run the risk of injuries to
the ankle ligaments when
landing (by courtesy of All Sport:
photographer, Stephen
Munday).

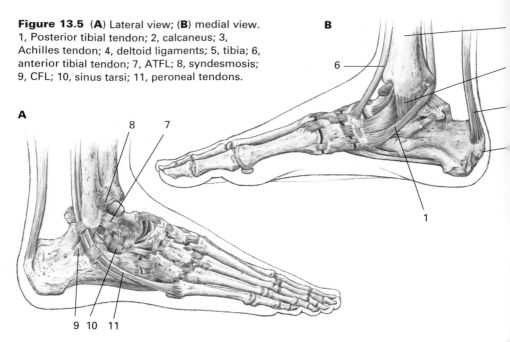

Figure 13.5 (**A**) Lateral view; (**B**) medial view. 1, Posterior tibial tendon; 2, calcaneus; 3, Achilles tendon; 4, deltoid ligaments; 5, tibia; 6, anterior tibial tendon; 7, ATFL; 8, syndesmosis; 9, CFL; 10, sinus tarsi; 11, peroneal tendons.

ankle joint positions are important in determining their potential f injury (Figure 13.5). The ATFL originates from the anterior inferi aspect of the lateral malleolus and courses anteriorly to insert laterally the neck of the talus. In the neutral position of the ankle this ligame is nearly parallel with the long axis of the foot. As the ankle moves ir full plantar flexion, it becomes parallel with the long axis of the tibia function as a primary ligament resisting ankle inversion. This ligame is the most often injured in inversion ankle sprains.

The CFL originates from the inferior aspect of the lateral malleol and is directed slightly posteriorly and distally to insert on the late aspect of the calcaneus. It contributes to the subtalar stability. In neutral position of the ankle the CFL is nearly parallel with the long a of the tibia providing lateral stability to the ankle. As the ankle moves plantar flexion, the CFL approaches a perpendicular position with fibula and, therefore, has less mechanical advantage for providing an stability.

The PTFL originates from the posterior medial aspect of the late malleolus and runs posteromedially to the posterior process of the tal This ligament assists in preventing posterior displacement of the talus relationship to the fibula. It is the least commonly injured ligament i lateral ankle sprain.

The *deltoid ligament* is a broad, fan-shaped ligament on the med aspect of the ankle expanding both the ankle and subtalar joints. It a superficial and a deep component. Functionally it resists eversion the talus in relationship to the tibia and of the calcaneus in relations to the talus.

The ankle *syndesmosis* comprises the anterior and posterior tibiofibu ligaments, the interosseous membrane, and the transverse syndesm ligament. This complex stabilizes the ankle mortise and may be inju in a lateral ankle sprain with the ankle in the dorsiflexed position.

Ankle ligament biomechanics

The ATFL, the CFL, and the PTFL function as a unit, and although one ligament may resist a specific motion, the primary stabilizing ligament is dependent upon foot position. Both the ATFL and CFL play a significant role in stabilizing the ankle, but in different positions.

The ATFL and CFL act synergistically when the foot is unloaded. With and without physiologic loading of the ankle the articular surface becomes an important stabilizer, accounting for 30% of stability in rotation and 100% of stability in inversion. Without loading, the primary and secondary ligamentous constraints vary with testing modes and ankle position. Ligament loads remain low within the functional range of motion (10° of dorsiflexion to 20° of plantar flexion). This supports the concept that ankle ligaments act as kinematic guides rather than primary restraints during normal activity. With external loading, however, the ATFL functions as a primary stabilizer against inversion and internal rotation for all angles of plantar flexion. The CFL and PTFL function as primary stabilizers against inversion and external rotation for all angles of dorsiflexion. The ATFL is the weakest ligament, having the lowest yield force and ultimate load. The CFL is the second weakest ligament, and the PTFL is the strongest lateral-collateral ligament.

Mechanism of injury

A *lateral ankle sprain* frequently occurs when a plantar-flexed ankle is inverted, completely rupturing one or more of the lateral ligaments. An isolated ATFL tear is present in about two-thirds of the cases. The second most common injury is a combined rupture of the ATFL and CFL, which occurs in about 20–25% of the cases. The PTFL is rarely injured except in severe ankle trauma.

A *medial ankle sprain* may occur when the foot is everted and externally rotated. Isolated ruptures of the medial deltoid ligament are rare, and usually occur in combination with fractures of the lateral malleolus and rupture of the syndesmosis.

The *syndesmosis* can also rupture, most commonly partially It is usually completely ruptured in combination with fractures and deltoid ligament tears. A complete rupture occurs in isolation in only 3%.

The risk for future arthrosis development and ankle instability is great if syndesmosis rupture is not recognized and treated correctly. It is, therefore, extremely important that the doctor is aware of the risk of this injury, and that it is diagnosed adequately through careful history taking, location of tenderness, stability assessment, and radiology.

Classification and grading

The classification of ankle sprains is based on the mechanism of injury. Excessive inversion motion of the tibiotalar joint in varying degrees of plantar or dorsiflexion results in an inversion or lateral ankle sprain. Excessive eversion motion of the ankle joint results in an injury to the medial aspect of the ankle and the deltoid ligament, and eversion ankle sprain. An ankle sprain is further stratified into grade I, II, or III based on the severity of the injury:

- grade I: ligament stretch without microscopic tearing, minimal swelling or tenderness, minimal functional loss, no mechanical joint instability
- grade II: partial microscopic ligament tear with moderate pain, swelling, and tenderness over the involved structures. There is some loss of joint motion and mild to moderate joint instability;
- grade III: complete ligament rupture with marked swelling, hemorrhage, and tenderness. There is a loss of function and severe joint instability. These patients have difficulties with full weightbearing.

Every sprain in which the range of movement of the ankle joint has been exceeded causes damage to the stabilizing tissues with bleeding, swelling and tenderness, and should be considered as a ligament injury. In cases of sprains and dislocations it is mainly the lateral and medial ligaments of the ankle joint that tear. Sometimes a small portion of bone is torn away at the point of ligament attachment, while the ligament itself remains intact. This type of avulsion injury is found in young, growing athletes with strong ligaments, and also in elderly individuals with brittle bones.

Ligament injuries in the ankle joint should never be neglected, as correct treatment often ensures complete recovery. A return to sporting activity should be deferred until there is no pain, and normal mobility and strength have been restored to the ankle joint. The injured athlete therefore should allow 4–12 weeks' break from training, depending on the degree of severity of the injury. When starting to strengthen the ankle joint by training, the joint should be supported by tape or bandage (p. 107). Gradually, proprioceptive training should be started.

When instability is present in the ankle joint after treatment has finished or after repeated trauma to the joint, surgery may be necessary.

Tear of the ATFL

The ligament in the ankle joint most frequently injured – the ATFL – runs between the fibula and the talus. Its main function is to prevent the foot from slipping forwards in relation to the tibia. In about 65–70% of ligament injuries of the ankle, this ligament alone is injured. In about 20% of cases there is a combination injury, with tears of the ATFL and the CFL. The mechanism of injury is usually a supination (inward rotation of the foot (Figures 13.6 and 13.7).

Symptoms and diagnosis
- Pain is felt on weightbearing and ankle motion.
- Swelling and tenderness occur anterior to the lateral malleolus.
- Effusion of blood later results in a hematoma, with bruising and skin discoloration around and distal to the injury.
- Instability in cases of a total ligament tear can be tested by pulling the foot forwards in relation to the tibia (*anterior drawer test*) (Figure 13.?). This test evaluates the integrity of the ATFL. The maximum amount

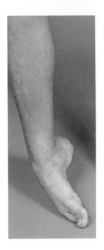
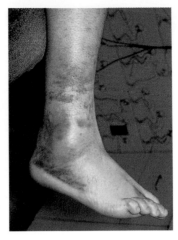

Figure 13.6 (Left) Mechanism of injury in ATFL tear. **(Right)** Injured ankle.

Figure 13.7 ATFL tear.

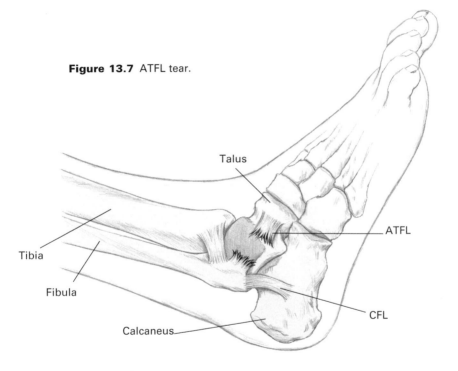

Talus

ATFL

Tibia

Fibula

CFL

Calcaneus

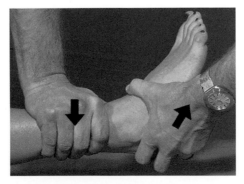

Figure 13.8 Examination of the stability of the foot in cases of suspected injury to the anterior talofibular ligament. The hand should grasp the calcaneus and talus as it is essential to test the stability of the joint between the tibia and fibula and the talus. The examiner should try to pull the foot forwards in relation to the lower leg.

of anterior displacement is produced when the ankle is in 10° of plant.
flexion; normal displacement is less than 3–4 mm (0.12–0.16 in).
comparison with the other side should be made.

- The *inversion stress test* (former talar tilt test, p. 370) evaluates the integri.
  of the CFL. With the ankle in neutral and the distal tibia stabilized, a
  eversion stress is placed on the heel and the tilt deformity of the hindfo.
  relative to the distal tibia is assessed. The normal range is 0–30°. Compa
  ison with the contralateral uninjured ankle is recommended.

- An evaluation of an acute ankle sprain is *optimally carried out 4–7 da.*
  after injury. It is then possible to detect the most tender areas by palp
  tion, indicating where the ligament injuries are. Stability will also t
  more reliable. Hematoma formation and spreading can be evaluated

- Stress X-rays during provocative testing of the anterior drawer ar
  talar tilt may aid in assessing ligament disruption. These tests are tod.
  mostly used for research purposes. Other tests such as MRI give
  good evaluation of the ankle ligaments (Figure 13.9), but are rare
  needed in the acute setting. Ankle joint arthrography, peroneal teno.
  raphy, and bone scans are seldom indicated.

Treatment

The treatment depends on the grade of the injury, but also on t.
functional capacity and whether there are recurrent 'giving wa.
problems.

The *athlete* should:
- avoid painful sporting activities;
- apply a compression bandage (see Figure 5.2), elevation, and cc
  treatment (see Chapter 5);
- start early *functional treatment* including early motion and weightbea.
  ing, using an ankle brace or other stabilizing support;
- start early rehabilitation with range-of-motion exercises, strength trai.
  ing, and functional activities (protocol on p. 521).

The *doctor* may:
- X-ray the joint in a grade III sprain or if an ankle gives persistent pa.
  in order to determine whether there is a fracture or an avulsion inju.
  (an X-ray is especially indicated if there is distinct tenderness over t
  tips of the malleoli and the posterior aspect of the fibula);

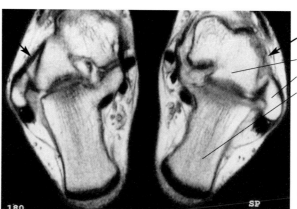

3
2
1

Figure 13.9 M
of normal ATFL
(**left**) and torn
ATFL (**right**).
1, Calcaneus;
2, distal fibular
(lateral) malleol.
3, talus.

– start proprioceptive training with a tiltboard. These exercises can usually begin within 2 weeks for grade I and grade II injuries, to improve balance and neuromuscular control, and should be continued for at least 10 weeks for maximum effect.

Surgery is seldom necessary, but may be indicated if there is a history of recurrent major and complete ligamentous disruption in a top athlete. After surgery the ankle is mobilized in a walking boot or a cast for 6 weeks, but motion outside the boot is allowed. Return to sport is possible within 10–12 weeks. If a large avulsion injury is present, surgery may be indicated, but functional treatment similar to that used for ankle sprains is the treatment of choice.

Healing and complications

The healing of a ligament injury in the ankle joint can take 1 week for a grade I injury, 2–3 weeks for a grade II injury, and 4–8 weeks for a grade III injury, depending on the severity of the impact and the extent of the injury. However, problems can remain for 8–10 months after the incident. When the injured athlete has no pain on moving the ankle joint and has good mobility athletic training—often with an ankle support—can start (p. 521).

Proprioceptive training is extremely important, otherwise the ligament is liable to be injured again. Strengthening of the tibialis anterior and peroneus longus and brevis should also be carried out. During the training period, which can extend over 6–8 weeks, the ankle should be protected from further overstretching with the help of an ankle brace, an adhesive strapping, an elastic bandage, or tape. An untreated ligament injury can result in stretching of the ligament which can lead to permanent instability with recurrent sprains.

If a ligament injury still causes problems with recurrent instability after 6 months, the ligament can be sutured together or surgically reconstructed (see p. 377).

Tear of the CFL

On supination and dorsiflexion of the foot an isolated injury can occur to the CFL (Figure 13.10). This is rare, however, and it is more likely to be injured in combination with the ATFL.

Symptoms and diagnosis

– Swelling and tenderness occur over the injured ligament, distal to the lateral malleolus.
– Pain is felt during weightbearing and when moving the ankle joint.
– Effusion of blood causes hematoma and bruising behind and below the lateral malleolus.
– The *inversion stress test* (former talar tilt test) shows increased supination compared with the undamaged ankle joint (Figure 13.11).
– A stress X-ray with inversion stress test provocation is occasionally used to confirm the diagnosis.

Treatment

The treatment is the same as for an ATFL tear, but in addition the *athlete* should consult a doctor if there is persistent pain or recurrent instability.

Figure 13.10 (Top) Mechanism of CFL tear. **(Below)** Rupture of the ligament between fibula and calcaneus.

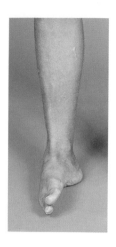

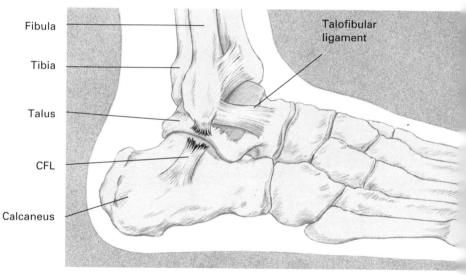

Fibula

Tibia

Talus

CFL

Calcaneus

Talofibular ligament

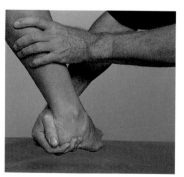

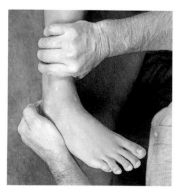

Figure 13.11 Inversic stress test. This tests both ATFL and CFL integrity.

The *doctor* may recommend supporting the ankle joint with an ank brace, an adhesive strapping, an elastic bandage, or a plaster cast about 2–3 weeks if the injury is serious. Surgery may be needed ir combination injury with the ATFL.

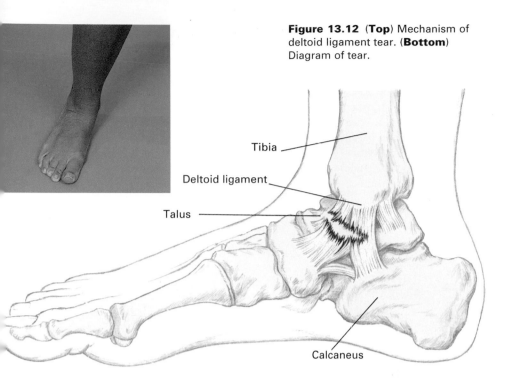

Tibia

Deltoid ligament

Talus

Calcaneus

Tear of the deltoid ligament

In less than 3% of all cases of ligament injuries in the ankle joint the deltoid ligament is damaged. Usually the tear is partial and injury occurs during pronation when the sole of the foot is turned outward. Tears of the deltoid ligament are most often located in the anterior aspect of the deltoid ligament (Figure 13.12).

Symptoms and diagnosis
- Pain is felt on weightbearing and on moving the ankle joint.
- Swelling and tenderness occur over the course of the ligament, usually in the anterior part of the medial malleolus.
- When the tear is complete, there is increased pronation in comparison with the range of movement of the undamaged joint.

Treatment

The *athlete* may:
- apply compression, elevation, and cold treatment (see Chapter 5),
- start early functional treatment;
- consult a doctor.

The *doctor* may:
- in cases of partial tear and maintained stability support the ankle joint with a brace, adhesive strapping, or an elastic bandage for 3–4 weeks;
- when it is difficult to decide if instability is present, examine the joint with the patient under anesthesia. The joint is rarely unstable. Surgery may be needed, followed by immobilization in a walking boot or a plaster cast for 4–6 weeks.

Injury to the syndesmosis

The syndesmosis comprises the anterior and posterior tibiofibular ligaments and the interosseous membrane. Diastasis (widening) of the syndesmosis occurs with partial or complete rupture of the syndesmosis ligament complex, including the tibiofibular ligaments and the interosseous membrane. About 10% of all ankle ligament injuries involve a partial tear of the anterior part of the syndesmosis. Partial tears of the inferior ATFL are more common in football players owing to the frequent occurrence of violent external rotation and plantar flexion trauma of the ankle.

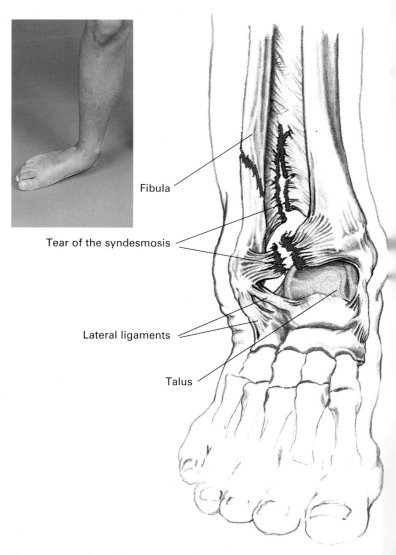

Fibula

Tear of the syndesmosis

Lateral ligaments

Talus

Figure 13.13 (Inset) Mechanism of injury to syndesmosis. **(Right)** A rupture of the syndesmosis is often combined with a fracture of the fibula and/or an injury to the deltoid ligament. The same stability examination is carried out as in cases of a rupture of the deltoid ligament, but in this case the foot is pushed straight out laterally.

Isolated complete syndesmosis injuries without fracture are rare; in a series of more than 400 ankle ligament ruptures, 12 cases (3%) of isolated syndesmosis rupture were identified. These ruptures occurred in various sports, such as skiing, motocross, skating, soccer and other ball sports, and seem to be increasingly more common in American football. Rupture of the syndesmosis is often associated with rupture of the deltoid ligament or the medial malleolus. This rupture is partial and often involves the anterior aspect. Major instability involves the middle, deep, and superficial part of the deltoid ligament.

The importance of an accurate history to ascertain the mechanism of injury and a careful clinical examination of the patient with acute ankle trauma cannot be stressed enough. The mechanism of injury may be pronation and eversion is combined with external rotation of the foot.

Symptoms and diagnosis

- Tenderness and swelling occur at the anterior aspect of the syndesmosis between the tibia and the fibula. Less sharp pain is felt at the posterior region of the syndesmosis.
- The athlete is unable to bear weight on the injured leg
- Active external rotation of the foot is painful. The *external rotation test* is carried out with the leg hanging and the knee in 90° of flexion; the foot is externally rotated while the tibia is fixed with the other hand (Figure 13.14). Pain around the syndesmosis during this test is a strong indication of syndesmosis injury.
- The *squeeze test* is considered positive if compression of the tibia against the fibula at the midportion of the calf proximal to the syndesmosis produces pain in the area of the interosseous membrane or its supporting structures (Figure 13.15).
- The *Cotton test* is carried out with one hand holding the calcaneus and talus while the foot is tested for motion in a medial-lateral direction with the tibia fixed (Figure 13.16). It assesses the medial–lateral motion of the talus in the ankle. A feeling of side-to-side play when the foot is in neutral position is considered an indication of possible diastasis.
- Anteroposterior lateral and mortise view radiographs are needed to exclude fractures and avulsions. Stress radiographs in external rotation in both dorsiflexion and plantar flexion can display the diastasis between the tibia and the fibula. This test still needs to be validated. A widening of the ankle mortise is a sign of syndesmosis tear.

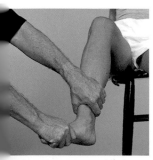

Figure 13.14 External rotation test.

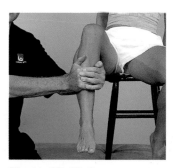

Figure 13.15 Squeeze test.

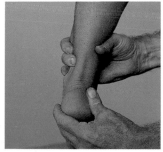

Figure 13.16 Cotton test.

- Bone scanning is a reliable procedure that can be used to guide initi
management when stress X-rays cannot be obtained because of pa
or swelling, or are unreliable.
- An MRI scan is sometimes needed to evaluate the extent of the inju
and is now considered the examination of choice.

Treatment

The *athlete* should:
- apply compression, elevation and cold treatment (see Chapter 5);
- consult a doctor as soon as possible.

The *doctor* may:
- in cases of partial isolated syndesmosis tears, treat the injury conser
atively, with an ankle brace and early functional treatment;
- in cases with complete tears of the syndesmosis, decide on surgery.
the syndesmosis is completely ruptured, the fibula can shorten a
rotate externally leading to ankle joint incongruency and degeneratie
A complete tear is managed by suturing the ligament and tempora
fixation of the tibia and fibula with a screw, staple, or cerclage (ste
wire). A walking boot or brace is applied for 6–8 weeks. Early moti
is encouraged. The syndesmosis screw is usually removed 8–12 wee
after surgery.

Complications

Late complications include incongruency of the ankle joint, late arthr
sis, and calcification of the interosseous ligament.

Tibiofibular synostosis

Tibiofibular synostosis (ossification of the syndesmosis) can occur af
an ankle sprain associated with a syndesmosis rupture. The rupt
produces periosteal damage and a hematoma, which later ossifies, lead
to partial or complete ossification of the syndesmosis.

The typical patient is an athlete with a history of an acute or recurr
ankle sprain in whom syndesmosis rupture was not considered; 3
months after the injury, the patient experiences pain during the sta
phase and the initiation of the push-off phase of running and cutting. T
pain occurs because the synostosis impairs the normal tibiofibular mot
by preventing fibular descent on weightbearing and by restricting
normal increase in width of the ankle mortise that occurs on dorsiflex
of the talus. Clinical examination usually reveals restricted dorsiflexior
the ankle. Radiographs show development of the synostosis.

Therapy is aimed at removing the synostosis and restoring nor
fibular motion. If the athlete is experiencing symptoms, surgical excis
and reduction of the diastasis are indicated after the synostosis
matured.

Inadequate rehabilitation syndrome

Many athletes return to sports before they are fully rehabilitated and o
incur a re-injury or an additional injury. Examination demonstrates los

range of motion, such as limited dorsiflexion or a plantar flexion contracture. Hypotrophy of the lower leg muscles is common. Ankle motion may be painful and stiffness is common, although the X-rays are normal.

To prevent this problem, adequate acute treatment of ankle ligament injuries is important. Functional treatment should be the method of choice for complete rupture of the lateral ankle ligaments. Initial treatment should include a short period of ankle protection by brace, bandage, or tape, and early mobilization and weightbearing. Rehabilitation exercises are the most important step in the treatment process, with the goal of re-establishing ankle range of motion, muscle strength, and neuromuscular control. Emphasis should be placed on strength training of the peroneal muscles, the anterior and posterior muscles, and the intrinsic muscles of the foot. Proprioceptive training on an ankle tiltboard should be combined with increasing agility and sports skills training. If functional treatment of an acute injury fails, surgery may be necessary.

Immobilization with a lower-leg cast for 2–3 weeks is still common treatment; however, immobilization will result in weakening of all tissues, as well as hypotrophy of the muscles and limitation of motion, although may give a better stability in the end.

Inadequate rehabilitation syndrome can be prevented by scrupulously continuing rehabilitation until the patient has achieved full range of motion, strength, and the ability to walk and run. Full rehabilitation often requires careful supervision and monitoring by an experienced physical therapist. Compliance by the patient is essential for success.

If the syndrome does occur, treatment is reinstitution of the rehabilitation program. This treatment is usually successful.

Chronic ankle instability

Recurring ankle injury is common: 50–75% of patients have recurrent sprains, and 25% report frequent sprains. If mechanical instability is documented radiographically 80% will experience recurrent sprains.

Certain sports create particular risks. Soccer players with previous injuries are 2–3 times more likely to sustain another ankle injury than those without any history of injury. Recurrent multiple sprains are reported by 80% of high-school basketball players with a previous sprain.

Chronic ankle instability can be characterized as mechanical or functional (Figure 13.17).

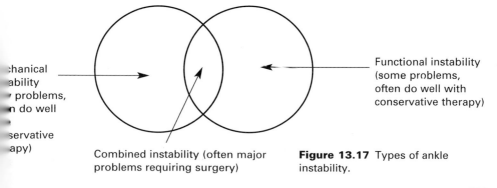

Mechanical ability problems, can do well conservative therapy)

Combined instability (often major problems requiring surgery)

Functional instability (some problems, often do well with conservative therapy)

Figure 13.17 Types of ankle instability.

Mechanical instability

Mechanical instability is characterized by ankle mobility beyond the phys
ologic range of motion, which is identified on the basis of a positive anteri
drawer and/or inversion stress test (talar tilt test). However, the criteria f
mechanical instability are variable. Most agree that mechanical instability
present when (1) there is more than 10 mm (0.4 in) of anterior translati
on one side or the side-to-side difference is over 3 mm (0.12 in), and/or (
the talar tilt is more than 9° on one side or the side-to-side difference
more than 3° on stress X-rays. However, pure mechanical instability of t
ankle is rarely the reason for the development of late symptoms.

Functional instability

Functional instability is signaled by a subjective feeling of the an
'giving way' during physical activity or during simple everyday routin
after a sprain. Frequent ankle sprains are associated with recurrent pa
and swelling. Functional instability can be described as mobility beyo
voluntary control; however, the physiologic range of motion is not nec
sarily exceeded. The diagnosis of functional instability is made prim
ily on the basis of a history of frequent and recurrent giving way, whi
is often associated with difficulty in walking on uneven ground.

The physical examination may show evidence of mechanical instab
ity, but this finding is not necessary to make the diagnosis. Functio
instability is frequently associated with muscle weakness and hypotrop
but this is often subtle. The incidence of functional instability after an
sprains has been reported to range from 15% to 60% and seems to
independent of the degree of severity of the initial injury.

The etiology of functional instability is complex, with important ro
for several types of factors—neural (proprioception, reflexes, and musc
lar reaction time), muscular (strength, power, and endurance), a
mechanical (lateral ligamentous laxity). Other possible factors have a
been considered, such as adhesion (scar) formation leading to decreas
mobility of the ankle, especially in dorsiflexion; peroneal mus
weakness; and tibiofibular sprain and articular cartilage damage.

An ankle sprain may be followed by complications, including mecha
cal instability, muscle hypotrophy, and functional instability. The mag
tude of disability correlates best with how many of these sequelae
present. The association between functional and mechanical instabi
remains unclear. Repeated sprains caused by functional instability r
later result in mechanical instability. Mechanical and functional instabi
may be sequential, but the two do not always occur together. Functic
instability is prevalent in 80% of patients with mechanical instability, :
in 40% of patients with mechanical stability. With continuing recurr
pains, the two instabilities tend to become coexistent. Chronic lateral ar
instability syndrome is most commonly a combination of mechanical
functional instability, regardless of the clinical manifestation.

Chronic ankle instability is often characterized by repeated episode
'giving way' with asymptomatic periods between episodes. In contr
athletes with other causes of chronic ankle pain usually experienc
constant aching discomfort in the ankle, although symptoms may v
This difference in history can often be an important key to the cor
diagnosis.

The *athlete* should:
– carry out functional rehabilitation including proprioceptive and muscle exercises (p. 520) such as tilt board training.
– use an ankle brace or tape to provide external stabilization.
The *doctor* may operate if there are recurrent 'giving way' episodes (see below).

Surgical treatment of ankle instability

Isolated mechanical instability without symptoms such as pain and 'giving way' is not in itself an indication for surgery. Rather, it is the combination of mechanical and functional instability that is the most commonly reported indication for surgery (see Figure 13.17).

It should be emphasized that repeated episodes of giving way do not seem to predispose to degenerative arthritis (loss of joint cartilage) in the ankle, but this may develop over a long period. The main reason for surgery is that the patient is not willing to accept the discomfort and functional loss that follows the recurrent 'giving way' episodes. The decision to operate is based on the history and clinical examination findings. Stress radiographs can sometimes be of value. Surgical procedures can be divided into nonanatomic reconstructions, in which another structure (such as the peroneal tendon) is substituted for the injured ligament, and anatomic reconstructions, in which the injured ligament is repaired secondarily with or without augmentation (reinforcement). With the anatomic techniques, usually both the ATFL and the CFL are reconstructed with the nonanatomic techniques, the normal biomechanics cannot be restored (Figure 13.18).

After an anatomic reconstruction, a posterior splint or brace should be used for 8–10 days to allow the wound to heal. Thereafter, a brace or walking boot should be used. The ankle can be taken out of the boot to

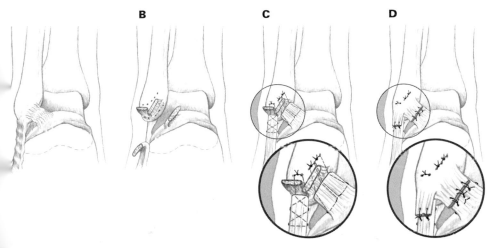

jure 13.18 Lateral ankle ligament reconstruction. (**A**) Ligament elongation after insufficient aling of ATFL and CFL, causing functional and mechanical instability. (**B**) Elongated ligament ided 3–5 mm from fibular insertion; drillholes through the lateral malleolus to roughened faces under ligament insertions. (**C**) Sutures through drillholes and distal ligament ends are ntened over bone bridges at the lateral malleolus (ankle in pronation). (**D**) Proximal ligament ls sutured back to reinforce the ligaments.

allow movement of the foot in 0–20° of plantar flexion. The healing time is 6 weeks, and return to full activity is possible after 10–14 weeks (rehabilitation protocol on p. 522).

The results of anatomic reconstruction are reported to be good or excellent in around 90%. Four factors may predict poor outcome: (1) history of 10 years or more of instability prior to surgery; (2) associated ankle osteoarthrosis; (3) generalized joint hypermobility and; (4) previous tendon reconstruction (tenodesis).

The anatomic technique is considered simple and allows early return to function. It should be the primary choice when surgery is indicated.

Subtalar sprain and instability

The subtalar joints consist of the talocalcaneal and talonavicular joints. The subtalar sprain has remained a mysterious and little-known clinical entity. The incidence is unknown, but it is widely accepted that most subtalar ligamentous injuries occur in combination with injuries of the lateral ligament of the ankle. Subtalar instability is estimated to be present in about 10% of patients with lateral instability of the ankle. A severe subtalar instability includes damage to the interosseous ligament.

An athlete with chronic subtalar instability usually describes 'giving way' episodes during activity and has a history of recurrent sprains and/or pain, swelling, and stiffness. There is a feeling of instability, especially when walking on uneven ground. Because the symptoms in subtalar and ankle instability are similar, athletes with a clinically serious recurrent ankle sprain should be carefully evaluated for subtalar instability. Localized tenderness on palpation over the subtalar joint is suggestive of involvement of the subtalar ligaments, but clinical evaluation of subtalar instability is difficult and unreliable. If a major sprain of a subtalar joint is suspected clinically, the diagnosis can be verified with subtalar arthrography, a subtalar stress view, or stress tomography. Although scientific studies proving the value of CT and MR imaging are not yet available, one or the other may ultimately be established as the best diagnostic modality.

The treatment is functional with exercises (as for ankle sprain, p. 51) and the use of an ankle brace. Surgery is occasionally indicated: anatomic reconstruction can be used.

Sinus tarsi syndrome

The sinus tarsi is located on the lateral aspect of the hindfoot (see Figure 13.5A). Sinus tarsi syndrome (pain at the lateral junction of the talus and calcaneus) is characterized by pain and tenderness over the lateral opening of the sinus tarsi, accompanied by a feeling of instability and giving way of the ankle. This is an uncommon injury: about 70% of affected athletes will have sustained trauma, usually a severe inversion sprain of the ankle. If the CFL is torn, the interosseous talocalcaneal ligament, which occupies the sinus, can be sprained as well. In most cases the ligaments heal quickly with little residual disability. However, because of the abundance of synovial tissue in the sinus tarsi area, synovitis may ensue.

| **Symptoms and diagnosis** | – Pain and tenderness at the sinus tarsi are often combined with a feeling of instability. |

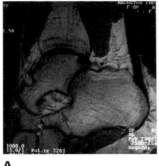 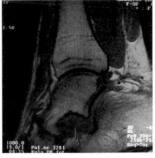

Figure 13.19 (**A**) MRI of normal sinus tarsi. (**B**) MRI showing sinus tarsi filled with edema.

- Pain on the lateral side of the foot is increased by firm pressure of the lateral opening of the sinus tarsi; this is a characteristic clinical sign.
- Pain is most severe when the patient is standing or walking on uneven ground.
- An MRI scan may demonstrate a rupture of the talocalcaneal interosseous ligament and signs of synovitis (Figure 13.19). The role of MRI in this case is, however, not fully evaluated.

reatment

The *doctor* may:
- give an injection of local anesthetic solution and corticosteroids into the sinus tarsi; this usually relieves the pain. Approximately two-thirds of patients respond to injections at weekly intervals (2–4 times). The number of injections should be limited because of the small amount of subcutaneous tissue in the area;
- carry out surgery with excision of the tissue filling the lateral half of the sinus tarsi. In refractory cases subtalar arthrodesis (stiffening of the joint) may be indicated.

Persistent ankle pain

Persistent ankle pain after an ankle sprain may be caused by incomplete rehabilitation, intra-articular injuries which include osteochondral or chondral lesions of the talus, loose bodies, arthrosis and impingement problems, as well as chronic tendon disorders involving the peroneal tendons and posterior tibialis tendons. Undetected fractures and nerve injuries may be present.

Osteochondral lesions of the talus

Osteochondral lesions, which involve injury to the bone (osseous) and articular cartilage (chondral) tissues, can be sustained during an ankle sprain. Osteochondral injury has been reported to occur in 6.5% of patients who have had an ankle sprain, and some form of chondral injury

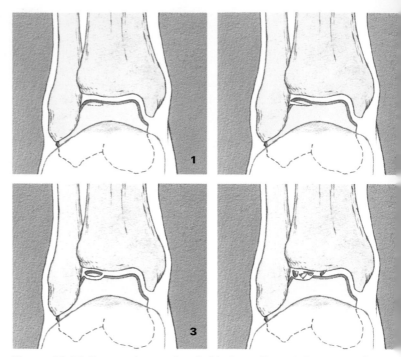

Figure 13.20 Stages of osteochondral lesions. *Stage 1:* A compression injury has caused microscopic damage to an area of subchondral bone. Pla X-rays appear normal. *Stage 2:* A partially detached osteochondral fragmen is detectable on X-ray. *Stage 3:* The osteochondral fragment is completely detached but remains in anatomic position. *Stage 4:* The detached fragmen is located elsewhere in the joint.

may occur in more than 50%. There are four stages of osteochond lesions (Figure 13.20).

Symptoms and diagnosis

 – There is often a history of ankle sprains with 'popping' sensations. ligament tear may mask the pain from an osteochondral lesion.
 – Pain is felt during and after exercise.
 – Swelling of the ankle occurs.
 – Tenderness may be present on the lateral side, occasionally on medial side. The lesions are most commonly located in the antero eral or posteromedial parts of the ankle.
 – A locking sensation of the joint is experienced.
 – Ankle movement is limited.
 – An X-ray will often confirm the diagnosis. Examination is made w anteroposterior, lateral, and mortise views in ankle flexion and ext sion. Mortise views in plantar flexion may disclose a posterome lesion, and corresponding views in dorsiflexion may disclose an ante lateral lesion;
 – Bone scan is indicated in patients with persistent pain if routine rays are negative (Figure 13.21).
 – Plain tomography, MRI, or a CT scan (Figure 13.22) can determ the exact location and extent of the lesion.

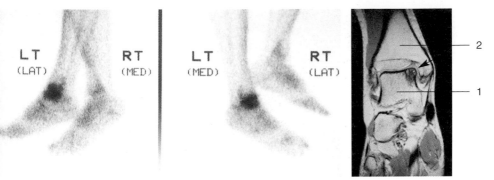

Figure 13.21 Bone scans of osteochondral lesion of talus. Dark areas show increased uptake.

Figure 13.22 MR scan of medial osteochondral lesion of talus (arrow). 1, Talus; 2, tibia.

Treatment

The *athlete* should:
– avoid pain-causing situations;
– keep up conditioning with cycling and other nonpounding activities.

The *doctor* may:
– treat stage 1 and stage 2 lesions conservatively; they often heal well and have a good prognosis;
– give an intra-articular injection of 10 ml of local anesthetic solution to help differentiate the pain caused by these lesions from that of other causes. If there is relief of pain, surgery can be considered;
– carry out early surgery on stage 3 and 4 lesions; delayed operative treatment of these lesions often fails. These injuries are treated by arthroscopic debridement. Drilling of the lesion bed may encourage repair with fibrocartilage. Open treatment is occasionally necessary, with bone grafting in large bony defects. Postoperative weightbearing is delayed for at least 2–6 weeks.

Healing and return to sports

The degree of success depends in part on the time between the occurrence of the injury and surgical treatment. Good results are reported in 40–80% of the cases if treatment is early. Advanced lesions for which treatment has been delayed for more than 1 year generally have a poor outcome. Return to sport depends on the healing.

Loose bodies in the ankle

Loose bodies originating from a stage 4 transchondral fracture of the talus should be suspected in patients with intermittent pain, swelling, and clicking. A few loose bodies may also originate from osteophytes (bony deposits) on the anterior distal rim of the tibia or the dorsal neck of the talus. Pure chondral loose bodies may cause the same problems; in these cases, plain X-rays will appear normal, and loose bodies can be detected with arthrography, CT, or MRI. Arthroscopy (Figure 13.23) will secure the diagnosis of osteochondral lesions. The treatment is arthroscopic removal of the loose bodies, sometimes with debridement and drilling of the lesion bed.

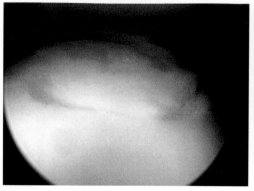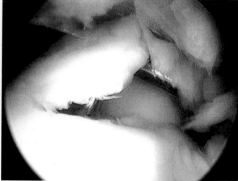

Figure 13.23 Arthroscopy of osteochondritis dissecans on medial aspect of talus. (**Left**) Fragment in place; (**right**) partially detached fragment.

Impingement problems

Bone impingement (footballer's ankle)

In cases of untreated acute or chronic overstretching of the ankle join changes can occur in the form of osteophytes anteriorly where the joi capsule is attached. The condition is not uncommon and mainly affec athletes who for many years have been participating in football, cros country running, orienteering, and so on. The cause may be hyperexte sion or hyperflexion of the ankle joint which causes traction in t attachment of the joint capsule or minor fractures due to impacts betwe the bone surfaces (Figure 13.24). The bony deposits can cause inflamm tion in the joint capsule and tendon sheaths.

Symptoms and diagnosis

– Tenderness is felt when pressing with the fingers over the front of t ankle joint. Sometimes the osteophytes can be felt.
– Pain occurs as a band across the ankle joint, e.g. when kicking soccer.
– Pain occurs when the foot is bent up or down.
– Mobility in the ankle joint is often slightly impaired.
– Osteophytes show up on X-ray.

Treatment

The *athlete* should:
– carry out strength and mobility training and also static stretchi exercises;
– try a heel lift (a build-up under the heel);
– use a heat retainer;
– apply brace or tape.

The *doctor* may:
– administer a steroid injection into the tender spot and prescribe re
– operate in cases of pronounced problems, with arthroscopic remo of the osteophytes. Postoperative recommendations include ea motion and return to physical activity, in most cases after 1–2 mont

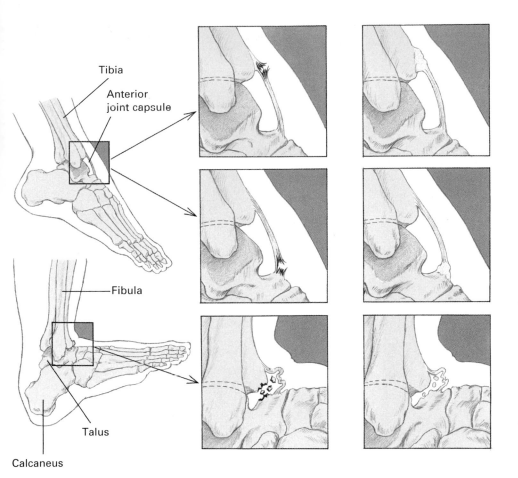

Tibia

Anterior
joint capsule

Fibula

Talus

Calcaneus

gure 13.24 Possible mechanisms of bone changes at the front of the ankle joint. (**Top left**)
·erstretching in passive plantar flexion. (**Bottom left**) Overstretching in passive dorsiflexion.
·e middle diagrams show alternative injuries in their acute stages, and the diagrams to the right
·ow chronic conditions.

Soft tissue impingement: meniscoid lesion, lateral gutter syndrome

An inversion sprain may result in post traumatic synovitis (inflammation
of the joint lining) with synovial thickening and an effusion. The term
'meniscoid lesion' has been used to describe entrapment of a mass of
hyalinized tissue between the talus and the fibula during ankle motion.
A ligamentous origin has been recognized. After an inversion sprain of
the ankle, ligament and capsule may impinge on the anterolateral aspect
of the talus. Meniscoid lesions may also be tears of the ATFL in which
the torn fragment becomes interposed between the lateral malleolus and
the lateral aspect of the talus—the lateral gutta syndrome.

mptoms   – The key to correct diagnosis is awareness of this lesion.
d diagnosis   – A long history of repeated ankle sprains is characteristic.

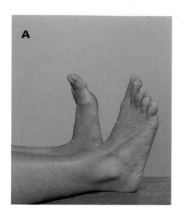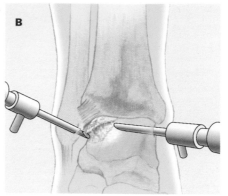

Figure 13.25
(**A**) Limited dorsiflexion is a very common finding in soft tissue impingement. (**B**) Arthroscopic surgery to remove the lesion.

- Occasional locking and catching sensations occur.
- A snapping phenomenon can be elicited when the foot is tested f inversion stability.
- Pain is experienced at push-off.
- Pain and discomfort occur at the anterior aspects of the ankle.
- Tenderness is felt just anterior to the lateral malleolus and discomfc in dorsiflexion, which often is limited.
- There is no evidence of mechanical instability, and X-rays are norm
- Often there is limitation of dorsiflexion of 5–10° compared with t other side. This is a diagnostic finding (Figure 13.25).
- Relief of symptoms after injection of 10 ml of anesthetic solution the point of tenderness supports the diagnosis.
- An MRI scan can help to establish the diagnosis.

Treatment

The *athlete* may:
- carry out dorsiflexion stretching;
- use a heel wedge;
- use an ankle brace.

The *doctor* may carry out arthroscopic examination to confirm t diagnosis and remove the lesion. Return to full activity is possible in weeks to 2 months.

Posterior impingement, os trigonum

Posterior impingement syndrome is most common in ballet dancers. occurs with weightbearing with the foot in plantar flexion. It is usually but not always—associated with an os trigonum, a small extra bone the back of the talus; however, an os trigonum can be present with causing pain. Impingement may also be caused by a fracture of the pos rior aspect of talus.

Symptoms and diagnosis

- tenderness is felt behind the outside of the ankle.
- Pain is felt at the outside back portion of the ankle when pointing toes downwards, especially with weightbearing.

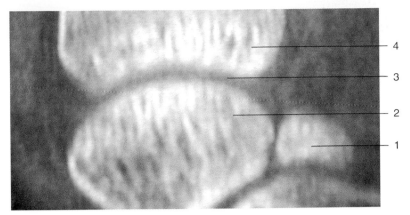

Figure 13.26 X-ray of os trigonum posterior to ankle joint contributing to posterior impingement. 1, Os trigonum; 2, talus; 3, ankle joint; 4, tibia.

- Pain is felt when the foot is passively placed with the toes pointing downwards.
- An X-ray will usually show a bone fragment (os trigonum) at the back of the ankle (Figure 13.26). Because the majority of these bone fragments are asymptomatic, its mere presence does not mean that it is the cause of the problem.
- Diagnosis is confirmed if injecting local anesthetic solution into the area temporarily relieves pain.

Treatment:

The *athlete* should:
- modify activities to avoid plantar flexion;
- begin physical therapy to strengthen ankle muscles for better support.

The *doctor* may:
- prescribe anti-inflammatory medication;
- in refractory cases, inject steroid into the area to reduce inflammation;
- in cases that do not respond to the above, operate to remove the bone fragment and soft tissue. This disorder only rarely needs surgery. Return to sport is permissible after 6-8 weeks.

Osteoarthritis: arthrosis of the ankle ('worn-out' joint)

The incidence of ankle arthrosis is low compared with that of arthrosis of the hip and knee joints. It is most commonly present after fractures about the ankle, especially when a fracture heals in a nonanatomic position. Other predisposing factors include stage 3 and stage 4 osteochondral lesions of the tibia or the talar dome. Long-standing ligament instability with chondral damage over a long time may cause osteoarthritis.

The treatment is symptomatic and includes unloading of the joint surfaces and reducing the reactive inflammation with nonsteroidal anti-inflammatory drugs. When 'catching' and 'locking' sensations are

present, arthroscopic debridement and removal of loose bodies may
warranted. Ankle arthrodesis is an option if conservative measures fa
The functional disability after an ankle arthrodesis can frequently be w
compensated for, especially in a young patient.

Chronic ankle tendon injuries

Peroneal tendon injuries

The peroneal tendons run behind the lateral aspect of the ankle a
midfoot to their insertions on the plantar side of the foot. The tendo
pass behind the lateral malleolus in the groove of the fibula and benea
the retinaculum, by which the tendons are held in position. Perone
brevis is the strongest abductor of the foot and functions as a second
flexor of the ankle and everter of the foot. The tendon functions to stal
lize the foot during gait, particularly in the final portion of the stance

In downhill skiing, the athlete can have a trauma of internal rotati
in combination with inversion. The retinaculum which holds the tendo
in their compartment can then tear or avulse from the fibula. This allo
the tendons to slip forward across the lateral malleolus (Figure 13.27).

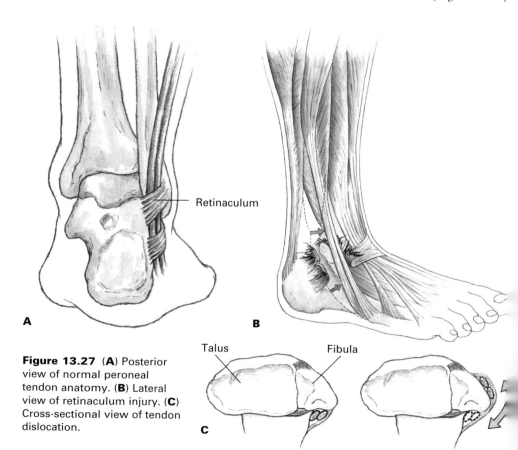

Retinaculum

Talus   Fibula

Figure 13.27 (**A**) Posterior
view of normal peroneal
tendon anatomy. (**B**) Lateral
view of retinaculum injury. (**C**)
Cross-sectional view of tendon
dislocation.

A

B

C

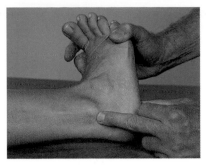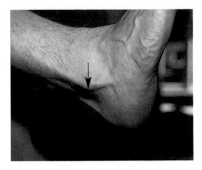

Figure 13.28 (A) Test to reproduce tendon subluxation. **(B)** Subluxation of the peroneal tendon.

subluxation or dislocation of the tendons can occur, as well as a tear. Recurrent dislocation of the tendon results in a inflammatory reaction, as well as degenerative changes causing a secondary tear, which may cause chronic problems. This injury can occur in athletes who have recurrent ankle sprains and unstable joints, as well as in downhill skiers, and in athletes who engage in jumping sports including football and basketball.

Symptoms and diagnosis

- Localized tenderness may be felt behind the lateral malleolus (see Figure 13.29).
- Pain is felt on active pronation of the ankle.
- The athlete can often reproduce a subluxation of the tendon by plantar flexing or dorsiflexing the ankle. This results in an often visible and palpable dislocation of the tendon anterior to lateral malleolus. This maneuver can cause pain. The tendon can also be dislocated by pressing from behind with the thumb against the lateral malleolus, which shows a defect behind the lateral malleolus (Figure 13.28).
- Swelling around the tendon is common.
- Occasionally a rim avulsion fracture of the lateral malleolus may occur (15-50%). These fractures are best seen on an ankle mortise view X-ray.

Treatment

The *doctor* may:
- apply a cast or a walking boot for 3-4 weeks in an acute injury;
- operate in order to deepen the groove and suture the retinaculum back to bone. A walking boot or a cast is applied for 4-6 weeks and return to sport is possible after 2-3 months;
- repair a tear (often longitudinal) if it is present.

Posterior tibial tendon injuries

The posterior tibial muscle arises from the back of the tibia and fibula, and merges into a tendon enclosed in a sheath which runs behind the tibia and the medial malleolus and is attached to the boat-shaped navicular bone on the inside of the foot. Increased pronation of the foot results in increased load and tension on the tendon of the tibialis posterior

muscle, leading to partial tears of the tendon and/or to inflammation
the tendon sheath. The tendon is subject to mechanical pressure behi
the medial malleolus where they run in a narrow groove. Inflammati
around the tendon is common, causing problems primarily in runni
but also in skating and skiing.

If inflammation around the tendon is not treated properly, comple
rupture of the tendon can occur. Complete rupture is not very comm
in athletes, occurring mostly in middle-aged women, but it can be deb
itating, and treatment is difficult, with variable results. The key is
recognize the symptoms and institute aggressive treatment prior
complete rupture.

Symptoms
and diagnosis

- Pain is felt when the tendon slides in the sheath during movement
- Pain is felt when the tendon is subjected to passive loading and act
  exercises.
- Tenderness can occur, as a rule, over the attachment of the tendon
  the navicular bone but also over the course of the tendon behind
  medial malleolus.
- Swelling sometimes occurs.
- Crepitations can be felt over the tendon when the injury is in its ac
  stage.
- Increased pronation of the foot is often present.
- In complete rupture a flat foot will develop, with the heel collaps
  towards the inside of the foot and the toes pushing to the outside
  the foot.
- In complete rupture the athlete will not reform the ankle when sta
  ing on the toes, and toe-standing may not be possible.
- An MRI scan will confirm the diagnosis.

Treatment

The *athlete* should:
- give up active sport and rest the foot for 1–2 weeks;
- apply cold treatment when the injury is in its acute stage and a
  that apply local heat, for example by using a heat retainer;
- apply tape or an ankle brace to the injured area;
- use a semifirm shoe orthosis (insert)—preferably custom-made—wh
  supports the longitudinal arch and reduces the pronation of the fc

The *doctor* may:
- prescribe anti-inflammatory medication;
- give a steroid injection into the tendon sheath—*never* into
  tendon—and prescribe rest;
- apply a walking boot or a plaster cast for 3–4 weeks;
- operate if the tendon sheath has become constricted so that the ten
  can no longer glide normally in it. The surgical exploration deals v
  whatever pathologic condition is present, whether it is a chr
  tendon sheath inflammation, tendinosis, or a tear along the tendo
- prescribe shoe inserts for cases of chronic rupture;
- operate in cases of acute complete rupture to repair the tendon;
- operate in cases of painful chronic rupture. Surgery cannot reform
  arch, but can reduce the pain. Return to activities after comp
  rupture is unpredictable.

Flexor hallucis longus tendon injuries

The flexor hallucis longus runs in a groove in the posterior talar process. At the level of the ankle joint the flexor hallucis longus passes together with the posterior tibial and flexor digitorum longus tendons under the flexor retinaculum. Injuries and overuse problems to the flexor hallucis longus tendon are not uncommon in activities such as ballet dancing, owing to frequent and forceful plantar flexion activities of the ankle and big toe. Repetitive push-off maneuvers transmit substantial forces across the tendon and sheath with possible irritation, swelling and malformation. Injury can also occur in other movements such as push-off and rotation in the tennis serve. Tendinitis of the flexor hallucis longus tendon is much more common than complete disruption.

The flexor hallucis longus can cause posterior ankle impingement due to os trigonum, an extra bone present in 20% of the population.

**mptoms
d diagnosis**
- Pain is reproduced with forceful ankle plantar flexion.
- Insidious pain can be located at the posterior medial aspect of the ankles behind the malleolus.
- Sometimes there is 'catching' or 'locking' of the tendon, caused by swelling of the tendon at an anatomically tight location behind the medial malleolus.
- Localized tenderness is felt over the tendon usually posterior or distal of the medial malleolus (Figure 13.29).
- At forceful active contraction of the flexor hallucis longus, there is a snap or pop, and crepitation over the posterior medial region of the ankle.
- MR can show fluid in the tendon sheath and sometimes tendinosis (Figure 13.30).

eatment

The *athlete* can:
- rest the area, with the help of crutches;
- apply cold treatment;

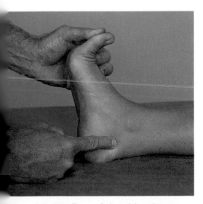

ure 13.29 Forceful ankle plantar
ion. Localized tenderness and pain
n posterior to the medial malleolus,
entuated by dorsiflexion of the big

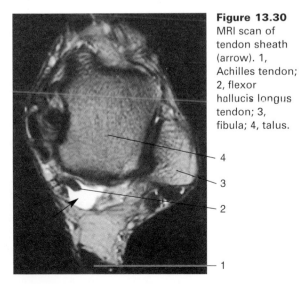

Figure 13.30
MRI scan of tendon sheath (arrow). 1, Achilles tendon; 2, flexor hallucis longus tendon; 3, fibula; 4, talus.

— 4

— 3

— 2

— 1

- apply tendon treatment principles (p. 45);
- dancers can continue working out, but should avoid dancing *en point*

The *doctor* may:
- prescribe anti-inflammatory medication;
- immobilize the joint with a walking boot for a short period;
- operate to release the tendon sheath, although this is rarely indicate
The scar tissue from surgery can sometimes be as incapacitating as t
tendinitis was prior to surgery. Dancers require at least 3 months of slo
progressive rehabilitation before they will be able to return to dancing
pointe.

Anterior tibial tendon injuries

The tendon of the anterior tibial muscle runs down the front of the low
leg and across the ankle joint, bending the ankle joint upwards. T
tendon and its sheath can become inflamed in any part of its course. T
inflammation can occur as a result of overloading or external pressu
often because of shoes or skating boots that are laced too tightly. The
can also be a rupture resulting in swelling, tenderness and weakness
dorsiflexion of the foot. The injury occurs in ice hockey, team handb
and basketball players, and also in runners and racket players.

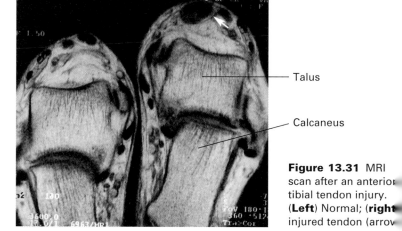

Talus

Calcaneus

Figure 13.31 MRI
scan after an anterior
tibial tendon injury.
(Left) Normal; **(right**
injured tendon (arrow

**Symptoms
and diagnosis**
- Pain is triggered when the foot is dorsiflexed at the ankle joint.
- Tenderness, swelling, and sometimes redness occur over the tendon
  the acute phase and function is impaired.
- Crepitus (creaking) can be felt if the foot is bent up and down wh
  the injury is in its acute phase.
- MRI will support the diagnosis (Figure 13.31).

Treatment
The *athlete* should:
- rest from painful activities, especially dorsiflexion of the ankle;
- apply ice massage in the acute phase (alternately with heat treatmen

390

- apply local heat and use a heat retainer after the acute phase;
- relieve pressure on the tendon by distributing the pressure of the shoe or skating boot over the surrounding parts of the foot, e.g. by putting foam rubber between the lacing and the tendon.

The *doctor* may:
- prescribe anti-inflammatory medication and ointments;
- prescribe an exercise program after the acute phase;
- apply a plaster cast or walking boot in severe cases when the injury is in its acute phase;
- operate in cases of complete rupture.

Ankle arthroscopy

Ankle arthroscopy is an increasingly useful technique for dealing with a wide range of ankle problems. It is used, not only for diagnosis but also as a valuable therapeutic tool. Indications include loose bodies, removal of osteophytes, debridement of osteochondral defects of the talus, removal of chronic enlarged synovial tissue, lysis of adhesions, and meniscoid lesions.

Arthroscopy is carried out with the patient supine and often with spinal anesthesia. This allows the patient to watch the television monitor, and the surgeon can explain the findings. A 4 mm, 30° arthroscope is used. If the joint is narrow, a smaller arthroscope is used.

The anteromedial and anterolateral portals are routinely used. The anteromedial portal is first established just above the tibiotalar joint. The skin incision is made just medial to the tibialis anterior tendon at the level of the tibiotalar joint. The wound is opened bluntly down to the capsule. The saphenous vein and accompanying nerve should be avoided. The anteromedial portal is more easily identified using transillumination. Before the skin incision is made, the intermediate dorsal cutaneous branch of the superficial peroneal nerve is identified and the course of the nerve is marked with a pen. It is easier to palpate the nerve when the ankle is plantar flexed and in some inversion. Posterior portals such as the posteromedial and posterolateral portals are not routinely used, but they can be suitable for the treatment of posterior medial osteochondral lesions. The anterior central portal has been described, but is seldom used. The authors prefer to work with the arthroscope in the anterolateral portal and use the instruments in the anteromedial portal, but this may be dependent on the location of the lesion.

Occasionally there is a need for an ankle joint distractor. It is not routinely used because most lesions can be reached through the anterior portals without distraction.

The portals are closed with tape or sutures, and a simple compressive dressing is used. The athlete can bear weight and carry out active range-of-motion exercises as tolerated. The patient can return to full activity 2–8 weeks following surgery except in the case of osteochondral lesions.

The indications for return to sports are pain-free range of motion a jogging without pain.

Patients with symptoms consistent with the above indications f arthroscopy are appropriate for referral if their symptoms have n improved or resolved after a reasonable course of conservative theraç Unfortunately, many problems of the ankle can be difficult to diagno and it is frequently difficult to decide when operative intervention indicated. Loose bodies and osteochondritis dissecans are clear indic tions for arthroscopic intervention. Athletes with anterior impingeme due to osteophytes are also relatively simple to diagnose. A great ma patients, however, present with symptoms of pain after an ankle spra and it can be difficult to distinguish whether their symptoms are due relative muscle weakness or imbalance, subtle instability, impingeme or possibly an injury to the syndesmosis, such as a supination– exter rotation injury, that may take more than 3 months to heal. The problems should be identified by detailed physical examination, streng testing, etc., but in practice it can be very difficult, even for physici who deal with these problems regularly, to establish a specific diagno Residual problems 3 months after an ankle sprain are often due to inco plete rehabilitation, but undetected trauma or intra-articular injuries n be present. Therefore, if there has been no response to conservat therapy after approximately 3 months, referral for arthroscopy should considered even if the specific indications listed have not been clea identified.

Bibliography

Ferkel RD, Kartzel RP, Del Pizzo W, et al. (1991) Arthroscopic tre ment of anterolateral impingement of the ankle. *American Journa. Sports Medicine* 19: 440–446.

Karlsson J, Bergsten T, Lansinger O, Peterson L (1988) Reconstruct of the lateral ligaments of the ankle for chronic lateral instabi *Journal of Bone and Joint Surgery [Am]* 70:581–588.

Peterson L (1991) Ankle ligament injuries and operative treatment pri ples. *Annales Chirurgiae et Gynaecologiae* 80:168–176.

Renström PA, Kannus P (1994) Injuries of the foot and ankle. In: De JC, Drez D (eds) *Orthopedic Sports Medicine: Principles and Prac* vol. 2, pp 1705–1767. Philadelphia: WB Saunders.

Renström P (1994) Persistently painful sprained ankle. *Journal of American Academy of Orthopedic Surgeons* 25: 270–280.

14 Foot

The foot (Figures 14.1–5) receives and distributes the body load when walking, jumping and running. Most sports contain elements of running or jumping, during which the strains on the lower extremities of the body increase sharply (see Chapter 3).

Anatomy and function

The lower extremities should be seen as functional units in which different parts cooperate. Deviations from the normal anatomy of the foot can cause problems in the knee and hip joints, and vice versa.

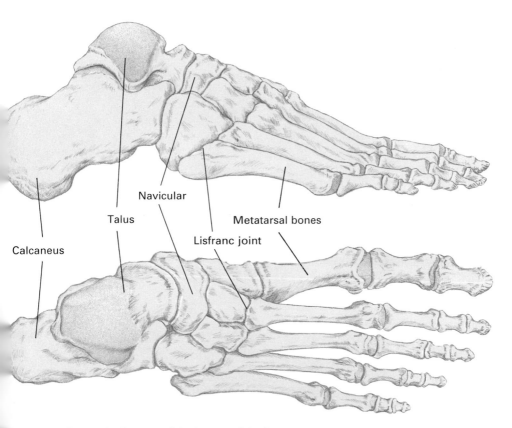

Navicular

Talus

Metatarsal bones

Lisfranc joint

Calcaneus

Figure 14.1 Anatomic diagram of the bones of the foot.

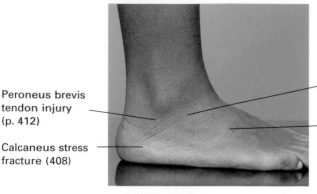

Figure 14.2 Lateral aspect of the foot and location of associated injuries.

Peroneus brevis tendon injury (p. 412)

Calcaneus stress fracture (408)

Talus fracture (p. 408)

Midtarsal sprain (410)

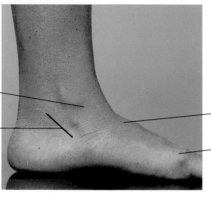

Figure 14.3 Medial aspect of the foot and location of associated injuries.

Talus fracture (p. 408)

Tarsal tunnel syndrome (405)

Spurs (p. 414)

Hallux rigidus (417)

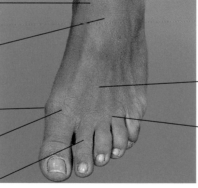

Tarsal navicular stress fracture (p. 410)

Inflammation of sheaths of toe extensor tendons (414)

Hallux valgus (415)

Hallux rigidus (417)

Hammer toe (416)

Figure 14.4 Anterior (superior) aspect of the foot and location associated injuries.

Metatarsal stress fracture (p. 412)

Morton's syndrome (421)

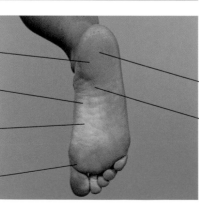

Plantar fasciitis (p. 402)

Entrapment of medial plantar nerve (407)

Digital plantar fasciitis (409)

Turf toe syndrome (419); sesamoid fracture (419)

Figure 14.5 Plantar aspect of the foot and location of associated injuries.

Heel fat pad pain syndrome (p. 400); heel pad bursitis (402)

Entrapment of first branch lateral plantar nerve (406)

The foot is composed of 26 different bones which are interconnected at approximately 30 joints and held together by ligaments and joint capsules. Some 30 tendons, including those of the muscles of the lower leg and those from the muscles of the foot itself, are involved when the foot moves. The foot can be divided into three parts. The hindfoot consists of the talus (ankle bone) and the calcaneus (heel bone). The midfoot consists of the navicular bone, four other bones (the cuboid and three cuneiform bones), and the metatarsal bones. The forefoot consists of the five toes. The big toe, like the thumb, consists of only two phalanges, while the other toes consist of three. The length and shape of the toes can vary considerably. When the toes are loaded, the big toe is pressed against the surface while the other toes make a grasping movement. Under the head of the first metatarsal bone there are two sesamoid bones.

There are two arch systems in the foot: a transverse anterior arch, and a longitudinal arch which follows the inside of the foot from the calcaneus to the metatarsophalangeal joint of the big toe. The front arch is held together by ligaments, including the plantar aponeurosis (the arch ligament), which runs along the arch from the calcaneus to the toes. In an unloaded state the ligaments maintain the shape of the arch, and in a loaded state they are stretched as the arch is pressed against the surface. The more the arch is loaded, the tighter the ligaments become.

Many movements of the foot and toes are controlled by muscles that have their origins in the lower leg and whose tendons are attached to the foot. Movements of more precision are controlled by muscles that have both their origins and insertions in the foot itself.

Foot movements

The foot has two axes around which movements can be made. One runs horizontally through the talus and is the axis for vertical movements at the ankle joint. The other axis runs diagonally, starting from behind the lower part of the calcaneus and extending forward and upward through the head of the talus. The movements the foot makes around this diagonal axis are known as pronation and supination. In pronation the sole of the foot is turned outward and the main part of the inside of the foot has contact with the ground, as in the position of a flat foot (Figure 14.6). In supination the sole of the foot is turned inward, so that the medial border of the foot is higher than the outer border.

Running and walking

During running, the foot is slightly supinated just before it is planted. The foot is usually placed on the ground with the outside of the heel touching first. During the supporting phase the arch is loaded and flattened and pronation begins which, together with contraction of the calf muscles, causes the forces generated to spread through the whole foot and leg. The flattening of the longitudinal arch continues until the arch ligament (plantar aponeurosis) is tightened. By this time the forces

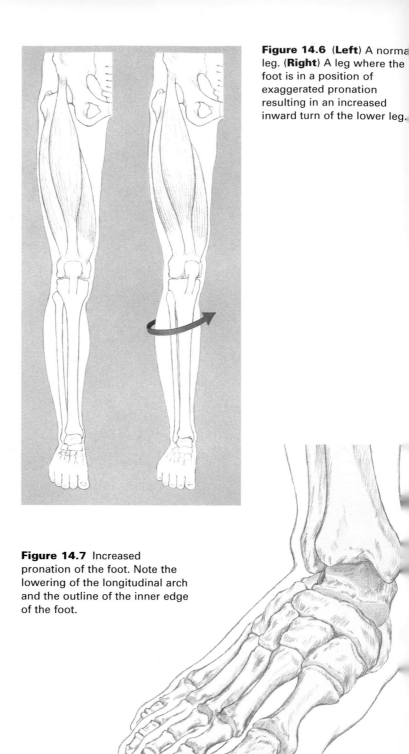

Figure 14.6 (Left) A normal leg. **(Right)** A leg where the foot is in a position of exaggerated pronation resulting in an increased inward turn of the lower leg.

Figure 14.7 Increased pronation of the foot. Note the lowering of the longitudinal arch and the outline of the inner edge of the foot.

generated by the body weight have passed through the foot, and preparations for push-off have started. The foot is in pronation for about 40–70% of the supporting phase and then gradually changes into supination, which stabilizes the front of the foot so that a better lever is available for push-off.

The angle of the foot

The angle of the foot in relation to the lower leg is important. The angle can be checked against skin markings which are made along the anterior tibia. The vertical axis through the talus and the calcaneus should be parallel to the tibial skin markings; it should also be at right angles to a line through the anterior transverse arch.

Causes of foot overuse injuries

The causes of foot injuries in running are multifactorial. Factors that influence the distribution of load include: anatomical features, body weight, shoe type, running surface, technique, and training program.

Anatomical factors

Significant deviations from the normal anatomical structure of the foot (e.g. excessive pronation and pes cavus) can cause injuries, but even minor variations can be sufficient to do so if subjected to prolonged or repeated loading.

Pronated foot
A certain degree of pronation is normal in a foot that is loaded, but excessive pronation is a compensatory movement caused by an incorrect relationship between the heel and the foot or between the leg and the foot (Figure 14.7). It is common for the relationship between leg and foot to be slightly imperfect, and the result can easily be inadequate balance. During weightbearing, the soles of the feet can be forced against the ground by excessive pronation.

During running, overuse injuries can recur because excessive pronation—or pronation maintained for too long in the supporting phase—causes increased stress on the supporting structures of the foot, and also causes increased work for the muscles. Excessive pronation may also be a mechanism by which the body compensates for other slight anatomical defects and deviations.

Excessive pronation, can be confirmed by the 'wet foot' test (Figure 14.8). The foot is dipped in water and footprints are made by walking on a smooth, dry surface. The footprints then show the load distribution across the foot. When the foot is normal the longitudinal arch does not leave a print, but if excessive pronation is present a print of the whole foot appears. Excessive pronation may cause increased load on the whole of the lower extremity, since it results in an increased inward rotation of

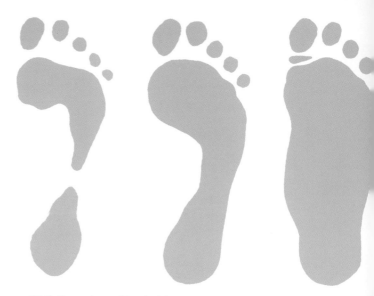

Figure 14.8 Footprints of loaded feet. (**Left**) A foot with a high instep (pe[s] cavus or claw-foot). (**Middle**) A normal foot. (**Right**) A foot with increased pronation (flat foot).

the lower leg. This can lead to a change of the biomechanical wo[rk] pattern of the thigh musculature so that the lower leg, the knee, and t[he] hip are subjected to increased load. This can be the cause of over[use] injuries or other painful conditions in these areas. Injuries associated w[ith] excessive pronation include chondromalacia patellae, tibialis poster[ior] syndrome, plantar fasciitis and trochanteric bursitis. It is, howev[er] important to stress that the anatomical changes—malalignment—bear[a] direct relationship to a specific diagnosis.

Cavus foot (claw foot)

A foot with a congenitally abnormal high longitudinal arch is calle[d a] cavus foot (Figure 14.9). Cavus foot is relatively inflexible and ha[s a] limited articular range of motion. It is often combined with tight c[alf] musculature and a tight plantar aponeurosis. The weightbearing surf[ace] is relatively small, so there is a risk of concentration of pressure resu[lt]ing in abnormal loading conditions.

Symptoms and diagnosis
- The foot is inflexible, and its arch is hardly flattened at all under lo[ad]
- Hammer toes can develop (the toes are bent and cannot be straig[ht]ened).
- The big toe is displaced downwards, which often leads to the form[a]tion of painful calluses.
- Pain on prolonged exertion. Cavus feet do not usually tolerate lo[ng] distance running very well.

Treatment
- Specially made arch supports with good shock-absorbing proper[ties] can be used. Shoes with 1 cm (0.5 in) heel wedges of a semiri[gid] material can be of value in relieving calloused areas.

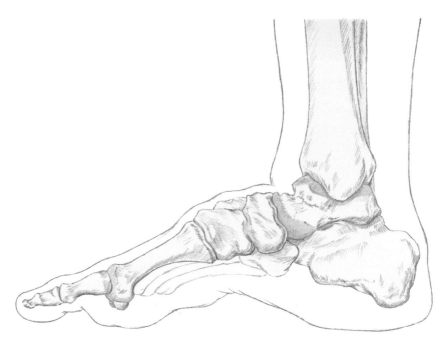

Figure 14.9 Pes cavus (claw-foot).

- Static stretching exercises can be carried out on a board inclined at an angle of about 35°. The athlete then performs alternate toe and heel raises.
- Any calluses should be pared down, and the shoes should be modified to relieve pressure and distribute the load over the sole of the foot.

Extrinsic factors

Extrinsic factors such as faulty training programs or slippery roads can cause foot injuries (see Chapter 3).

Hindfoot problems

Hindfoot discomfort can be localized to the heel or to the medial and lateral aspects of the calcaneus. Medial symptoms can be caused by nerve entrapments or injuries to the flexor tendon groups. Tarsal tunnel syndrome (p. 405) can be caused by entrapment of either the posterior tibial nerve or one of its branches, or of the medial and lateral plantar nerves under the flexor retinaculum. A tear or tendinosis of the tibial posterior tendon (p. 387) can also cause proximal arch pain. Pain can radiate distally into the longitudinal arch and may be associated with swelling and thickening of the tendon. A tear or tendinosis of the flexor hallucis longus tendon (p. 389) can also cause pain on the medial side of the hindfoot.

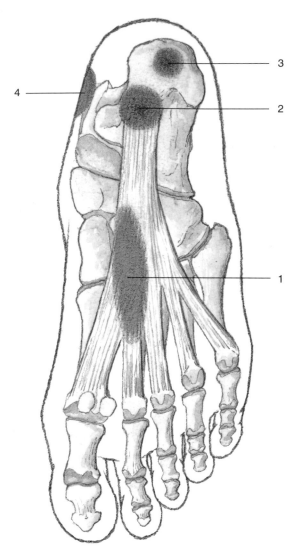

Figure 14.10
Plantar aspect of the foot, showing common painful areas.
1 Distal plantar fasciitis
2 Proximal plantar fasciitis
3 Heel fat pad pain syndrome
4 Nerve entrapment

Heel pain has many causes, including nerve entrapment, plantar fas injury and stress fractures. Heel pain can also be caused by painful h pad syndrome, plantar fasciitis (see below), or rupture of the plan fascia (Figure 14.10). A calcaneus stress fracture can cause pain weightbearing and is characterized by distinct tenderness elicited compression of the medial and lateral aspects of the heel. Nerve entr ments are not uncommon.

Heel fat pad pain syndrome (fat pad hypotrophy)

The heel cushion is composed of elastic adipose tissue surrounded b fascia of connective tissue attached to the skin. The fascia forms a sp fibrous septum with U-shaped compartments oriented vertically, creat

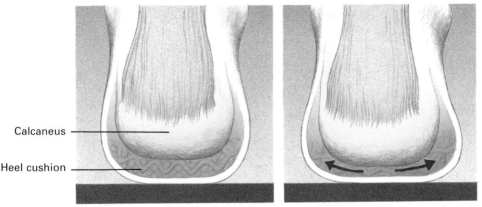

Calcaneus ——————

Heel cushion ——————

Figure 14.11 (Left) Normal heel cushion. The bone is protected by fatty tissue. **(Right)** Heel fat pad pain syndrome. The fatty tissue is pressed out towards the sides of the heel impairing the protection for the heel bone.

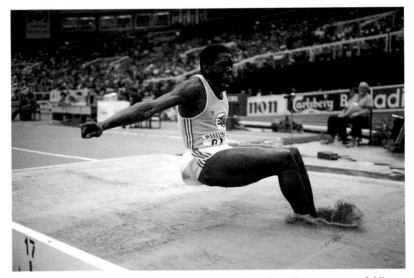

Figure 14.12 Triple-jumper landing on a soft surface (by courtesy of All Sports: photographer, Gray Mortimer).

a multiple array of small compartments containing fat. The resulting structure is designed to resist compressive loads (Figure 14.11). Unlike the skin on the dorsum (top) of the foot, the skin on the sole of the foot cannot slide backwards and forwards over the tissues beneath. Repeated jumps landing on the heels, on a hard surface—as performed by hurdlers, long-jumpers, and triple-jumpers (Figure 14.12)—can rupture these connective tissue bands. The fat in the compartments is pressed outwards from the area of the heel that contacts the running surface, reducing the protective effect of the fat cushion. With less protection, the skin becomes more sensitive to pain during loading. After the age of 40 years the adipose tissue often gradually deteriorates, creating a softer, thinner heel pad.

The athlete often complains of diffuse plantar heel discomfort that is worse when running on hard surfaces. There is no radiation of this pain.

If the ruptures in the connective tissue bands are minor and recent, the
is only local tenderness in the heel cushion; however, in long-standi
cases the underlying bone can be felt beneath the skin, and the cond
tion is then very difficult to treat. It must therefore be prevented. Part
relief can be achieved by using shorter steps when running to decrea
the load on the heel; but the mainstay of prevention is the use of sho
that are suitable for the surface and have a heel that absorbs most of t
shock and distributes the forces well. Supportive cushions may
inserted under the heel. Shoes with a heel cup can contain and centr.
ize the remaining fat tissue to enhance its protective ability. An ar
support can also reduce the pressure on the heel.

Heel pad inflammation and bursitis

Trauma to the foot or overuse can cause inflammation of the heel pa
Between the calcaneus and the heel cushion there is a small bursa whi
can become inflamed and painful after impact loading, as in basketb
or running. Owing to this inflammation the fat pad can become so tenc
that it cannot withstand weightbearing loads.

This condition most often occurs in middle-aged adults and athlet
but can occur in at any age. It may be bilateral in 10–15% of cases. Lor
distance runners with cavus feet seem to have this injury more often

On examination the heel pad is tender and firm. This injury is gen
ally self-limiting with conservative treatment. Heel cups or an a
support with a notch for the painful area may be effective.

Plantar fasciitis: heel pain syndrome (heel spur)

The arch ligament or plantar aponeurosis is a fibrous band that ru
forwards from the plantar medial aspect of the calcaneus to blend w
ligaments attached to the toes. When the heel is lifted during take-off
running on a hill, the angle between the toes and the metatarsals increa
and the aponeurosis is stretched (Figure 14.13). As the toes are b
more, the aponeurosis becomes more stretched and the longitudinal a
is thereby stabilized. However, a taut aponeurosis also becomes a pot
tial injury site. During a vigorous take-off, a rupture can occur in
origin of the plantar aponeurosis or in the short flexors of the to
Injuries can also occur during a fast turn which causes increased load
the tissues of the sole of the foot.

Athletes who have excessive pronation of the foot are more likely
develop an overuse injury or a tear in the origin of the plantar aponeu
sis. When, as a result of the pronation, the arch is stretched and the t
spread out, the aponeurosis is subjected to increased strain. Prolon
sporting activity in shoes that do not provide sufficient support for
arch can also contribute to plantar fascial pain. However, no clear
between heel pain syndrome and flat foot (pes planus) or claw foot (
cavus) has been established, and the cause of plantar fasciitis is still uncl
This explains why so many names have been given to this condition.

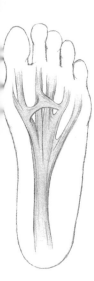

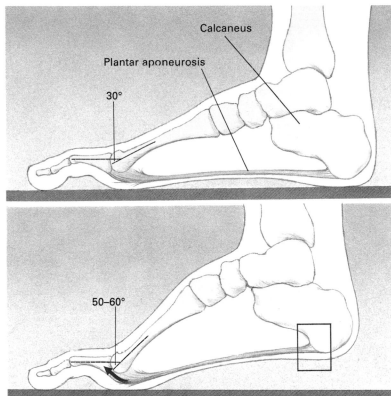

Figure 14.13 (Top) The foot and plantar aponeurosis (fascia) when the whole foot is loaded against the surface. **(Bottom)** The plantar aponeurosis is stretched during take-off. The lined area indicates the seat of inflammation at the origin of the plantar aponeurosis from the heel bone. **(Far left)** The plantar aponeurosis seen from underneath.

Plantar fasciitis also occurs in the midfoot (see Figure 14.10).

mptoms
d diagnosis

– The discomfort is insidious at onset.
– During initial activity, pain can be experienced at the calcaneal origin of the aponeurosis, but tends to disappear with continued activity. At rest the problems abate.
– Morning stiffness and a painful limp when the athlete gets out of bed and starts to walk are common. This stiffness goes away after a short warm-up.
– These athletes may experience pain when standing on their toes and walking on their heels.
– Occasional numbness may be experienced along the outside of the sole of the foot.
– Focal tenderness and sometimes swelling of the medial aspect of the calcaneus where the aponeurosis inserts may be present (Figure 14.14).
– Associated tightness of the Achilles tendon is common.
– Heel pain is more commonly seen in the shorter leg of athletes with a leg-length discrepancy.

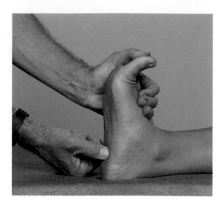

Figure 14.14 Focal tenderness and swelling at medial aspect of calcaneus.

- An X-ray sometimes shows edema and/or a bony outgrowth (heel spur) which arises as an irritant reaction to the stretching of the aponeurosis attachment at the calcaneus. The heel spur originates from the origin of the flexor digitorum brevis muscle and is directed distally and sometimes in the plantar direction. Only 3% of patients with plantar fasciitis have a plantar heel spur, compared with 15% of asymptomatic patients; the exact relationship between plantar fasciitis and the heel spur has therefore not been defined.
- A triple-phase bone scan can be helpful to support the diagnosis. The delayed phase of the bone scan may be abnormal with a mild focal uptake at the level of the insertion in about 60% of the patients. The diagnosis is, however, mainly clinical.

Treatment

The *athlete* should:
- cool the heel with ice if the injury is acute;
- support the injured foot with crutches if there is pain on weightbearing;
- learn about the injury: it is important to note that the injury is usually self-limiting;
- modify training to avoid abuse: pounding activities should be avoided and cycling and swimming can be substituted for running;
- carry out static stretching exercises as a preventive and rehabilitation measure; this stretching should include the Achilles tendon as well as the plantar fascia.
- use taping to unload the area, or apply a heat retainer sock or insert
- check if the sports shoes may be causing an increased load on the aponeurosis (the shoes may be too stiff or too soft);
- use a shock-absorbing heel cup in the shoe;

The *doctor* may:
- educate the patient about the injury, its chronic (but self-limiting) nature, and its extended healing time;
- prescribe an orthotic arch support with a notch (unloading area) corresponding to the painful area;
- prescribe a heel cup. Heel cups can be of different types:
  (1) a viscoelastic material that deforms slowly on cup compression load;

(2) a harder plastic cup that surrounds the heel and compresses the fat of the pad to allow the padding to absorb the impact load better; or

(3) soft felt or hard plastic materials forming a heel cup and medial longitudinal arch support combination to help unload the plantar fascia;

- prescribe a night splint or molded plastic ankle orthosis (a foot orthosis with the ankle fixed in 5° of dorsiflexion). This will hold the fascia in a stretched position throughout the night to decrease morning stiffness;
- prescribe anti-inflammatory medication;
- prescribe physical therapy, including one or more of the following: contrast baths, whirlpool, phonophoresis, iontophoresis, and massage. These can often give some short-term relief but their long-term effects are limited;
- give a cortisone injection. This should be given from the medial side and injected close to the bone, between the bone and the fascia. A direct injection in the heel pad should be avoided since it may cause heel pad fat hypotrophy;
- operate if problems persist despite adequate conservative therapy of more than 6–12 months. Surgery can involve different procedures. The most common procedure is the plantar fascia release, where the plantar fascia is cut away from its insertion on to the calcaneus. Endoscopic techniques are being developed but are still experimental.

Healing and complications

The injury should be treated early to avoid prolonged problems. Even with proper treatment return to sports activity after a chronic injury may take 6 months or more. After surgery the return to sports activity is usually 2–3 months but can be longer. Some tenderness at the wound site may remain for a long time. An occasional complication of surgery is injury to the medial calcaneal nerve, which can result in a painful neuroma or heel pad numbness. The athlete needs to be aware of the risks before undergoing surgery.

Entrapment of nerves

The most common entrapment of nerves is the tarsal tunnel syndrome which is caused by increased pressure either on the posterior tibial nerve or one of its branches, or on the mediolateral plantar nerves. Heel pain can also be caused by entrapment of the first branch of the lateral plantar nerve (Baxter's nerve).

Tarsal tunnel syndrome

Just below the medial malleolus lies a passage through which the medial and the lateral plantar nerves pass (Figure 14.15). Excessive pronation of the foot increases the load on tissues surrounding the flexor tendons, and can cause inflammation and swelling, resulting in entrapment of these nerves (the tarsal tunnel syndrome). Inflammation may also occur from pressure by a posterior bony prominence of the talus.

The affected athlete feels pain arising from the area of entrapment. It radiates distally along the inside of the foot and along the sole towards the toes; this is the area that the nerves supply. There is direct focal

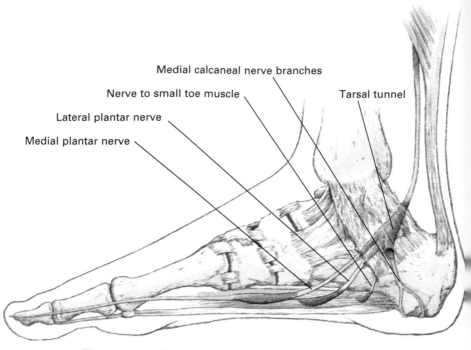

Figure 14.15 The posterior tibial nerve and its branches (medial aspect).

Medial calcaneal nerve branches

Nerve to small toe muscle

Lateral plantar nerve

Medial plantar nerve

Tarsal tunnel

tenderness over the nerve as it passes beneath the flexor retinaculum. Tapping the nerve at that area can cause a burning, tingling sensation which radiates out to the plantar aspect of the foot. The diagnosis can be verified by electromyographic (EMG) and nerve conduction studies. However, a normal study does not exclude the diagnosis.

Treatment of this injury is by an arch support with a medial heel wedge, which will decrease the tension on the nerve. Steroid injection into the tarsal tunnel can be beneficial temporarily. Surgical release of the tarsal tunnel can provide relief of the symptoms in 90% of cases. Return to sports is possible within 6–8 weeks.

Entrapment of the first branch of the lateral plantar nerve (Baxter's nerve)

Some doctors estimate that entrapment of the branch of the lateral plantar nerve accounts for approximately 20% of chronic heel pain. This entrapment occurs as the nerve changes from a vertical to a horizontal direction around the medial plantar aspect of the heel (Figure 14.16). This nerve entrapment occurs most often in athletes such as sprinters, and in ballet dancers who are often on their toes. The medial calcaneal nerve branches that innervate the plantar medial aspect of the heel are not involved with entrapment of the first branch. Inflammation and spur formation at the insertion of the flexor digitorum brevis muscle into the heel can cause swelling and compression of the nerve along the plantar fascia.

This injury may cause pain towards the end of the day, or after prolonged activity. The clearest diagnostic sign is maximal tenderness where the nerve is compressed. As plantar fasciitis may predispose to the injury, there may be some tenderness over the proximal plantar fascia where it inserts into the calcaneus. Some weakness may be experienced.

The treatment includes rest, anti-inflammatory medications, and physical therapy. Steroid injections can be given. A shock-absorbing heel cup can decrease the inflammation in the area. In athletes with excessive pronation, a longitudinal arch support can decrease compression of the nerve. In athletes with prolonged symptoms, surgery gives relief in 85% of cases, with return to sports activities within 3 months.

Entrapment of the medial plantar nerve (jogger's foot)

The medial plantar nerve crosses deep to the adductor hallucis muscle, passing through the 'knot of Henry' and continuing along the medial border of the foot. Entrapment occurs at the 'knot of Henry', especially in athletes with hyperpronation of the foot (Figure 14.17). Athletes who have a forefoot that is pointed outward (abduction), or have the heel externally

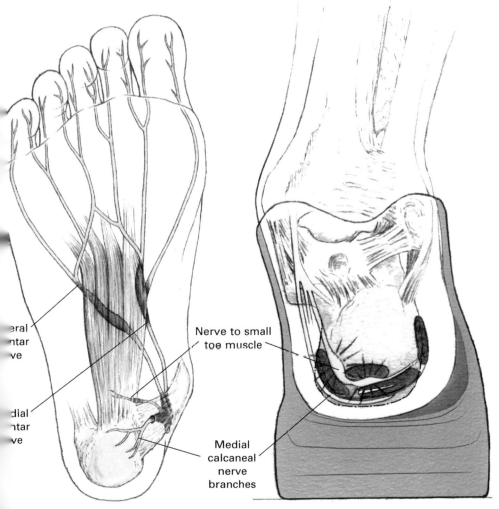

Figure 14.16 The posterior tibial nerve and its branches (plantar aspect).

Figure 14.17 Nerve entrapment around the heel in a shoe.

rotated (valgus), also have a predisposition to this problem. An athlete with previous ankle injuries or chronic ankle instability can have this problem. The pain radiates distally into the medial toes, and also may radiate proximally into the ankle. The pain is worse with running on curves and uphill. Tenderness occurs at the medial plantar aspect of the arch. Decreased sensation on the medial aspect of the foot can occur after running.

Conservative treatment is by the use of a medial longitudinal arch support or a heel lift. Surgery can be successful, with return to sport within 6 weeks.

Stress fractures of the calcaneus

Stress fractures are found in otherwise healthy individuals from the age of 7 years onwards (p. 8). Stress fractures of the calcaneus are relatively uncommon.

Symptoms and diagnosis	– Pain in the heel occurs during activity. – There is very distinct tenderness and local swelling. Diffuse pain can be elicited by compression of the heel from both medial and lateral sides. Pain is not localized only to the plantar aspect of the heel. – An X-ray of the injury shows no fracture in about half the cases. If there is still a suspicion that the injury is a stress fracture, another X-ray may be taken 2–3 weeks later when healing tissue (callus) can be seen around the fracture. – If the X-ray does not prove the existence of a fracture, a bone scan can confirm the diagnosis.
Treatment	– Weightbearing is permitted as tolerated; crutches are usually needed initially. – A shock-absorbing heel pad can be beneficial. – Treatment otherwise is as described on p. 11.
Healing	The injured athlete can resume sporting activities to the full extent when free of symptoms. This usually occurs 6–8 weeks after symptom onset.

Fractures of the talus

The talus (ankle bone) can be fractured in motor sports, parachuting, football, downhill skiing, ski-jumping, high-jumping, and indoor sports. This injury is rare and difficult to treat, and is likely to be complicated by injuries to the blood vessels that provide nutrients to the talus. The loss of blood supply can prejudice healing, and complications are common.

Fractures of the calcaneus

In traumatic injury and falls from a height, fractures of the calcaneus occur. The injured person finds it difficult to stand on the foot because of pain and severe swelling. The treatment consists of rest with a variety degree of relief from weightbearing; sometimes surgery is considered. A fracture of the calcaneus can cause prolonged—and sometimes permanent—disability.

Tarsal coalition

Tarsal coalition is a condition of abnormal union of two or more bones in the foot. The coalition may be by bony, fibrous, or cartilaginous tissue. The union of bones may cause symptoms by restricting the motion of one of the joints in the subtalar complex, imposing strain on the other joints and producing pain. Coalition sites are between the talus and the navicular bone, and between the talus and the calcaneal bone. Union may also occur between other bones. Talonavicular coalition is unusual and can be seen at a very early age.

The calcaneal coalition, which is uncommon, can give symptoms of pain, stiffness and decreased pronation/supination in children aged 8–12 years. The diagnosis can be confirmed by X-rays if there is a bony union; sometimes a CT or MRI scan is needed. Treatment includes the use of an orthosis or a brace to decrease painful subtalar motion. Often surgical treatment is needed. Prolonged rehabilitation is required before return to sport is possible.

Midfoot problems

The midfoot consists of the tarsal and metatarsal bones: the navicular, cuboid, three cuneiforms, and five metatarsal bones. Dense ligaments between these bones create marked stability and a rigid structure. Most motion occurs in the 'sports joint', the transverse tarsal joint. Isolated injuries of the midfoot are rare and atypical, requiring high-energy forces. Conditions affecting the midfoot involve sprains of the ligaments as well as arthrosis of the joints. The accessory navicular, an extra bone, can cause pain on the medial midfoot. Stress fractures of the navicular can also occur.

Distal plantar fasciitis

Distal plantar fasciitis presents with localized pain and tenderness of the midportion of the plantar fascia in the midfoot. It is much less frequent than conventional plantar fascitis. The pain can radiate proximally or distally, but is most pronounced in the midfoot. This injury occurs more frequently in sprinters and middle-distance runners, who use their toes more during running. On physical examination there is often a tenderness of the midfoot of the plantar fascia that is a little more diffuse than in conventional plantar fasciitis. Dorsiflexion of the toes can increase the patient's symptoms as the fascial fibers are stretched.

Treatment can include: circumferential taping, anti-inflammatory medication, physical therapy, and plantar fascia stretching. A medial heel wedge or orthosis may decrease tension on the plantar fascia, but can

sometimes increase the athlete's problems. This injury is usually sel
limiting and can heal with conservative therapy. The prognosis is goo

In some cases a tear of the aponeurosis may occur. Most of these tea
occur in athletes who have been treated with local steroid injection
These tears are most commonly treated conservatively but occasional
surgery is required.

Midtarsal sprains

The midtarsal joints hold a key position in the medial–lateral longitud
nal arches; they also act together with the subtalar joints during inversic
and eversion. Injuries range from nondisplaced ligamentous injuries an
subluxations, to dislocations. Conservative treatment is indicated fe
undisplaced ligamentous injuries, with a short immobilization period an
active mobilization of the ankle and the foot thereafter. All displace
midtarsal dislocations need anatomic reduction with internal fixation.

Tarsal navicular stress fracture

Tarsal navicular stress fractures occur most commonly in athlete
especially runners and jumping athletes. The pain is insidious and loca
ized to the arch. There is increased pain in the midfoot with motion an
weightbearing, and limited dorsiflexion of the ankle. The condition
vague and uncharacteristic, and diagnosis is difficult. There may
tenderness localized to the navicular bone, but this is not always preser
Plain radiographs are often normal. The diagnosis is made by a positi
bone scan. A CT scan or plain tomography will show the extent and t
nature of the fracture. The fracture is usually sagittally oriented at t
midpoint of the medial–lateral dimension of the bone.

These fractures are treated by avoidance of weightbearing and use of
walking boot. They usually heal in 6–8 weeks. If there is some displaceme
surgery is indicated; however, there is a high complication rate with delay
union, nonunion, or recurrence of the fracture requiring new surge
Return to sporting activity is possible 3 months after conservative treatme
and 3–6 months after surgical treatment, depending on the type of surge

Diagnosis of this injury is often delayed, with an average time fro
onset to diagnosis of 4 months. A failure to begin treatment early m
result in prolonged pain and complications.

In patients with vague arch pain on physical activity, a bone scan is
indicated.

Injury to Lisfranc's joint

Lisfranc's joint is the joint between the five metatarsal bones and th
corresponding midtarsal bones—the three cuneiforms and the cuboid bo

(see Figure 14.1). The keystone that provides stability to the Lisfranc joint is the second metatarsal base. The Lisfranc ligament extends from the base of the second metatarsal to the medial cuneiform; injury to this ligament is uncommon, but must be well treated or severe deformity and chronic pain may result.

There are two mechanisms of injury. The direct mechanism is a simple crush injury to this region of the foot. The indirect mechanism, which is more common, is longitudinal compression with the foot in plantar flexion, typically in a backward fall with the foot trapped by the dorsum of the toes; similar injuries occur in road traffic accidents, falls from a ladder, tobogganing accidents, or mis-stepping off a kerbstone. A dancer may sustain this injury by overbalancing when *en pointe*, allowing the whole weight of the body to fall on the ligaments and capsule of the tarsometatarsal joints. These injuries can also occur in American football, when the player is kneeling on the ground with toes and ankle dorsiflexed, and somebody lands on his heel.

The diagnosis is reached by clinical examination and X-rays; a CT scan is often helpful.

The treatment can sometimes be conservative, including early closed manipulation with maintenance of position by a plaster cast. Most commonly, however, surgical fixation with pins or screws is the treatment of choice to maintain anatomic reduction. Complications after tarsometatarsal dislocations are common and often serious, and many athletes are unable to return to demanding sports activities. Even if there are no complications, a return to sport is rarely possible before 9–12 months after the injury. Before a return to sport is contemplated, the athlete must demonstrate a full, painless range of motion of the foot and ankle with no signs of chronic inflammation or arthrosis. Swimming and cycling can start earlier than pounding activities such as running.

Metatarsal fractures

Fractures of the metatarsal bones are common. The injury mechanism is often a direct blow to the dorsal aspect of the foot caused by a heavy object falling (or a person jumping) on to the foot. Direct trauma results in a transverse neck fracture of the second, third, or fourth metatarsals. Indirect forces often result in spiral shaft fracture. The symptoms from these injuries are characterized by pain on weight-bearing. The diagnosis is suggested by marked tenderness on palpation of the metatarsal bones or pain with compression of the foot, and confirmed by X-rays.

Treatment of the majority of isolated metatarsal shaft and neck fractures is nonoperative. Displacement in the plantar or dorsal direction should be avoided as this will result in areas of increased weightbearing load with the potential for developing skin problems. Early weightbearing in a rigid boot or cast is recommended. Return to sports is often possible 3 months after a conventional metatarsal fracture. The prognosis is good.

There are three distinct types of fracture at the base of the fifth metatarsal. *Jones' fracture* is a transverse fracture of the base of the bone

caused by forefoot adduction and plantar flexion. For *stress fractures* se
below. The third type is an *avulsion fracture*. This is caused by a force
ful contraction of the peroneus brevis tendon in response to a sudde
inversion injury of the foot. These fractures can be treated symptomati
cally in a cast or a walking boot. In widely displaced fractures and delaye
union, surgery may be indicated.

Metatarsal stress fractures

About 20% of all stress fractures of the lower extremity are located i
the metatarsals, with the second metatarsal being the most common si
(march fracture, p. 9). The symptoms are insidious and gradual, and
can take 1–2 months or more before a stress fracture can be verified t
X-rays (see Figure 2.5). Bone scans within a week or two could confir
the diagnosis. These stress fractures are treated nonoperatively wit
limitation of activities for 4–6 weeks; however, running in water may t
beneficial.

Stress fractures of the proximal fifth metatarsal require special attentio
These fractures are localized to the proximal part of the bone distal
the tuberosity and the peroneus brevis insertion. The majority occ
because of repetitive stress, with a high incidence among basketb
players. There is marked discomfort along the lateral border of the foc
which may occur 1–2 weeks before a true stress fracture develops. The
is a significant incidence of late union, nonunion, and refracture; wi
consequent long-term problems for athletes.

For the acute fracture, a non-weightbearing cast or walking boot f
6–8 weeks can be tried. Union must be radiographically confirmed befo
this treatment is stopped; it is then followed by 6 weeks of limited acti
ity. Because of the high rate of failure to heal, there is an increasi
indication for early internal fixation with an intramedullary screw; tl
markedly decreases the healing time. The surgery is limited and exposu
of the fracture site is not necessary. A gradual return to weightbeari
can be possible in 2 weeks, with return to sports as soon as pain a
tenderness are gone, usually in 4–8 weeks.

Chronic or delayed union can also be treated by screw fixation or oth
internal fixation techniques. If there is sclerosis (bone thickening), op
curettage and bone grafting are recommended. Return to sports can th
be possible at 3 months.

Overuse injury or tear of the peroneus brevis tendon

Inflammation and partial tears at the site of the fifth metatarsal bo
attachment of the tendon of the peroneus brevis muscle are not unco
mon in soccer players. Sometimes the tendon sheath can be inflam
resulting in crepitus. Pain is felt over the upper part of the fifth metatar
bone. When the injury is in its acute stage, anti-inflammatory medicati
are used. If necessary, a plaster cast or a walking boot is applied. In ot
respects the injury is treated according to the advice given on p. 45.

Insufficiency of the longitudinal arch (flat foot)

Feet show many individual differences. The longitudinal arch may be flat, but the foot can still be functional. However, if the foot is under excess load because of incorrect loading, excess body weight, or prolonged standing, the arch can collapse to a greater degree and result in a flat foot. In cases of very low arches, the medial edge of the foot is lower than the lateral edge. This causes the metatarsal bones and toes to rotate outwards.

Symptoms and diagnosis
- Often there are no problems at all.
- Pain can occur due to overuse, causing aching in the feet and lower legs.
- When there is repeated load, e.g. during running, pain can occur in the foot, lower leg, knee, and groin.
- A feeling of fatigue in the feet can occur.
- Calluses can form on the sole of the foot at areas of increased load.

Preventive measures
- Flexibility training and static stretching of the ankle joints and calf muscles should be performed.
- Foot and toe strengthening exercises may be helpful.
- The athlete should use shoes with good construction of the outer sole, inner sole, and heel counter.

Treatment

Treatment includes:
- arch supports;
- taping;
- rest from painful activities.

In certain cases the affected athlete must take a break from running, but can still maintain physical fitness by crosstraining activities such as swimming and cycling.

Insufficiency of the anterior transverse arch

The anterior transverse arch functions to provide elastic support to the forefoot. The middle metatarsal bones and the toes flex down towards the floor when the anterior transverse arch is loaded during the supporting and take-off phases of gait. A slackening of the ligaments between the metatarsal bones can occur. If this happens, the arch loses its shape and load-absorbing ability. The foot then becomes broader, and the metatarsal bones and toes acquire a fan-like spread.

Symptoms and diagnosis
- Pain is felt when the anterior transverse arch is loaded.
- Calluses form under the ball of the foot as a result of the skin being exposed to increased pressure.
- Eventually the big toe can deviate and come to lie across the other toes (hallux valgus, p. 415).

- Pressure can cause a bursa and a bony outgrowth to form on the medial side of the big toe. Continued pressure, such as that from poorly designed shoes, can lead to inflammation in the bursa (bunion).
- The condition can cause 'hammer toe' deformities: that is, all the toes except for the big toe lie in a permanently bent position. This can cause increased pressure on the nerve supplying the cleft between the third and fourth, and the second and third toes (Morton metatarsalgia), and/or painful calluses (corns) can form on top of the toes.

Treatment
- A shoe orthotic device with a pad for the anterior transverse arch should be fitted.
- In cases of hallux valgus with bursitis and hammer toes, surgery may be necessary.
- Gripping exercises with the toes are prescribed.
- A general exercise program should be started.

Spurs on top of the foot

Sometimes spurs (bony prominences or exostoses) occur on the top sides of the foot. A spur can increase in size or become inflamed. They are usually caused by pressure from shoes that are too narrow or laced too tightly. The spurs most often appear on the dorsum of the foot anterior to the ankle, and are sometimes composed of separate bone. Foot mobility is often normal, but the affected person cannot wear shoes. Tenderness can be caused by inflammation in a bursa which has formed over the spurs. An X-ray shows either a small bony prominence or sometimes an extra bone.

The treatment for a painful spur is an alteration of the shoe. Sometimes the bony prominence can be removed surgically.

Inflammation of the sheaths of the extensor tendons of the toes (extensor peritenonitis)

The long muscles that straighten the toes are attached to the anterior aspect of the tibia along with the muscles that dorsiflex the foot. The tendons from these muscles cross to the foot at the ankle, with the extensors along the dorsum of the foot to the toes. These tendons and their sheaths can be subjected to increased pressure from sports shoes that are ill-fitting or laced too tightly. They can also be overused running in hills or in sand. Inflammation of the area causes pain on top of the foot, which worsens during running. Tenderness can be elicited along the course of the tendons. In acute peritenonitis, crepitus can sometimes occur.

– The athlete should rest actively, and avoid abusing the foot.
– Anti-inflammatory medication may be helpful.
– The shoes should be altered. Sometimes a piece of felt or foam rubber with a notch to unload the painful area can prevent pressure from being applied by the tongue of the shoe.
– When the problems are prolonged, a steroid injection along the sheath of the tendon may be helpful. This should be followed by 2 weeks of rest.
– In chronic cases surgery is an option.

Forefoot and toe problems

Toe fractures, claw toes, hammer toes, and hard and soft corns are common forefoot problems. When an athlete complains of forefoot pain, the examiner should check for the presence of associated callosities. If no callosities are present, the examination should focus on possible neurological problems. If neither of these conditions is present, joint problems such as instability or arthrosis should be looked for.

Hallux valgus

The big toe (hallux) can normally be angled laterally away from the midline by up to 10°. If the angle is greater than 10°, the condition is called hallux valgus (Figure 14.18). In such cases of displacement, a bony

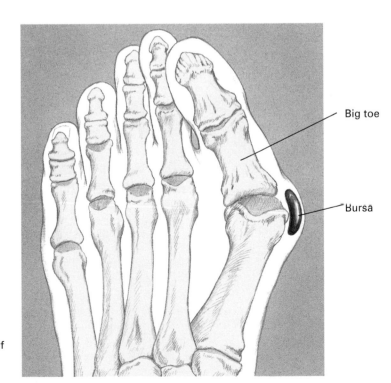

Big toe

Bursa

Figure 14.18
Hallux valgus with a bursa over a bone outgrowth on the inside of the foot; this is where the outward angle of the big toe is greatest.

415

growth forms on the medial side of the foot where the angle is greates
This exostosis is covered by a bursa which can sometimes becom
inflamed and extremely painful as a result of exposure to abnorma
pressure (a bunion).

One cause of hallux valgus is a depressed anterior transverse arc
Another is excessive pronation, with imbalance and contracture of th
muscles of the big toe. Other contributory factors are thought to be il
fitting shoes, and displacement of the first metatarsal bone.

<table>
<tr><td>Symptoms
and diagnosis</td><td>– The big toe is angled more than 10° outwards and may be presse
against the second toe. The second toe may in turn be presse
against the third toe, so that an increasingly faulty foot posture
present.
– A callus often occurs on the sole of the foot under the secor
metatarsal bone.
– There may be problems with shoe wear.
– Skin redness and tenderness can occur on the medial edge of the fo
where the angle is greatest.</td></tr>
<tr><td>Treatment</td><td>The athlete should:
– wear shoes with a wide toe box;
– put a piece of soft felt or a rubber pad between the big toe and t
second toe.
The doctor may:
– prescribe arch supports with pads under the anterior transverse arc
– prescribe shoes shaped to match the exostosis;
– operate only when the problems are severe. The operation c:
consist of removal of only the exostosis and bursa, or if the ang
between the first and second metatarsals is large, a wed
osteotomy, where the bone is cut to change the angle. The heali:
time for the former procedure is 4–6 weeks and for the osteoton
3–4 months.</td></tr>
</table>

Hammer toe

Hammer toe is characterized by a flexion contracture (Figure 14.1'
which is an inability to extend the toe at the proximal interphalange
joint (the joint between the toe bones). In the early phases the deform
is flexible (i.e. can be passively corrected), but with time it will becon
fixed. This contracture can be caused by insufficiency of the anter:
transverse arch (p. 413) or by wearing shoes that are too small. Pain
corns and calluses will appear over the prominent joint. Occasiona
there can also be a painful callus at the tip of the toe.

The treatment includes relieving pressure over the painful area,
wearing shoes with a larger toe box. Support for the transverse arch n
be indicated if it is flattened. Padding can be used as necessary. Shav:
of painful calluses can temporarily relieve discomfort. Sometimes sur
cal intervention is necessary. After surgery return to jogging can be po:
ble after 8 weeks.

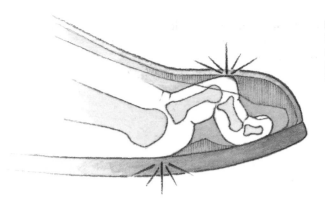

Figure 14.19
Hammer toe: the different possible pressure areas are indicated.

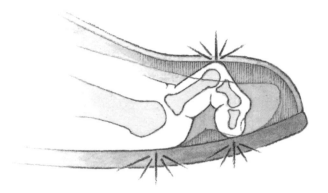

Hallux rigidus (stiff big toe)

Hallux rigidus can occur after repeated minor injuries to the articular surfaces of the metatarsophalangeal joint of the big toe. Early degenerative arthritis, with chronic pain and discomfort, can then develop. The mobility, especially dorsiflexion, of this joint is then impaired. The affected athlete finds it difficult to run or walk normally. Long-distance runners may complain that pain from the big toe makes them unable to run the required distances. The lack of dorsiflexion (Figure 14.20) means that the athlete is forced to compensate by rolling off the lateral aspect of the foot, which will result in other areas of injury. The diagnosis is mainly made by clinical evaluation—specifically, limitation of dorsiflexion of the first metatarsophalangeal joint.

Forced dorsiflexion will usually reproduce the athlete's discomfort. Palpation can often demonstrate a rigid bone on the dorsolateral side of the metatarsal head (Figure 14.21). Sometimes swelling can be present. An X-ray of the metatarsophalangeal joint or the big toe can often show limited changes, but may demonstrate dorsal spurs (osteophytes) due to degenerative arthritis (p. 25).

The treatment includes the use of a larger toe box to relieve the pressure. Sometimes a stiffer shoe with a steel shank or rocker-bottom sole can be used. A build-up to allow a 'rolling off' motion can be helpful;

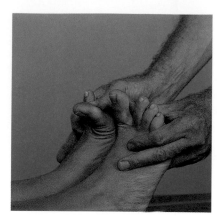

Figure 14.20 Lack of dorsiflexion.

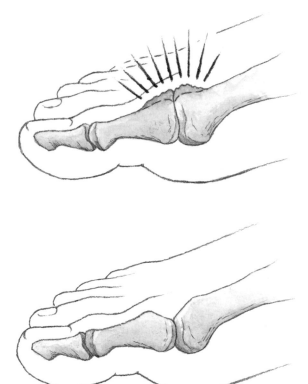

Figure 14.21 Hallux rigidus (stiff big toe). (**Top**) Bone spurs on top of joint. (**Bottom**) Surgery removes the bone spurs.

however, this is difficult for athletes to use. Occasionally nonsteroi[...] anti-inflammatory medication can be helpful. Sometimes the athlete [...] to change to another sport, like cycling or swimming, to relieve the jo[...] Operative treatment of hallux rigidus is sometimes necessary. In athlet[...] removal of dorsal spurs can sometimes restore motion and prolong [...] athlete's active life, but it will not remove the cause of the injury. M[...] extensive surgical procedures are available, but the results vary. Ther[...] no reliably effective treatment for this injury.

Turf toe syndrome

Turf toe syndrome occurs when a player's shoe grips the surface during a sudden stop, and the foot slides forward in the shoe, causing a vigorous dorsiflexion of the big toe (Figure 14.22). The ligaments under the first metatarsophalangeal joint (the joint at the base of the big toe) and the joint capsule are stretched, and the articular surface is injured. It is a common injury in American football, especially on artificial all-weather surfaces, and may occur in squash, badminton, and tennis. These injuries are common and are responsible for a large number of missed practice sessions.

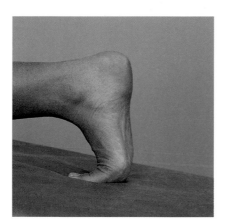

Figure 14.22 Position causing turf toe syndrome.

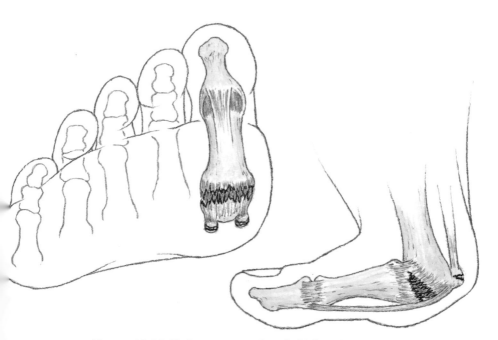

Figure 14.23 Turf toe, as seen (**top left**) from below, and (**bottom right**) from the side

419

The symptoms are swelling and tenderness at the base joint of the big toe, with pain on stretching and bending the toe (Figure 14.23). The athlete localizes the area of maximal pain to the undersurface of the big toe. Radiographic examinations must be done to exclude a fracture.

The immediate treatment includes cooling, compression, bandaging, elevation of the foot, and relief from weightbearing. After 2–4 days the injured athlete can again bear weight. Unrestricted motion is allowed except that a walking boot is used to immobilize the toe when walking. The injured joint can also be stabilized by taping, and a firm-soled shoe can be helpful in limiting joint motion. The injured athlete should allow at least 2–4 weeks of rest from sporting activities; although in running sports rehabilitation may take 2–3 months. Some athletes have persistent symptoms for many years, but can still continue their sport.

Fracture of the sesamoid bones

The two sesamoid bones under the metatarsophalangeal joint of the toe are the most vulnerable to fracture. These bones lie within the tendon of the flexor of the big toe. A fracture can occur either by direct impact or when the big toe is forced to bend vigorously upwards, as in take-off or landing on the flexed toe (Figure 14.24). Sometimes inflammation can occur in the tendon sheath surrounding the sesamoid bones due uneven pressure distribution in the area.

Symptoms and diagnosis
- The athlete cannot run on the toes and has pain on take-off.
- Local tenderness and swelling occur.
- Pain occurs when the toe is bent upwards.
- If there is a fracture, an X-ray may confirm the diagnosis. However these fractures are often difficult to see on plain films.

Treatment
- A walking boot or a plaster cast should be worn for several weeks.
- If the injury does not receive medical attention until a late stage and the fracture has not healed, surgery may be considered. Surgery may consist of removal of all or part of the sesamoid bone.
- The injury often affects athletes with high arches and a tight arch ligament. Surgical measures can sometimes be taken to reduce tension in the arch ligament.

Morton's syndrome

When the foot plantar flexes and the toes dorsiflex during push-off, the nerves between the second and third metatarsals, and the third and fourth metatarsals, can be compressed by the ligament between the bones (Figure 14.25). Additional compression can come from the metatarsal bones as a result of ill-fitting shoes or a depressed anterior arch. The plantar digital nerves that join between the metatarsal heads can become irritated by this compression and form a local nerve swelling (neuroma). This occurs most commonly between the third and fourth metatarsals. Each nerve transmits the sensitivity and pain from

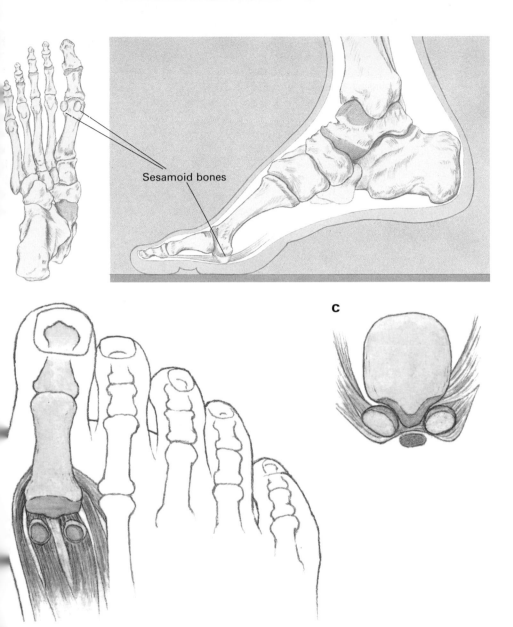

ure 14.24 Sesamoid bones, as seen (**A**) from below and from the side, (**B**) from above (where the first metatarsal bone has not been shown, to allow the sesamoid bones to be ualized), and (**C**) in transverse sectioning.

lateral side of one toe and the medial side of the adjacent toe, where the athlete may feel pain and numbness. This condition is known as Morton's syndrome.

nptoms — The injured athlete usually complains about recurrent pain from the
l diagnosis lateral side of one toe and the medial side of the next. It is generally the third and the fourth toes that are affected.

- The symptoms are often compared to an electric shock.
- Sensitivity can be impaired on the adjacent sides of the two affected toe
- The pain is sometimes relieved by walking barefoot.
- By compressing the metatarsal bones, pain can be triggered in t
  affected toes (see Figure 14.25).
- Local tenderness may be elicited between the toes (metatarsal head
  when a thin object, such as the back of a pen, is pressed against the ski

Treatment

The *athlete* should:
- rest and relieve pressure on the toes;
- wear wide-fitting shoes;
- avoid activities that include pushing-off; swimming and cycling a
  good alternatives.

The *doctor* may:
- prescribe anti-inflammatory medication for 1–2 weeks;
- prescribe an orthotic arch support with a metatarsal pad to spread t
  metatarsal bones and thereby ease the pressure on the nerve;
- prescribe physiotherapy;
- give an injection of local anesthetic solution and a small amount
  cortisone;
- operate to remove the neuroma from between the metatarsal hea
  Return to sports is possible within 2–3 months. This is a very eff
  tive treatment, but there will be a permanent loss of sensation to t
  adjacent sides of the affected toes.

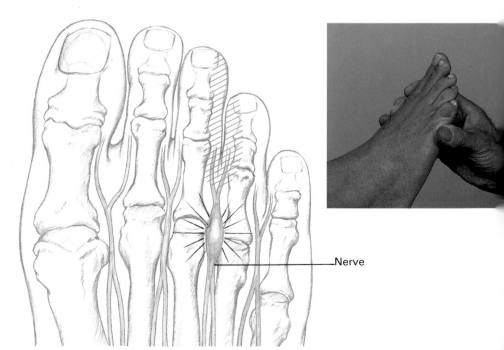

Nerve

Figure 14.25 When the front arch is weak, a nerve can get trapped between the bones. The nerve then swells, increasing pressure which in turn may cause radiating pain and numbness the toes (shaded areas). (**Inset**) Compressing the forefoot can elicit pain.

Fracture of the toes

Fractures of toes occur frequently in many sports, especially kicking sports. Fractures of the big toe are the most serious, especially if a joint is involved. If there is displacement, the bone ends must be realigned, after which the injury is treated with immobilization for about 4 weeks. Fractures of other toe bones heal without any treatment other than rest, provided there is minimal displacement. A 3–5 week break from training that involves the toe is necessary. Swimming, skiing, and weight training of the rest of the body may be continued.

Toe-nail problems

Ingrowing toe-nails

An ingrowing toe-nail is a common complaint amongst athletes, usually caused by ill-fitting shoes pressing the skin against the edge of the nail. The big toe, which has a broad nail, is most often affected.

Preventive measures are essential. Shoes should be big enough, well-fitting and comfortable, and tight socks should not be worn. Careful foot hygiene is necessary. The toe-nails should be cut regularly, at least once a week, and cut off straight, as they can grow down into the nail fold if the sides of the nail bed are trimmed to a curved outline. Nails that are too thick should be thinned.

In cases of ingrowing toe-nails, bacterial infections can invade the cuticles and cause extreme discomfort. Such infections should be drained and the area kept dry and treated with a local antiseptic and possibly an antibiotic powder. Antibiotics taken by mouth may also be of value. If ingrowing toe-nails cause persistent problems, surgery can be resorted to. A number of different approaches may be used, but it is usual for either a 'wedge' of nail or the whole nail to be removed, depending upon the length and severity of problems and on previous treatment. Excision of the nail bed (from which new nail growth arises) ensures that the nail does not regrow.

Black nails ('tennis toe', 'soccer toe')

Black (bruised) nails can occur as a result of a blow to the nail, being trodden on, wearing shoes that are too narrow, or the toe-nails being left too long. Bleeding occurs in the nail bed and appears as a black spot or patch under the nail. Bruised nails occur in most sports; in running they can be caused by the toe-nails being pressed against the front part of the shoe, especially when the shoes are too small, or when the athlete is running downhill.

Bleeding in the nail bed tends to be painful because the blood gathered under the nail exerts pressure on the tissues. This pressure can be released (after cleaning the nail), by making a hole with a clean, sharp knife, a red-hot needle, or a straightened paperclip (Figure 14.26). This is by no means as alarming as it sounds. The blood drains out spontaneously through the hole which is then protected with a dressing to prevent the nail bed becoming infected. This procedure preserves the nail, which would otherwise fall off after 2–3 weeks

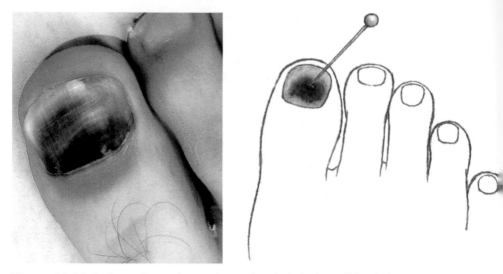

Figure 14.26 A pin or clip can be used to make a hole in the nail for drainage.

because of disruption of its blood supply. Once an injured n
becomes loose and begins to separate from its attachment to
cuticle, there is a risk of infection occurring and it is wise to se
medical advice.

Anyone who has had a bruised nail should consider how the inj
occurred, and if the shoes are at fault, should change them.

Subungual exostosis

In cases of repeated impact to a toe, for example when a basket
player's toe is trodden on repeatedly, an exostosis (bony outgrow
sometimes develops under the nail at the outer extremity of the affec
toe and impinges on the nail bed. This usually affects the big toe,
is very painful and highly sensitive to pressure and further impact.
many cases the nail has to be removed to relieve the pressure, an al
native being to remove the exostosis surgically.

Skin conditions

Calluses

The skin thickens in response to pressure to form a callus. Pressure
the feet can be caused by shoes that are laced too tightly or are
narrow, or by some anatomical variation. Calluses can occur at m
different sites, the most common being:

– the heel;
– the ball of the foot, especially in those who push-off with the sec
  toe;

- the top surface of 'hammer' or otherwise bent toes;
- the medial side of the big toe where there is an exostosis at that point.

Calluses on the foot are treated by relieving pressure. If necessary they can be trimmed with a sharp knife or filed with a foot file by an athletic trainer (Figure 14.27). Sometimes calluses are recurrent, and then treatment is a question of removing the triggering cause, for example an exostosis, or altering or replacing faulty shoes. This usually prevents further problems.

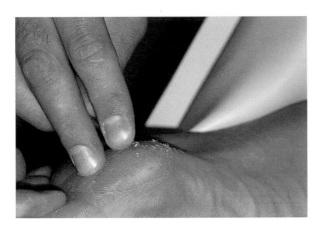

Figure 14.27
A callus under the big toe in a tennis player is being trimmed.

Skin outgrowths

Skin outgrowths are a kind of callus that forms between the toes, usually the fourth and fifth toes, as a result of pressure from shoes that are too narrow. Treatment consists of wearing shoes with a wider fitting at the same time as protecting the affected area from further pressure, e.g. by the use of rings of felt or foam rubber placed around the outgrowths.

Athlete's foot

When foot hygiene is inadequate, and when the feet are not dried thoroughly after showers or baths, fungal infections may develop (Figure 14.28). The fungus causes the skin between the toes to become soggy, cracked, and whitish in appearance, and often to smell offensive. The condition is infectious and can spread from one individual to another via floors on which people walk barefoot such as those of locker rooms, showers, and swimming baths. Preventive measures include:
- regular washing of the feet with soap and water followed by thorough drying;
- regular, frequent changes of socks;
- porous shoes that allow circulation of air and evaporation of moisture;
- avoidance of walking barefoot in locker rooms, etc.

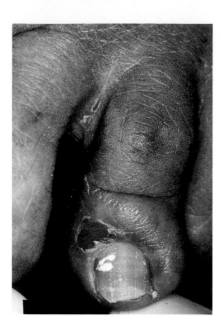

Figure 14.28 Tinea pedis interdigitalis infection (by courtesy of Baran et al 1996).

The *doctor* may prescribe a fungicidal preparation. The applicati... should be used regularly as directed and treatment continued for 2 wee... after the skin appears to have returned to normal.

Verrucas or warts

Verrucas (warts) are caused by a virus and can be transferred from o... individual to another via the floors of showers and locker rooms wh... people walk barefoot. The incubation period is 1–6 months. Verru... are most often located on the sole of the foot, are round or oval ... shape, and have a crack or dark spot in the middle. They can gen... ally be distinguished from calluses, although this may be difficult wh... a verruca appears in a weightbearing area and both conditions ... present.

Verrucas cause pain when pressed against underlying tissue, and ... also be painful when pressed from the sides. They may become infec... by bacteria, and rarely this infection may spread to the bloodstream.

Verrucas will disappear spontaneously after 2–4 years, but treatm... should be commenced as soon as they are discovered in order to prev... spread.

Any unusual lump or bump that appears on the skin, especially if... diagnosis is not obvious and the skin is discolored or bleeds, sho... prompt a consultation with a doctor.

Treatment

The *athlete* should file or rub down the verruca with an emery board... far as possible, perhaps after soaking the foot in hot water for 10... minutes, and then treat the verruca with a proprietary wart preparat... containing salicylic acid. The instructions for use should be followed w...

care and the normal surrounding skin protected. Treatment may have to be continued for several months.

The *doctor* may cut or burn away the verruca if necessary.

Bibliography

Baran R, Dawber RPR, Tosti A, Hancke E (1996) *A Text Atlas of Nail Disorders*, London/St Louis: Martin Dunitz/Mosby.

Baxter DE (1994) *The Foot and Ankle in Sport.* St Louis: Mosby.

Renström P, Kannus P (1993) Injuries to the foot and ankle. In: DeLee JC, Drez D (eds) *Orthopaedic Sports Medicine*, vol. 2, pp. 1705–67. Philadelphia: WB Saunders.

Head injuries

Head injuries occur in most sports, particularly in contact sports and riders, downhill skiers, and boxers (Figure 15.1). There is also a risk injury when heading a soccer ball, especially if faulty technique is use A kicked ball in flight can reach a speed of 100 km/h (60 mph) and wei about 450 g (1 lb) (even more if it is wet), so considerable forces can transmitted from the ball to the head.

Although serious injury can occur without any loss of consciousne in general the severity of the injury is related to the degree of memo loss and the period of unconsciousness. An attempt should therefore made as soon as possible after an incident involving a blow to the he to determine the patient's cognitive ability and to decide whether uncc sciousness has indeed occurred. The easiest way to assess the situati is to ask the injured person what happened before, during, and after accident, and to set a cognitive task such as counting backwards in sev from 100.

After a head injury, the following situations may develop:

1. *Head injury without unconsciousness (concussion).* Injuries in t category have a broad range of severity. In general the severity of injury is graded by the degree and period of cognitive impairment a by the period of memory loss. Athletes with concussion may compl of confusion, headache, nausea, and/or dizziness.

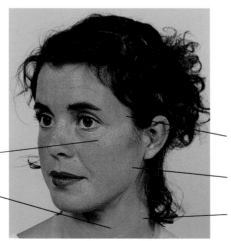

Figure 15.1 Location of injur to the head.

Maxilla fracture (p. 432)

Larynx injuries (437)

Zygomatic bone fracture (p. 4

Mandible fracture (433)

Neck wounds (437)

Athletes who have a brief period of confusion and return to a normal cognitive state within 5 minutes, with no memory loss and no symptoms (i.e. no headache, nausea, dizziness, etc.), may be able to return to play after an evaluation by a trained individual.

Athletes who have memory loss or symptoms for longer than 5–10 minutes should not return to play. They should be kept under observation, must not be left alone and should consult a doctor for advice.

2. *Head injury with unconsciousness of short duration (less than 5 minutes).* If there has been a short period of unconsciousness and the injured person is complaining of symptoms such as headache, nausea, vomiting and/or dizziness, and is generally upset, a serious injury may well have occurred. The injured person should be transported to a doctor or hospital for further management. As a rule, the symptoms settle without any further problems, and observation in hospital, if it is felt necessary, will be unlikely to last for much longer than 24 hours. A CT scan can assist in evaluation.

3. *Head injury with unconsciousness of long duration (more than 5 minutes)* is very serious. The injured person should be taken to hospital as soon as possible for diagnosis, observation and treatment.

Unconsciousness

Whether or not the injured person is unconscious at the time of examination, head injuries should always be regarded as potentially serious because grave complications can ensue.

A distinction should be made between unconsciousness caused by head injuries on impact (for example, a fall or collision) and those triggered by some other cause, such as inadequate circulation during long-distance running. It is up to the person providing assistance to determine the cause and act accordingly.

Measures at the scene of injury

It is important to note that head injuries are associated with a high incidence of cervical spine injuries. Therefore all maneuvers must protect the cervical spine. In all unconscious patients it must be assumed that the patient has a neck and spinal cord injury.

It is of vital importance to ensure immediately that the unconscious person has *free air passage* and is breathing normally. Obstruction of the airways in an unconscious individual due to any condition can cause death, and if breathing or heart activity stops for longer than 3–5 minutes, permanent brain damage occurs.

An injured person who is breathing unaided should not be moved except to remove anything that may obstruct the airway. If a safety helmet is worn, do not attempt to remove it—removal risks further injury to any neck

problems. Access to the face can be obtained by removing any fac
guards.

If the injured person is not breathing, artificial respiration must
commenced, using mouth-to-mouth resuscitation. The injured person
placed in a supine position. Care must be taken to protect the neck whi
moving the patient; this requires several people, with one person
charge of holding the head to keep the neck and spine aligned correctl
Once the patient is supine, artificial respiration is started:

- the mouth cavity is cleared of objects such as dentures, loose teet
  soil, or vomit.
- the lower jaw is pulled up and the head tilted slightly backwards. Tl
  tongue of an unconscious person can fall against the back wall of tl
  throat and obstruct breathing. Slight backward tilting of the injure
  person's head and support of the chin is usually sufficient to free tl
  air passages. One hand is put on the injured person's forehead whi
  the other supports the chin to pull the jaw forward. Care must
  taken to avoid excess neck extension that could cause further injury

Mouth-to-mouth resuscitation

To administer mouth-to-mouth resuscitation (the 'kiss of life'), take
deep breath, open your mouth wide and press it as closely as possible
that of the injured person (Figure 15.2). If it is an adult, pinch t
nostrils closed and breathe out strongly into the mouth at the same tin
(The patient's chest should heave if this is done correctly.) Then lift yo
head, turn it sideways and breathe in while the patient breathes out. Blo
in at a rate of about 12 times a minute for adults, that is, once every
seconds. If the patient is a child, blow in more frequently, more gent
and preferably through the patient's nose and mouth simultaneously.
not stop until the patient begins to breathe independently.

In addition, after two breaths, the patient's pulse should be check
If no pulse is present, cardiac chest compression should begin, followi
the guidelines from the American Heart Association for basic cardiop
monary resuscitation.

- *The unconscious person should be taken to hospital as soon as possible.*
- While waiting for transport *the patient should be kept covered* a
  something warm, such as a blanket, should be placed beneath
  person's body.
- *Give nothing to drink* to a person who is or has been unconscious.
- *Never leave anybody who is or has been unconscious alone.*

Mouth-to-mouth resuscitation is the only effective method of artificial respiration when no aids are at hand. The method should be
mastered by everybody.

Complications

In cases of head injury, it may take hours or days for evidence of com
cations to appear. *Internal bleeding* from ruptured blood vessels may oc
even if there is no bony injury to the skull, and unless controlled

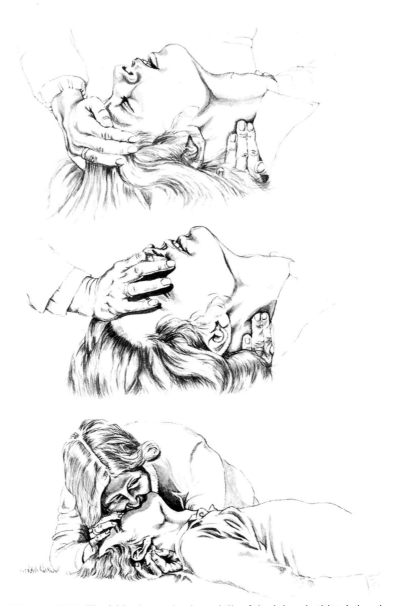

Figure 15.2 (**Top**) Maximum backward tilt of the injured athlete's head supporting the neck. (**Middle**) Pinch the nostrils together. (**Bottom**) Blow air into the athlete's mouth.

gradually compress the brain (Figure 15.3). The increased pressure on the brain tissues can affect the breathing center, and breathing may stop. Only an immediate operation to stop the bleeding and relieve the pressure will give the injured athlete a chance to recover.

Bleeding from the ears or bleeding with a simultaneous flow of fluid from the nose suggests that a fracture of the base of the skull may have occurred. This may indicate a very severe injury and requires emergency room evaluation. A variety of different techniques may be used for investigation, including X-rays, specialized scans and ultrasonography.

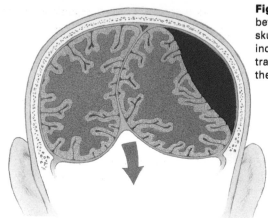

Figure 15.3 Bleeding between the bones of the skull and brain. The increased pressure is transmited down towards the base of the skull.

Facial injuries

Open wounds

Wounds on the forehead and scalp may occur in association with injuri to underlying tissues. Such injuries often occur in contact sports, suc as ice hockey, rugby, and soccer, as well as in riders, downhill skiers, ar others. When there is copious bleeding, face lacerations that requi suturing, or a risk of skeletal injuries, the injured person should see doctor. For general treatment of wounds see p. 57.

Fractures

Fracture of the maxilla

Fractures of the maxilla (upper jawbone) occur in contact sports such football, ice hockey, rugby, handball, and boxing. This injury should suspected if:
– the upper jaw has been subjected to a blow;
– the teeth are out of alignment and there is pain on clenching the teet
– one half of the cheek feels numb;
– a tender irregularity can be felt in the bone edge along the low border of the eye socket;
– there is double vision.

Fractures of the upper jaw are most often treated surgically and heal 6–8 weeks.

Fracture of the zygomatic bone

The zygomatic bone runs between the cheek and the ear, and a fractu should be suspected if:
– the zygomatic bone or the upper jaw has been subjected to a blow;
– there is tenderness with swelling over the zygomatic bone;
– chewing is painful.

If an X-ray shows that the fractured zygomatic bone is pressed inwards, the injury is operated on and heals in about 4 weeks.

Fracture of the mandible

A fracture of the mandible (lower jawbone) should be suspected if:
- the chin has been subjected to a blow, for example a punch in boxing;
- pain occurs on opening the mouth or clenching the teeth;
- the teeth are out of alignment;
- there is local tenderness in front of the ear.

Surgery is necessary if displacement has occurred. The lower jaw is fixed to the upper jaw by wiring the teeth for 6–8 weeks.

Nose-bleeds

A nose-bleed is caused by rupture of one or more blood vessels in the nose, and is common in contact sports such as handball, ice hockey, football, and boxing. Note that a broken nose should be suspected when bleeding occurs after a blow and/or there is deformity or crepitus.

Treatment

The *athlete* should:
- sit upright if possible;
- place thumb and index finger over the nose and pinch the nostrils together for about 10 minutes, after which bleeding will stop in 9 out of 10 cases. Keep the head bent forwards rather than backwards;
- put a ball of cotton wool or a compress in the nostril for about 1 hour. Make sure that it cannot be inhaled and do not forget to remove it;
- see a doctor if the bleeding continues in spite of the above measures or if there is deformity.

The *doctor* may:
- insert a compress with vessel-constricting agents;
- insert a pressure balloon in cases of severe bleeding;
- cauterize the ruptured blood vessel;
- perform a delayed reduction if deformity is present. Acute reductions can cause increased hemorrhage and are not advised.

Ear injuries

Injuries to the outer ear

Injuries to the outer ear are not common in sport. Repeated blows or repeated pressure against the ear, as in boxing and wrestling, can, however, cause bleeding that if untreated can result in a 'cauliflower ear' (Figure 15.4). A similar acute injury is seen in rugby players.

Emergency treatment with cooling and compression should be applied in order to reduce the swelling to a minimum. Bleeding in the outer ear can be treated by aspiration and packing, or suturing to prevent later

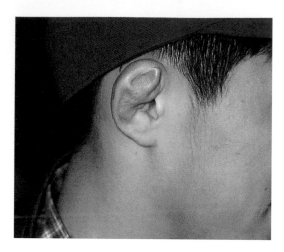

Figure 15.4
'Cauliflower ear'
occurring in wrestling

deformity. Treatment is not very effective, however, so prevention wi
protective headgear is preferable.

Injuries to the middle and inner ear

If a blow to the side of the head is followed by pain from the ear, sligl
bleeding, or impaired hearing, a rupture of the eardrum should b
suspected. These symptoms should always lead to a medical examinatic
since injuries to the eardrum can result in permanently impaired hearin
However, the majority heal spontaneously.

Those involved in shooting should always use effective ear defende
to avoid permanent hearing loss from damage to the inner ear.

Eye injuries

The area around the eye is constructed in such a way as to give the e
the greatest possible protection against external impact. Direct impa
against the eye from a large object, such as a football, can result in blee
ing and swelling in the eyelid and surrounding soft tissues, but seldo
injures the eye itself. However, blows from small or pointed objects, su
as elbows, fingers, sticks, rackets, squash balls, and pucks, can cau
direct injuries to the eyeball. Most eye injuries are minor, but serio
injuries need immediate attention to avoid loss of vision. Indications f
which immediate contact with a physician is advised include:
– severe eye pain;
– double vision;
– loss of visual acuity;
– decreased field of vision;
– blood or blurring at the pupil or iris;
– abnormally shaped pupil;
– suspected penetrating injury or tear;
– decreased eye movements.

Inflammation and bleeding in the conjunctiva

The eye is relatively resistant to irritation, but swimmers can be affected by inflammation of the conjunctiva (which covers the whole of the eyeball) because of the chlorine in swimming-pool water. The complaint can also be triggered by oversensitivity or overexposure to sunlight. It is harmless, and the problems can be relieved by eye drops. Swimmers can prevent the complaint by using protective goggles.

Subconjunctival hemorrhage is probably the most common eye problem. It can occur from trauma to the eye or by spontaneous rupture of blood vessels due to a sudden increase in blood pressure from exertion. So long as no visual symptoms or prolonged photophobia are present, this injury will resolve spontaneously and no treatment is required. Subconjunctival hemorrhage can sometimes mask other, more serious problems; if these are suspected, a doctor should be consulted immediately.

Lid lacerations

Lacerations of the eyelids, especially those that involve the tear system at the inside corner of the eye, require meticulous repair. A doctor should be consulted immediately.

Corneal abrasions

One of the most common eye injuries in sport is a small scratch on the cornea (the clear central part of the eye covering the iris). The wound can be caused by a finger-nail, a foreign body in the eye, or a contact lens. The affected person complains of pain and a gritty sensation in the eye, especially in bright light and when blinking. Increased tear flow is a common symptom. If a wound on the cornea is suspected, a doctor should be seen for advice since the injury can affect the sight. The treatment is usually ointment or eye drops and rest; an eye pad may be applied for a day or so.

Bleeding into the anterior chamber of the eye

A blow to the eye with a blunt object can cause bleeding in front of the iris (hyphemia). The blood forms a fluid level between the iris and the cornea at the bottom of the anterior chamber of the eye. The treatment of immediate bed rest, and sometimes bilateral eye bandaging for 5–6 days to control additional bleeding. The injured person should see a doctor for examination and observation. The condition often heals without any permanent disability, but secondary glaucoma and blood-staining of the cornea are worrisome complications that may impair sight.

Detached retina

The retina can be partly detached by a hard blow to the eye, and th should be suspected if the injured person has impaired sight within limited field of vision. The injury should be examined by a doctor.

Injuries to the mouth

Tongue injuries

The tongue can sometimes be bitten accidentally during sporting acti ity, leaving a bleeding wound which is painful but not serious. A ga that is less than 0.5 in (1 cm) long does not need any treatment. Mo extensive wounds may need careful stitching by a doctor.

Dental injuries

Dental injuries are especially common in children. A quarter of all den injuries in children occur during physical training or sporting activiti Collisions with opponents during contact sports are the most comm cause, but direct blows from equipment such as hockey sticks or cricl balls may be to blame.

In the majority of cases it is the front teeth of the upper jaw that a affected, and in half of these cases more than one tooth has be damaged. Dentists usually classify dental injuries in the following wa
- fracture of the crown of the tooth affecting the enamel only;
- fracture of the crown of the tooth affecting both enamel and denti
- fracture of the crown of the tooth with exposed pulp;
- injury of the attachment of the tooth in the jaw;
- injury of the root of the tooth;
- combination of fracture of crown and root;
- a lost tooth.

It is rare that a dental injury heals spontaneously without treatme Dental injuries in children are serious, since injuries to teeth and ja that are not fully developed can adversely affect them for life.

Treatment

The injured person should see a dentist *immediately* (the progn worsens with every hour's delay) in cases of the following types of der injuries:
- a broken tooth;
- a tooth that is knocked out;
- a tooth that is loose and bleeding.

A tooth that has been knocked out should be kept, since it sometimes be reimplanted successfully. The likelihood of this occurr depends on the length of time for which the tooth has been out of socket and the degree to which the periodontal membrane has dried c During the journey to the dentist the tooth should be kept moist, i

436

suitable medium so that drying of the periodontal membrane is minimized. Suitable media include sterile saliva or cold milk; it can also be kept under the tongue or in a saliva-soaked handkerchief.

Different types of gum shields (mouth guards) for athletes have been constructed, including those suitable for use in ice hockey and boxing (p. 83). Unfortunately in some sports there is resistance among top-level players to using these shields; this sets a bad example for young people. It should be a matter of course that all athletes in contact sports use this form of protection.

Neck injuries

With all neck injuries care must be taken to evaluate the cervical spine (p. 209). Spinal injuries can sometimes be masked by pain elsewhere. If there is any suspicion of spinal injury, the neck should be immobilized and the athlete transported to hospital immediately.

Injuries to the larynx

The larynx (voice box) is hollow and is composed of elastic cartilage lined with mucous membrane. Air passes between the vocal cords to reach the lungs. When a blow to the anterior neck is sustained (as in a chop to the neck by an arm, stick, or ball), the cartilage of the larynx can be depressed quite sharply. When the impact ceases, the cartilage springs back owing to its elasticity; when that occurs the mucous membrane may be torn loose. Bleeding can then occur between the cartilage and the mucous membrane and can spread to affect the vocal cords, which become swollen and cause hoarseness of the voice. The swelling can gradually increase until it obstructs the opening between the vocal cords to impede breathing. Children are particularly prone to this injury.

Blows against the front of the neck followed by hoarseness should prompt an emergency visit to hospital, since complications can be catastrophic.

Injuries to the larynx usually, however, heal with no treatment other than rest and observation.

Wounds to the neck

Wounds to the neck can involve the large blood vessels running to and from the heart. Injuries of this type are uncommon but serious. They

437

can occur in ice hockey when a skate hits the neck, or during acciden
in motor sports. Profuse bleeding occurs and must be stopped immed
ately by pressing a towel against the wound and applying constant ha
pressure. The injured person should be transported to hospital immed
ately. Protective collars are mandatory in ice hockey.

Chest injuries

Fractured rib

Fractured ribs are common, especially in contact sports. They can occ
after a direct blow with a blunt object, such as the handle of a stick,
as a result of forceful compression of the chest during a hard body tack
as in rugby or ice hockey.

Symptoms and diagnosis
- Pain is felt over the fracture area, especially when breathing deep
  coughing or sneezing.
- Tenderness and swelling occur over the fracture area.
- Compression of the whole chest causes pain over the fracture area.
- An X-ray of the chest confirms the injury and excludes underlyi
  lung damage.

Treatment
Fractured ribs generally do not require any treatment other than pa
relief; they heal spontaneously. Binding or strapping is discouraged as
prevents complete expansion of the lungs. Very occasionally, if seve
ribs are fractured and there is a possibility of interference with norm
respiration, the injured person may be admitted to hospital for obser
tion (Figure 15.5).

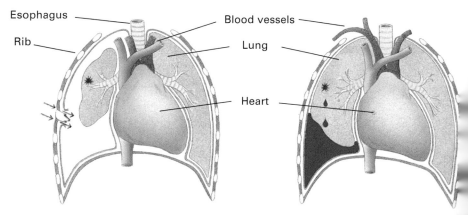

Figure 15.5 (**Left**) An open injury where the sharp end of a broken rib has punctured the lun
and caused leakage of air and at the same time collapse of the lung (pneumothroax). (**Right**) A
injury which has caused bleeding from the lung to pass into the pleural sac (hemothorax).
Pneumothorax and hemothorax can occur together.

In cases of a fracture without complications the injured athlete can resume sport as soon as symptoms allow.

Occasionally the sharp end of a fractured rib can puncture the lung and cause leakage of air (pneumothorax) or bleeding (hemothorax) into the pleural sac surrounding the lung. Increasing breathing difficulties should arouse suspicion that one of these complications has occurred. If it has, treatment will include draining the pleural cavity by means of a tube inserted through the chest wall.

Abdominal injuries

Injuries to the abdomen are rare in sport, but their outcome can be catastrophic (Figure 15.6). They can be the result of falling off or being kicked by a horse, and also occur in contact sports and among cyclists, downhill skiers, and others.

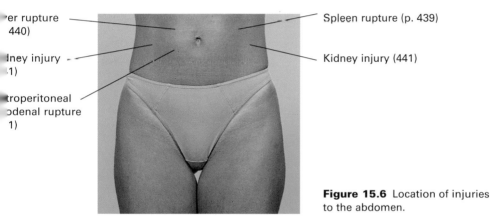

er rupture
440)

Iney injury
1)

troperitoneal
ɔdenal rupture
1)

Spleen rupture (p. 439)

Kidney injury (441)

Figure 15.6 Location of injuries to the abdomen.

Rupture of the spleen

The spleen is located in the upper left part of the abdomen (Figure 15.7), and its rupture is the most common cause of death among athletes with abdominal injuries. The injury may result from a direct blow to the abdomen, e.g. when a cyclist falls and the handlebar strikes the upper left part of the abdomen. Rupture can also occur, albeit rarely, in cases of fractured ribs. It is important to remember that a ruptured spleen can result from any violent blow to the left side. Athletes who have had infectious mononucleosis (glandular fever) recently are more at risk.

A rupture of the spleen and its surrounding capsule causes bleeding into the abdominal cavity with ensuing pain, nausea, and tenderness and tenseness of the abdominal muscles. The injured person is at first affected only by pain, but after perhaps an hour signs of shock appear: a fast, weak pulse, sweating, paleness, and sometimes drowsiness or loss

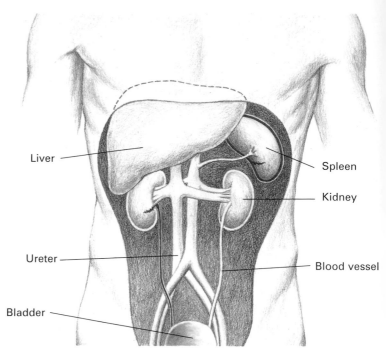

Figure 15.7 (Right) Rupture of the spleen within its surrounding capsule **(Left)** Rupture of a kidney. The bleeding caused by the rupture can pass blood into the urine.

of consciousness. If the capsule remains intact, bleeding from damaged organ will occur more slowly, with gradual distension a weakness of the capsule. There is then a risk that rupture will triggered by physical activity about 1–2 weeks after the initial injury; t occurs in 10-20% of cases.

If symptoms such as nausea, fatigue, or pain in the left upper abdom or left shoulder tip persist after a blow, a doctor should be consulted

Treatment   The course of events and the results of the doctor's examination and inv tigations will determine the length of stay in hospital. A CT scan and deep peritoneal lavage are helpful in confirming the diagnosis. Except severe cases, attempts are made to preserve the spleen because of its imp tance in the immune response; treatment includes rest, surgical suturi and local coagulants, depending on the degree of injury. In severe inju the spleen is removed. Following splenectomy the patient should rece polyvalent pneumococcal vaccine and should be monitored closely infection. Patients will have a lifelong impaired immune response.

Rupture of the liver

The liver is located in the upper right-hand part of the abdomen be the rib cage (see Figure 15.7). Its tissue is frail and it can rupture result of blows to this area. The injury occurs only rarely in sports, and most liver injuries are minor and self-limiting. Large ruptures can occur, however, causing shock with nausea, vomiting, lightheadedness, fainting, and drowsiness, with severe pain and distension of the abdomen. With any of these symptoms the athlete should be taken to hospital immediately. Almost all liver ruptures can be controlled with either rest and observation or surgery. A CT scan and/or deep peritoneal lavage are useful diagnostic tools.

Major ruptures of the liver can also result in bile leaking into the abdominal cavity. This can be more of a problem than the bleeding, since chemical or bacterial peritonitis can occur, which can damage all the organs in the abdominal cavity. A careful evaluation with surgical inspection and repair of bile leaks is essential.

Kidney injuries

Kidney injuries in sports are rare. The kidneys are located above the pelvic girdle, one on each side of the spine. As a result of a violent impact to the flank, a kidney can rupture, causing blood to appear in the urine. The bleeding often stops spontaneously and causes no further problems, but if disruption of a kidney is severe, and bleeding continues, surgery may be needed to repair or remove the kidney.

Blood in the urine after a blow to the kidney area should lead the athlete to seek medical advice. Diagnostic studies that can assist in assessing the degree of damage include CT and ultrasound scans, and intravenous pyelography.

After sustained, vigorous physical exertion without impact, a small amount of blood can appear in the urine, causing a faint red discoloration. This does not necessarily indicate a kidney injury, but should be investigated by a doctor.

Retroperitoneal duodenal rupture

Retroperitoneal duodenal rupture is rare, but can be caused by a blow from a blunt object, such as the knee of an opponent, in the upper abdomen. The intestines generally are not injured because they are mobile; however, the duodenum is fixed to the retroperitoneum and can be injured. The injury is characterized by severe upper abdominal pain and vomiting occurring several hours after the injury, owing to obstruction of the gastrointestinal tract and retroperitoneal leakage or bleeding from the injury. If the injury is severe enough, part of the duodenum may necrose several weeks after the injury and leak into the abdomen to cause peritonitis and even death. A CT scan is essential in diagnosing and monitoring the injury. Duodenal drainage and observation in hospital may be necessary. If necrosis of the duodenum is occurring, it must be removed surgically, preferably before rupture, to avoid peritonitis.

Injuries to the lower abdomen

A blow to the testes can cause bleeding and swelling that can disrupt the blood supply to the testes and cause sterility. The injury can be prevented by using a cup, especially for goalkeepers and catchers in ball sports.

Blows to the penis can cause a painful cramp in the sphincter of the bladder, which can make it difficult to urinate. The pain usually ceases once urination takes place.

Gynecological injuries, such as forced vaginal douche and hematoma of the vulva, can occur in water skiers, especially when an inexperienced skier falls in a squatting position. Wearing a wet-suit prevents such problems.

Acute winding

After blows to the abdomen it is not unusual for the athlete to be winded and remain lying doubled up on the ground. The athlete will recover more quickly if allowed to crouch, so that the abdominal and respiratory muscles can relax.

Bibliography

Kelly JP, Rosenburg J (1987) Practice parameters: the management concussion in sports. *Neurology* 48: 581–585.

16

Children and adolescents

Regular training of children and adolescents is becoming more common in sport, and competitive sports are indulged in with ever-increasing intensity at ever-decreasing ages. In certain sports, such as figure skating, swimming and gymnastics, children start regular training when they are 5–6 years old, and even in contact sports, such as soccer, training and competition they are beginning to train at earlier ages. In certain sports training for 2–4 hours, 5 or 6 days a week, is not unusual.

Are there any long-term advantages in allowing children to start regular training and competitive activity at such an early age? Children's play has always included running and jumping, which form a natural basis for sporting activity, but the increased demands and increased intensity of regular training can have a negative effect on an adolescent, and caution is needed. In some sports, swimming and tennis for example, studies have shown that very few winners of junior competitions become successful seniors—in other words, it is difficult to predict future development. Many young people give up their sporting activities too early because they are no longer enjoying themselves. Children and adolescents should be given the opportunity to try different sports rather than concentrating exclusively on one.

In principle, sports for children and adolescents should be fun and should not mean painfully hard training. The principles adults use in training cannot be directly applied to youngsters but must be adapted to their development. The risks of allowing adolescents to train and compete regularly can be looked at from different angles—physiological, psychological, and orthopedic—and the effects of sport on the latter can be divided into three groups:
– effects on the development of the musculoskeletal system;
– injuries due to accidents (traumatic injuries);
– injuries due to overuse.

Effects on development

The development of the musculoskeletal system in adolescents is governed by their ability to adapt in response to a changed or recurrent load, during training or following injury. Adaptation as a result of prolonged one-sided training can cause permanent changes, exemplified by the tennis player who, at an early stage, begins asymmetrical training and loading of the racket arm. This can result in development of a 'tennis shoulder', with an increase in the size of bones and muscles and increase laxity of the joint capsule, ligaments, and tendons around the shoulder of the racket arm. This causes dropping of the shoulder and a relative lengthening of the arm. In extreme cases an S-shaped curve (scoliosis) can develop in the thoracic spine.

Another example of the effects of training can be seen in young gymnasts. Long training increases the range of movement in the vertebral column, bringing about permanent changes in vertebral bodies and in the pelvis with increased mobility between the bones that form the pelvic girdle. We do not yet know with certainty what these changes will lead to in the long run, so it is essential that intensive regular training in children and adolescents takes place under medical supervision. At the same time, one-sided and repetitive training must be avoided and rules that reward abnormal mobility, as in scoring gymnastic competitions should be changed.

The training of children and adolescents should be comprehensive.

Traumatic injuries

Children and adolescents are injured more often than adults, but the injuries are usually less serious. This may partly be due to the fact that children are physically smaller than adults, so that less force is involved in the injury. Children's tissues are significantly different from those adults: their bone structure is more resilient and adaptable, and the muscles, tendons, and ligaments are relatively stronger and more elastic. Unlike the situation in adults, the articular cartilages have some blood supply, enabling injuries in those areas to heal to some extent.

The skeleton is the most vulnerable structure in adolescents. Though the bones are adaptable to various stresses, and in this respect are superior to those of adults, they are not as adaptable as the cardiovascular system and the muscles. In children and adolescents who participate in regular training, the musculature can develop more rapidly than the skeleton, which may be hazardous because of the unusual stress imposes. Because of the resilience of the tissues, overuse injuries are relatively rare in children and young people, although in recent years their incidence has been increasing noticeable, probably because of more intensive training in younger children.

Injuries to the growth zones

Growth in length of the skeleton takes place in the growth zones epiphyseal cartilages. In the femur 70% of the growth occurs in the lower epiphysis and 30% in the upper. Corresponding figures for the lower

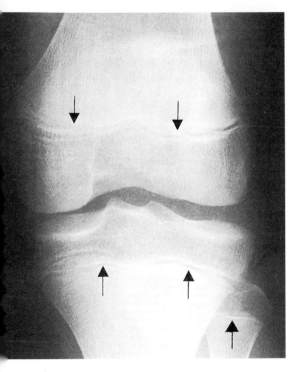

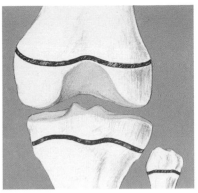

Figure 16.1 (**Left**) X-ray of a knee joint in which arrows indicate the growth zones of the femur, tibia and fibula. (**Above**) The corresponding growth zones. The main growth of the lower limbs takes place in these zones.

are 55% and 45% respectively. The epiphyseal cartilages are weaker than the rest of the skeleton and are susceptible to injury.

The age of the skeleton has a role in determining the effect of physical training on the epiphyseal cartilages. Hormone factors are also important. The epiphyseal cartilages are at their weakest during puberty and towards the end of the growth period when they are beginning to lose their elastic properties.

Epiphyseal cartilages are weaker than normal tendons and ligaments in adolescents, and an impact that would cause a total tear of a major ligament in adults, tends in adolescents to cause an avulsion of the epiphysis. So an impact against the side of the knee joint in children and adolescents may cause an epiphyseal injury, while a similar impact in an adult would tear the medial collateral and anterior cruciate ligaments. When tears of major ligaments are suspected in adolescents, X-rays should be taken so that the epiphyseal cartilages can be checked and any skeletal injuries discovered.

The epiphyseal cartilage (growth zone) is weaker than the connective tissue joint capsules, so that dislocations of major joints resulting from accidents are less common than injuries to the epiphyseal cartilage in children and adolescents.

In 10% of cases, injuries to the growth zone can disturb normal growth in length. The effects vary. While an injury to an epiphyseal cartilage is healing, bone growth on the affected side is halted, but the undamaged bone on the opposite side continues to grow. In cases of injury to the growth zone of the lower part of the femur this can mean a difference in length of more than 25 mm (1 in) between the two sides. Sometimes

445

an injury is partial and only the undamaged part of the cartilage grow. causing the leg to be crooked or angulated.

Growth zones can slip in relation to the bone (epiphysiolysis) (p. 258 The injury is not uncommon in the hip joint, in which the femoral hea can gradually or suddenly slip from the shaft. Epiphysiolysis should t treated by surgery.

Common fractures

Bone tissue is softer in adolescents than in adults, and the younger tl person the less likely it is to break. For this reason, fractures in childre show different characteristics (Figure 16.2). The skeleton also has a bett

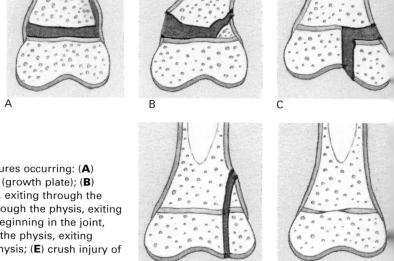

A   B   C

D   E

Figure 16.2 Fractures occurring: (**A**) through the physis (growth plate); (**B**) through the physis, exiting through the metaphysis; (**C**) through the physis, exiting into the joint; (**D**) beginning in the joint, extending through the physis, exiting through the metaphysis; (**E**) crush injury of physis.

blood supply in children than in adults which reduces the time need for fractures to heal. Treating fractures in children and adolesce involves principles different from those in treating adults.

– The fractures heal better and fewer visible signs remain in children a young people than in adults. An X-ray of a fracture taken 18 months af the injury will show perfect healing and no sign of a fracture in an adol cent, while a change in the shape of the bone is often seen in an adul

– Fractures heal faster in adolescents than in adults, and therefo children and young people do not have to wear a cast for so long.

– Adolescents sustain different types of fractures from adults. Bones tl are still growing are resilient, and can therefore be bent quite vigorou before breaking. An example of this is the 'greenstick' fracture, wh can occur in the lower arm in children.

Avulsion fractures

In adolescents the strength of the tendons, the ligaments, and the muscles is greater than that of the bones, while this situation is reversed in adults. This means that children and adolescents usually suffer skeletal injuries as a result of accidents or overuse. The bony attachment of the ligament or muscle is torn away from its origin, instead of the muscle or ligament itself tearing. Such avulsion fractures are often located in the growth zones of the flat bones and are most common in the front of the pelvis and also in the ischium where the posterior hamstring muscles have their origins (Figure 16.3). Avulsion fractures often occur suddenly during hard, rapid loading of the muscles.

When an adolescent has suffered accidental injury, and tenderness, swelling, and effusion of blood are present in the injured area, an X-ray should be taken. If bone attachments have been torn away and displaced to such an extent that they cannot reattach to their original site, surgery should be considered in order to reposition the fragments. A large displacement of the fragment can impair future functioning of the ligaments or muscles if the injury is not treated correctly.

Sometimes it is not fragments of the bone that are torn away but only the periosteum to which the tendon or ligament is attached. This can cause a loss of function in the muscle or ligament, but is not visible on X-ray. For this reason, functional testing of muscles and joint stability is of the utmost importance to make the correct diagnosis and choose the correct treatment. Magnetic resonance imaging can be helpful.

An injury caused by avulsion can be more serious than a straightforward rupture of a muscle or tendon, since it has the same implications

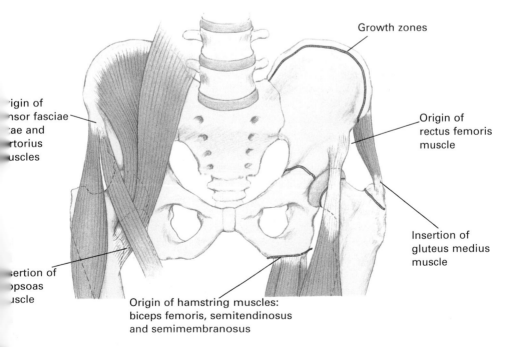

Figure 16.3 Common sites for avulsion fractures.

Growth zones

Origin of rectus femoris muscle

Origin of tensor fasciae latae and sartorius muscles

Insertion of gluteus medius muscle

Insertion of iliopsoas muscle

Origin of hamstring muscles: biceps femoris, semitendinosus and semimembranosus

447

as fracture. Injuries due to avulsion should therefore be distinguishe from the muscle ruptures that often occur in adults who have bee subjected to similar violence. Healing times are longer for avulsio fractures than for ruptures of a muscle and can be anything from 1 mont to 6 months depending on treatment. It is essential that avulsion fracture are diagnosed at an early stage so that adequate treatment can be startec If these injuries are neglected, the result can be chronic pain and impair ment of joint or muscular function resulting in instability or impaire mobility.

Adolescents who have tenderness, swelling and effusion of blood in the injured area after an accident should be X-rayed.

Injuries due to overuse

Injuries resulting from overuse in adolescents usually affect the apophy ses, the parts of the skeleton that constitute the attachments of tendon ligaments, muscles, or joint capsules.

Apophysitis

In a muscle and tendon unit there are certain areas at high risk of injur these are the attachments of muscle and tendon to bone, the muscle ar tendon tissue itself, and also the point at which muscle and tendon merg (the muscle–tendon junction). In adults, the muscle or tendon tissue itse is often injured by trauma, while the corresponding trauma in adole cents causes injuries to the attachments of the muscle or tendon to bon Studies have shown that physical training increases the strength tendons and ligaments faster than that of their attachments.

Apophysitis (inflammation of an apophysis) resulting from overu occurs mainly in specific sports, such as soccer, football, long jump, ar high jump, that involve a great deal of jumping and bending of the knee thus exposing the apophyses to great tensile stress and overloadir (Figure 16.4).

The site at which apophysitis most often occurs is that of the attac ment of the patellar ligament to the tibia (Osgood–Schlatter disease, 323). Overloading of the apophysis causes inflammation in the attac ment of the tendon which manifests itself as pain, tenderness, ar swelling. An X-ray shows fragmentation of the bone under the attac ment of the tendon. Apophysitis also often occurs in the attachment the Achilles tendon to the calcaneus (apophysitis calcanei, p. 359).

In cases of apophysitis it is essential that the affected athlete rests an early stage, avoiding the movements that trigger pain, until no mc

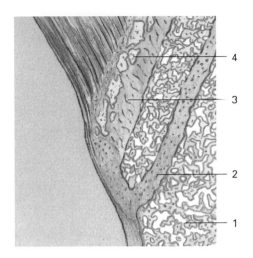

Figure 16.4 Apophysitis under magnification: 1, metaphysis of tibia; 2, growth plate; 3, separation filled with fibrous tissue and fibrocartilage; 4, bone fragment.

pain and discomfort are felt. The condition can otherwise be of long duration.

The most common cause of apophysitis is one-sided training. Here it is appropriate to warn against excessive strength training by young, growing people. When strength training is carried out with a heavy load, the strength of the muscles develops faster than the strength of the skeleton and can result in apophysitis and also in avulsion fractures. Growing youngsters should therefore practice strength training using only their own body as a load.

Stress fractures

One-sided loads on the skeleton can, when intensity and load are too high, lead to stress fractures or fatigue fractures if the adaptive ability of the body is insufficient to cope. Stress fractures can affect children who begin athletic training as early as the age of 7 years. The frequency of stress fractures in adolescents is increasing. The injury can be caused by frequently repeated movements under normal load, e.g. long-distance running, or by movements of a lower frequency but with a higher load, e.g. weightlifting. The most dangerous combination, however, is a high load and a high frequency. In principle, stress fractures can occur in any bone of the body, but are most common in the lower limbs. They occur mainly in the metatarsal bones, and in the tibia, fibula, femur, hip and pelvic bones, and vertebral bodies. Stress fractures should always be suspected in people who are subjected to repeated movements or heavy loads and who complain of pain on exertion. Usually there is no pain or discomfort at rest. Local tenderness and swelling over the painful area are found and a clinical examination usually leads to the diagnosis. If no fracture is discovered on X-ray examination, it should be repeated 3–4 weeks later if the symptoms persist. The diagnosis can then be confirmed. A bone scan can confirm the diagnosis at an early stage.

The risk of stress fracture can be reduced primarily by increasing training gradually but also by varied training alternating with regular rest so that the body has time to recover. The surface that athletes use in training can also be of importance, and the construction of the shoes is vital. Anyone running on a hard surface should always wear shoes with good shock-absorbing properties. When there is a change from a hard to a soft surface or vice versa, the intensity of training should be reduced during the transition period.

Articular cartilage injuries

The collagen tissue of the articular cartilage has less tensile strength in adolescents than in adults; thus children and young people can injure the articular cartilage more easily than adults as a result of sprains and direct blows. A prolonged extreme load on the knee joint, e.g. in downhill skiing or sailing, can result in injuries to the articular cartilage of the patella. In this condition, the patellofemoral pain syndrome (p. 310), pain arising from the inner surface of the patella or around the patella is triggered mainly by running uphill and downhill and by squatting. The articular cartilage of the patella softens and debris gathers. Since the cartilage does not contain any nervous tissue it is not clear why pain is triggered, but it may originate from the synovial membrane or subchondral bone. The causes of chondromalacia patellae are not known for certain either, but the condition responds to heat therapy and isometric training of the anterior and posterior thigh muscles.

Another cartilage injury that occurs in adolescents is osteochondritis dissecans (p. 306) in which a part of the articular cartilage and bone that has been damaged breaks away and can become free, moving inside the joint where it causes problems.

The diagnosis of these cartilage injuries is made with the help of arthroscopy.

Training young athletes

The most decisive stage of an athlete's life from a medical and orthopedic point of view is probably the moment of decision to concentrate on a particular sport, with all that that entails in the way of prolonged and planned intensive training. It would be desirable for a young athlete's physiological qualifications for the sport in question to be analyzed, but unfortunately there is as yet no sound medical basis for a reliable judgment.

Regular, targeted training is now starting at younger and younger ages. Training methods that have been developed for adults are directly applied to children without adapting them either to suit their age or to suit individual variations. With regard to training and competitive activities for adolescents, the trainer and the coach must be aware of the risk that exist for children in the long term as well as in the short term. Sport must remain play for children and a means of maintaining physical health for adults. Training activities must therefore be questioned: is it really right to train as hard as athletes do today in order to reach the top level, and are the right training methods being used?

Children are not miniature scale models of adults. They mature at different rates, and puberty can occur any time within a span of about 4–6 years. This physiological inequality in development is often forgotten by coaches and managers.

Physical fitness training

Physical fitness training is no more effective for young people aged 10–20 years than for any other age group. The anaerobic energy-producing capacity—the ability to produce energy in the absence of oxygen—is lower in children aged 10–12 years than in teenagers. Regardless of age and this capacity, however, young people can benefit from taking part in activities that demand anaerobic energy, and children do not seem to feel tiredness in the same way that adults do. However, recent findings indicate that adolescents do not lose anything by delaying systematic physical fitness training until they are in their late teens.

Strength training

In growing children the internal organs are able to adapt to great loads while the musculoskeletal system can easily be damaged. The effects of training in children and young people are seen mainly in the muscles, the cells of which increase in size. This increase in size is directly related to the length and intensity of the training program. The muscles become stronger when they are trained and lose their strength rapidly when the training ceases.

Children and young people respond to muscular strength training because there is relatively more effect on the musculature than on the skeleton. Under normal circumstances their muscles are not used for strength-requiring activities to the same extent as those of adults, and strength training in growing youngsters therefore has a more obvious effect on their musculature. In adolescence great increases in strength are characteristic of both men and women, but in the early teens the increase in strength is distinctly less than the increase in body size. Athletes in their early teens are therefore not quite as strong as their body size might indicate.

In strength training with heavy loads, muscular strength develops faster than the strength of the skeleton, which can lead to avulsion fractures.

There are a number of different types of strength training. In isometric training the ability of the muscle to exert power increases but its stamina does not increase as much as in dynamic training. In adolescence the attachments of tendons and muscles in particular are vulnerable, and therefore children and young people should be cautious about isometric work with a load, which means that the muscles are working without appreciably changing their length. Light dynamic work, such as running and walking, when the muscles are working by lengthening and shortening, is in most cases sufficient.

Training with heavy weights should be avoided by individuals who are still growing. The load on the vertebral column during weight training for example, can be so great that the vertebrae are affected. Only the weight of the body should be used as a load in strength training, and only when the skeleton has stopped growing, which in girls happens about the age of 16 years and in boys at 17–18 years, should systematic strength training with heavy weights be permitted. Before that a growing youngster can perhaps use light weights, but the training intensity should only be stepped up by increasing the number of exercises carried out.

A strength training program should be drawn up according to the growing youngster's age, maturity, body build, physical fitness, and sex. Time for tissue recovery is very important.

The International Federation of Sports Medicine (FIMS) has issued a position statement on resistance training for growing individuals. recommendations are given here with permission.

The available evidence suggests that resistance training can result in significant strength improvements in both children and adolescents, and that such programs can be performed safely if several important safety aspects are adhered to.

1. No resistance training program should be started without the proper supervision of a certified strength and conditioning professional.
2. The child should be taught the proper technique for each exercise.
3. Exercise equipment being used should be safe and suitable for the child's size.
4. High training intensities should be avoided, and maximal intensities should not be performed before the child reaches 16 years of age, or Tanner Stage 5.
5. All progressions in training intensity should be made very gradually.
6. Resistance training should be used as a supplemental form of physical activity and should not be used in place of the child's normal activity.

7. Resistance training programs for children should be designed to meet the needs of the particular sport of the child or adolescent.
8. All exercises should be performed throughout the full range of motion of each muscle in a controlled manner.
9. Fast, sudden, and ballistic movements during the exercise should be avoided.
10. Warm-up and cool-down exercises should be performed prior to and after all training sessions.

General mobility training

A considerable part of an adolescent's mobility training consists of basic movements which are carried out more or less automatically, such as moving the body and maintaining the balance. This type of movement is hereditary and is controlled by instincts which are passed on genetically and gradually develop during childhood. Balance, for example, is not fully developed until the age of 9–10 years. Whether physical training can influence development in a positive or negative direction is not known. In most sports there are complex patterns of movement which have to be learned with the aid of the pre-existing instinctive knowledge. When such a pattern has been developed it is difficult to change, so it is important to learn it correctly from the start. The nervous system can incorporate new patterns right into the teenage years. It is undesirable to incorporate incorrect information into the nervous system before it is fully developed, as it would subsequently be difficult to alter. Technique training should be carried out during the latter part of the period of growth.

Training in different age groups

7–9 years: play, technique, and all-round training

Training of children aged 7–9 years should above all be full of variation and fun, that is, the play element should predominate. Light fitness training including different ball games is suitable. All-round training should be the aim. Technique training should be introduced now, as children of this age are very receptive to learning.

10–11 years: general basic training, technique training, and all-round training

Training of children aged 10–11 years should include technique and coordination exercises, since this is an excellent time for improving

reflexes and mobility technique by training. Play elements are importan
features in the training, but systemic fitness training and anaerobic train
ing are not meaningful during this period.

12–14 years: general fitness training, learning of technique and tactics

During the age period 12–14 years, which partly coincides with pubert
there are rapid changes in growth and maturity, both physically an
mentally. The training must be adjusted to the maturity of the individ
ual youngster. *The body is, both physically and mentally, in a sensitive sta*
of development, and this must be taken into account. The play eleme
should be given ample scope. Technique training can also be carried o
since the ability to learn continues to be high during this period
growth. Some specialization can begin in the sports for which the you
athletes have shown talent. They can be introduced to tactical metho

15–16 years: preparation for specialized training

In young people aged 15–16 years basic physical fitness must be bu
up, and therefore regular fitness training should become a habit. Anae
obic training can now begin. Comprehensive gymnastics and flexibil
training are of great importance during this period, since growth oft
makes young people stiff and unsupple. Strength training can start wh
the muscles and skeleton allow an increased load. At this age you
people can start to learn the correct lifting technique, but should o
use light weights. *A heavy load should not be used, as the skeleton has*
yet stopped growing. The strength training should be intensified
increasing the number of times an element of exercise is carried out,
by increasing the load. It is important that the athletes spare their bac
from overload by using the correct lifting technique.

During this period, specialization in different sports can be und
taken.

Over 16 years of age: specialized training

Young people who are over 16 years old can participate in specializ
training which does not differ appreciably from that of adults. Grow
in girls tends to be complete by the age of 16–18 years while the dev
opment of boys continues up to the age of 18–20 years.

The role of training

When it comes to training and competition for adolescents there has
be an awareness of the risks these entail, both in the short and in

long term. Knowledge of the special characteristics of the musculoskeletal system in growing youngsters is therefore of great importance. There is a need to question training methods which make such hard, monotonous, and regular demands that sport becomes agony rather than the enjoyable pastime it should be. The aim should be to encourage a large number of young people to become active athletes so that a vast pool will be available from which top athletes can be produced in the long run. A lasting interest in sports should be founded in adolescence so that in adulthood sport is regarded as a means of maintaining physical health and fitness for the whole of one's life. During the years when adolescents are at their most receptive and find it easy to learn, the stress should be on technical training which can be made interesting and stimulating. Hard physical training and specialization, for those who have the ambition to go far, should start at a later stage.

Adolescents are different from adults, and it is important to remember this when harder and harder training of young children is beginning to be the norm. Age groups create a classification which is purely chronological and ignores the complete physiological picture of a growing youngster. It is quite common for there to be a difference in maturity of more than 5 years between young people in the same age group. Thus, a group of children aged 11–12 years can include youngsters whose biological maturity is on the same level as that of a 16-year-old. All training of children and young people must therefore be individual. Coaching courses must be mandatory so that those who train and manage growing young people are well prepared for their task.

In the world of sport there is a widespread opinion that training has a better effect the earlier in life it starts. Scientific studies have been unable to verify this theory. The question is rather whether too hard and intensive training at an early age can have any adverse effects in later life. Apart from anything else, such training is one reason why many young people give up sport.

– Intensive training of children and young people with the aim of making them into top-level athletes should not begin without a medical examination, and should then be supervised by a doctor.
– Anyone involved in training growing young people should have a sound knowledge of physical development in adolescence.
– Training programs for children and young people must be drawn up individually. Development (biological maturity) can vary by 4–5 years in youngsters of the same chronological age.
– The training should be adjusted to the individual, not the individual to the training.

Bibliography

Sewell L, Micheli LJ (1986) Strength training for children. *Journal of Pediatric Orthopedics* 6: 143–146.

17

Extreme environments

Prolonged activity in the open air such as hill walking or climbing especially in winter, places heavy demands on individuals who may be exposed to exertions they are unused to or are unprepared for.

Preventive measures

Basic physical fitness

Anyone traveling into remote places should first achieve basic physical fitness. A long hike should not be attempted before practicing its unfamiliar aspects, such as carrying a full backpack.

Equipment

The equipment carried must be carefully chosen to meet the demands of the hike. Shoes should always be well worn-in and the backpack should fit well. Comfortable and appropriate equipment is a prerequisite for an enjoyable stay out in the open, and a change of clothes should always be carried.

Health

A strenuous hike not only may fail to restore health and strength, it may demand more than it gives in return. Anyone who has recently suffered a bad cold, bronchial infection, or similar infection should not indulge a long, demanding hike. In such circumstances, staying in the area and taking short day trips with rests is more likely to be beneficial.

Body heat

It is vital to learn to conserve body heat, particularly in winter. Body heat is maintained by metabolizing food and by muscular work. During stays out in the open, demands are increased, and a hungry person feels the cold more easily, so a high-energy food intake is recommended. Alcohol and tobacco should be avoided. Damp clothes should not be allowed to dry on the body, as this causes heat to be lost by evaporation.

Blisters and wounds

Blisters are a perennial problem on long treks. The treatment of blisters is given on p. 59, wounds are discussed on p. 57.

Insect bites or stings

Insect bites cause itching, but the urge to scratch them should be resisted. A locally applied steroid cream usually works well to prevent irritation, and if the reaction is severe a doctor may prescribe an antihistamine. If an allergy is in question, consult a doctor before the trip.

Sprains of the knee and ankle

Ligament injuries to the knee and ankle joints often occur during outdoor activities. These injuries are discussed in Chapters 12 and 14 Anyone who sprains an ankle while far from help *should not remove the shoe to examine the injury*, particularly in winter. Generally, nothing can be seen but swelling, and it is usually then impossible to replace the shoe because of the swelling and discomfort. High boots are an excellent support for the ankle joint.

Injuries due to overuse

During prolonged exertion such as hill walking, overuse problems can occur, especially when the person is unfamiliar with the type of activity that is involved. Walking downhill may cause pain around the kneecap (patellofemoral pain syndrome, p. 310), while long walks uphill and running on sandy beaches can result in Achilles tendon problems (p. 359). If a heavy backpack is carried on a long walking tour, the straps can press against the shoulders and exert increased pressure on the suprascapular nerve (Figure 17.1) (p. 145).

Before any activity of this sort, careful preparations are essential. Equipment should be chosen carefully and well worn-in, and unfamiliar activities such as carrying a full backpack should be practised.

Fractures

For general symptoms and treatment, see p. 7. Fractures should always be treated by a doctor, so during remote outdoor activities, it is usually the responsibility of the injured person's companions to arrange transport.

Fractures should be immobilized by splinting. Skis, sticks, or straight branches can be used in the absence of anything better. The splinting

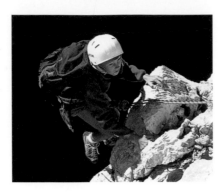

Figure 17.1 A heavy backpack may press upon the shoulders (by courtesy of All Sport: photographer, Didier Givois).

should include the joints on either side of the fracture. If the femur fractured, for example, the hip and knee should be stabilized, and tł splint should extend from the armpit down to the foot. If a suitable spli: is not available, a broken leg can be supported by strapping it to the oth leg, and a broken arm can be strapped to the body. If it is badly displace it may be necessary to realign a broken leg by straightening it longitud nally before transporting.

Apart from the splinting, as little as possible should be done fractures out in the open, and transfer to a hospital should not ł delayed.

General rules for care and transport of injured people

If a severe injury occurs in a remote area, the injured person should placed in a sheltered position and kept warm. Something warm, like anorak or survival bag, should also be placed *underneath* the perso body. If it is likely to take more than 4 hours to reach a hospital, t patient should be given something hot to drink and, if necessa something to relieve the pain, and kept calm while waiting for transpo

It is difficult to move a seriously injured person, and the transp should be carefully prepared. If a stretcher, sledge, or boat is availat it should be brought to the scene of the injury, and during the move t injured person should be made as comfortable as possible. Do not hesit to call for helicopter help in cases of severe injury, such as fractures. a neck or spinal cord injury is suspected, appropriate immobilization a cervical spine transport precautions are necessary.

Frostbite

'Frostbite' is a collective name for injuries that are caused by exposure low temperatures, which may mean temperatures above as well as bel freezing point. The extent of the frostbite depends on the temperatu the length of exposure, and the wind-chill factor. In temperatures ab

Table 17.1 Wind-chill factor

	Temperature in °C (°F) at increasing wind speeds			
In still air	5 m/s	10 m/s	15 m/s	20 m/s
0 (32)	−5 (24)	−15 (6)	−18 (1)	−20 (−5)
−10 (14)	−21 (−7)	−30 (−20)	−34 (−28)	−36 (−33)
−20 (−5)	−34 (−28)	−44 (−51)	−49 (−58)	−52 (−64)

freezing, dampness is also a factor. 'Lifeboat foot', 'air-raid shelter foot' and 'trench foot' are conditions caused by sitting still in cold and damp conditions.

Increased wind speed increases the likelihood of frostbite. The true temperature at different wind speeds is shown in Table 17.1.

When the outside temperature is −10 °C (14 °F) and the weather is calm, it is tempting to go out skiing; but if the wind force is 10 m/s, the effective temperature is −30 °C (−20 °F). Note that the same effect is exerted by wind rush in motorcycle racing. Simply turning one's face into the wind gives a good idea of wind speed.

Local frostbite

**ymptoms
d diagnosis**
- The skin becomes white and numb, though the victim does not always notice what is happening.
- Usually a gradual onset of local stinging pain occurs, but this may be absent if the cold is extreme.

reatment
The *injured person* should:
- shelter behind a companion, in a survival bag or in something similar;
- use body heat to warm the affected area. A warm hand can be placed against a frostbitten cheek or nose. A chilled hand can be put in the armpit or on the warm skin of the abdomen. A chilled foot can be placed against a companion's abdomen;
- never use snow to rub or massage frostbitten skin;
- never warm up in front of an open fire as the sensitivity in the frost-bitten part may have been impaired and severe burns can result.

A *companion* or *leader* should:
- provide the injured person with dry, warm clothing and a hot drink;
- force the injured person to keep moving to increase body temperature;
- take the injured person indoors, or, in cases of extensive frostbite, to hospital.

Frostbitten feet should not be rewarmed until evacuation from the area is possible. It is possible to walk on frostbitten feet without much further damage; but once the feet are rewarmed, the pain makes walking impossible.

In cases of local frostbite the injured person can be warmed in a hot bath (40 °C, 104 °F) if this is feasible. This treatment should not be used, however, in anyone suffering from general hypothermia.

Complications If blisters appear a few hours or days after the skin has suffered a local cold injury they should be left untouched. The surface of the blister the best protection against infection. The long-term effects of frostbite can be extreme sensitivity to cold in the skin that has been damaged together with stinging pains and sweating.

Hypothermia

People suffering from hypothermia become progressively weaker and more indifferent. They are overcome by tiredness, and can fall asleep and ultimately die because of their reduced body temperature: it may seem much more pleasant to submit and fall asleep than to fight and overcome the cold.

Treatment If the patient is *conscious* the following rules apply:
– The patient should be provided with dry, warm clothes.
– The patient should be *forced* to move about and activate the muscle
– A warm, sweetened drink should be given. Too hot a drink causes the blood vessels of the skin to dilate so that even more heat is lost, the core temperature is lowered further and the heart may be damaged
– The patient should, if possible, be taken indoors as soon as possible
– Warming should be carried out slowly at normal room temperature. Heating packs and warmed blankets can help to rewarm the patient mild cases.
– The patient should be taken to hospital as soon as possible.

If the patient is *unconscious* the following rules apply:
– Do not attempt to give anything to drink.
– Remove wet clothes.
– Warm the patient slowly at room temperature with the head at a lower level than the feet. Breathing and pulse should be checked.
– Warm blankets and heating pads can be used until the patient is transported to hospital.
– The patient should be taken to hospital as soon as possible when warming can be carried out under controlled conditions.

Sport in hot climates

Training and competition in hot climates can cause great problems for athletes, and anyone training or competing in such environments should be aware of the risks and preventive measures (Figure 17.2).

The temperature of the body, generated by muscle work and metabolic heat, is regulated by evaporation, radiation, and convection. Evaporation

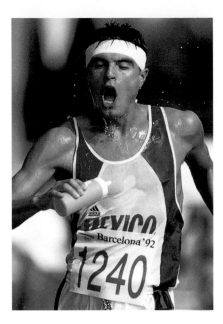

Figure 17.2 Hot climates can pose problems for athletes (by courtesy of All Sport: photographer, David Leah).

is the most important method of heat loss. For effective control of body heat by evaporation, the athlete must drink sufficient amounts of liquid. Heat loss is dependent on environmental conditions, such as the temperature of the air, humidity, wind speed, solar radiation, and solar reflection from objects in the environment. Heat convection will cease in air temperatures above 38°C (100°F); evaporation will cease when water vapour pressure is over 40 mmHg (5.3 kPa); the slower the wind speed, the slower the rate of sweat evaporation.

An increase in body temperature has both physiological and psychological consequences for athletes and may affect their ability to perform. Heat injury may occur in three forms: heat cramps, heat exhaustion, and heat stroke.

Heat cramps

Heat cramps are associated with prolonged exercise. They are intermittent, of short duration, and often excruciating. Heat cramps affect the muscles that work most intensively. In runners and soccer players, the calf muscles are most commonly affected, and in racket players, the arm muscles are affected. The exact mechanism of heat cramps is unknown, but they may be due to intracellular water and electrolyte disturbances. Cramps are extremely painful and can make further activity impossible.

Heat exhaustion

There are two forms of heat exhaustion: water depletion and salt depletion, the former being the major threat to athletes. During strenuous muscle work in warm environments, the athlete may lose 1–2 l (2–4 pints) of body water per hour in sweat. If this loss is not replaced by water intake, dehydration will occur. Intracellular fluid volume decreases and the osmolarity of the extracellular fluid increases, drawing water from the cells into the extracellular space. Severe dehydration may cause circulatory collapse and kidney failure.

Symptoms

The athlete experiences fatigue, dizziness, and muscle uncoordination and may become delirious or (in severe cases) comatose.

Treatment

In the early stages, the athlete should drink water; in advanced cases of dehydration, fluid should be given intravenously. It is not necessary to give electrolyte solutions during the early stages of dehydration.

Heat stroke

Heat stroke may occur if the rise in body temperature is unchecked. will cause tissue damage, including inactivation of enzymes, and damage to cell organelles and cell membranes. Distinctive features are serious central nervous dysfunction and multiple organ failure. Heat stroke can occur in long-distance runners, cyclists, tennis and soccer players, and especially in American football players, who wear protective padding that interferes with evaporation.

Symptoms

The athlete may become confused and delirious; this may be followed by convulsions and coma. The body temperature will increase to 41–42 °C (104–109 °F) and the skin may look and feel dry and hot, owing to the cessation of sweating. There is a 50–90% mortality rate associated with this condition.

Treatment

Cool the athlete as soon as possible with tepid water and air movement. Ice packs can be used to assist with cooling. Send the athlete to a doctor or a hospital to continue the cooling process and to restore the water and electrolyte balance.

Complications

Complications of heat stroke include:
– damage to the liver, with jaundice;
– damage to the kidney, with renal failure and acidosis;
– minor myocardial injury; arrhythmia may be present;
– hypotension and collapse of the circulatory system;
– watery diarrhea resulting from electrolyte imbalance;
– damage to the brain.

Prevention

It is important to prevent heat injuries. Strenuous sporting activity in high temperatures should not be allowed, especially when the vapor pressure exceeds 40 mmHg (5.3 kPa). The real danger is dehydration, which can be prevented by a sufficient intake of water.

Risks at high altitudes

Air density and barometric pressure decrease at high altitudes. The partial pressure of oxygen in the air decreases in proportion to the barometric pressure. Those taking part in endurance sports must be aware of this relationship. At an altitude of 3000 m (10 000 ft) and above, the partial pressure of oxygen falls to a level at which intellectual function may be affected, and at much lower altitudes the ability to do aerobic work is reduced. Anaerobic work and pulmonary ventilation increase, and lactic acid production will begin sooner.

These negative effects of high altitude can be decreased by acclimatization, which increases the hemoglobin concentration in the blood. The optimal time for acclimatization varies depending on the altitude but usually athletes should allow about 2–4 weeks before competition at high altitude. In some sports the high altitude may improve the performance of the athlete, especially in sports such as long jump and sprinting in which air resistance is normally a hindrance in achieving better results. This is not the case with technical sports and other sports in which performance is limited by the need for oxygen.

Skin injuries from solar radiation

The solar radiation that the skin is exposed to during stays in high altitude and in the summer is far more intense than the average athlete is used to. To avoid sunburn it is necessary to become accustomed to the sun gradually. Sunscreens or sun filter lotions with a high protection factor should be used for the skin, and salve for the lips. Exposed parts such as the forehead and nose can be protected with a peaked cap or a piece of paper.

Degrees of burns

- *First degree*: the skin is red. Damage is confined to the superficial layers of skin. This heals in a couple of days without treatment.
- *Second degree*: blisters form on the skin. If they burst, a sterile bandage and possibly a medicated compress should be applied. If the burn covers a skin area greater than $10 \, cm^2$ ($2 \, in^2$) a doctor should be consulted.
- *Third degree*: all the layers of the skin are destroyed, and the victim should definitely consult a doctor. During the early stages of a burn it can be difficult to judge whether it is second or third degree.

Sun or snow blindness

Sun or snow blindness is caused by ultraviolet rays, and is manifested as an inflammatory reaction in the conjunctiva and cornea of the eye. Visible sunlight and ultraviolet radiation are not the same; ultraviolet rays penetrate even when the weather is hazy and cloudy. As a preventive measure, tight-fitting, preferably dark-colored, sunglasses with side shields should be used. The sunglasses should be used at all times, as the eyes never grow accustomed to the strong ultraviolet radiation encountered during visits to snow-covered regions or when sailing (Figure 17.3).

Symptoms

– The affected person feels 'gritty' discomfort, swelling and pain in the eyes towards evening.
– The whites of the eyes become red, and the victim is disturbed by strong light.
– When the injury is severe, the affected person has to be led as if blind.

Treatment

The injured person's eyes must be protected from light. This is achieved by fitting a pair of sunglasses with small pieces of cardboard in which holes have been made for the pupils, so that the wearer can only just see to move about. Eye drops or eye ointments that have a relaxing effect on the ring muscle of the iris may be prescribed.

Generally sun or snow blindness lasts for 2–4 days and does not result in any lasting disability.

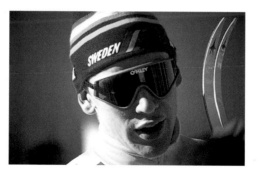

Figure 17.3 The eyes should be protected from intense sunlight.

Athletes with disabilities

Disability may be classified as follows:
- disability resulting from amputation; paralysis following birth injuries or injuries to the back or nervous system;
- defects of sight and hearing; mental disability;
- medical disability, such as heart disease, respiratory disease, diabetes, hemophilia.

Although disabled people may have received excellent training in a hospital or special center, they are still likely to have significant limitations and may lose some of their acquired skills when they return to the community. Sporting activities, graded according to level of skill and type of disability, offer a chance to continue training and acquire new skills outside the hospital. Sport also offers enormous benefits in social and psychological terms (Figure 18.1). Sports activities for disabled people are arranged in most countries, and participation is generally free of charge. Most of the sports involved have been adapted to suit disabled athletes and competition takes place up to international level.

Sports injuries in disabled athletes do not differ substantially from those suffered by other athletes. The most common injuries are pressure sores and blisters, crushing injuries, and ligament, muscle, and skeletal injuries.

The disabled athlete's chances of avoiding injury depend on the nature of the disability. Certain disabilities, such as wasted muscles with impaired muscular strength, or paralysis with loss of sensation, make recognition and diagnosis of injuries more difficult.

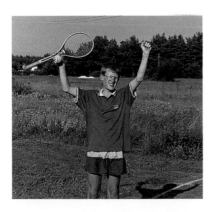

Figure 18.1 Sport and physical activity are extremely important for disabled people of all kinds.

All disabled persons should have the opportunity to take part in sporting activities, according to their capabilities and qualifications, under appropriate medical supervision and in cooperation with physical therapists or trained sports coaches.

Pressure sores

People with paralyzed legs often are dependent on crutches or a wheel chair and often have impaired sensitivity over the buttocks. Sitting for long time causes pressure that can result in the development of pressure sores. These start as small red spots that do not look particularly ominous but if overlooked because of impaired sensitivity, may progress rapidly create a deep sore which takes a long time to heal.

Prevention is of paramount importance. The athlete should not remain sitting for too long but should regularly be lifted out of the chair. *Before each competition or training session the coach should examine the athlete and look for signs of pressure sores.* If any skin redness is detected, the area question should be relieved from pressure, by using a rubber ring or by using alternative sitting positions. The skin area should be washed with soap and water, dried thoroughly, rubbed with surgical spirit, and exposed to the air. If a sore has appeared a doctor should be consulted.

Blisters

Many disabled athletes have to use aids such as corsets, artificial limbs and various types of bandages (Figure 18.2). The pressure from the

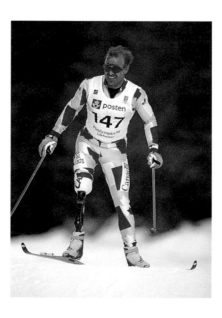

Figure 18.2 Cross country skiing (by courtesy of All Sport photographer, Clive Brunskill).

aids can cause redness and blisters, and the athlete should be examined for these conditions before and after training and competition. General principles concerning the treatment of blisters can be found on p. 59.

Contusion injuries

In wheelchair sports, basketball in particular, the wheelchairs come into close contact with each other and rapid maneuvers are necessary. The athlete's fingers can be jammed both in and between the wheelchairs. Such injuries are characterized by swelling and tenderness, and abrasions may be present. The swelling should be treated as soon as possible by applying ice and then bandaging.

Injuries caused by wheelchairs are difficult to prevent, but changes in their construction, such as protective frames fitted at the same height as the handle and situated on the same level regardless of wheelchair model, might be beneficial. The skin injuries from crushing or jamming incidents can be prevented if the athlete wears gloves or applies nonirritant tape to exposed areas.

Fractures

Impaired mobility or paralysis is inevitably accompanied by some degree of weakening of the skeleton (Figure 18.3). Furthermore, in such cases the muscles are often so wasted that they provide little protection for the bones. Fractures can therefore occur relatively easily, especially when unexpected loads are applied. Such fractures are often extensive with considerable splintering in the fracture area. Minor fractures may not be discovered immediately if the athlete has impaired sensitivity.

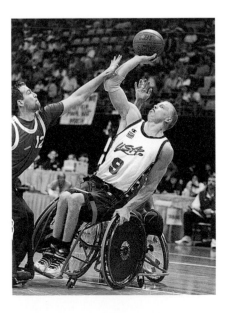

Figure 18.3 Wheelchair basketball (by courtesy of All Sport: photographer, Adam Pretty).

Athletes who wear support braces should loosen them during sportin
activities in case they act as levers and contribute to a fracture. The trea
ment of fractures is described on p. 7.

Injuries to muscles, tendons, and ligaments

As muscles affected by paralysis become hypotrophied, their functior
are taken over by other muscles that as a result become stronger fror
increased use. Arm and shoulder muscles are often remarkably wel
developed in people who depend upon wheelchairs. The risk of overus
of tendons and tendon attachments is increased by the addition
demands made upon specific muscle groups. Guidelines on treatment ar
given on p. 45. Impaired muscle strength often places greater loads c
ligaments and increases the risk of ligament injury.

Back and shoulder problems

Anyone who is confined to a wheelchair spends a large part of the tin
sitting, and back problems with more or less constant aching a
common. A corset can often be beneficial but can be uncomfortable
wear for any considerable period, especially in summer.

People in wheelchairs often suffer from shoulder pain as a result
one-sided repetitive movements in the shoulder joint.

Urinary tract infection

A great number of disabled people have problems with urinary tra
infections because of paralysis, impaired bladder sensation, and consta
sitting. The symptoms of a urinary tract infection can be slight or abser
so regular bacteriological checks on the urine should be made.

General medical complaints

General medical conditions, including heart disease, high blood pressur
asthma, diabetes, and hemophilia, do not preclude sporting activity, b
it should be undertaken only with the advice and supervision of a doct
and/or physical therapist. Those suffering from these disorders ha
tended to hold back from participating in physical exercise because o
belief that it could be dangerous for them, but it is now known that
can in fact be beneficial. It is likely that the numbers who indulge
sport despite their medical history will increase in the future.

19

General risk factors

The human body is built for physical activity, not for rest. Throughout the ages humans have had to expend great physical effort simply to survive; today, however, much of our life is sedentary. A human heart at rest pumps out blood at 4–5 l/min (8–11 US pints per minute); during physical effort the volume might increase to 10–40 l/min (21–84 pt/min). When breathing normally at rest 6 l (0.2 ft^3) of air is exchanged per minute, but the volume can increase to over 100 l/min (3.5 ft^3/min) if necessary, and a well-trained athlete can exchange up to 200 l/min (7 ft^3/min).

Available evidence indicates that even very moderate physical activity, provided it is regular, is valuable in preventing cardiovascular disease.

Pains in the chest and abnormal fatigue during sporting activity are serious warning signals. If they appear, the sporting activity should be stopped immediately.

Sports competitions should never be run in very hot or very cold conditions. Competitors should always be given the chance to warm up properly in cold weather. Sport should be carried out regularly, the extent and intensity of training being increased gradually.

Infections

Respiratory tract

The word 'cold' is used in everyday speech to cover a variety of respiratory infections. These are usually transmitted by direct contact or by airborne spread, e.g.when an infected person sneezes.

The warning signs of an impending upper respiratory tract infection include feeling feverish, tired, and generally unwell. There may be aches and pains in the muscles, similar to the stiffness felt after training; headache, runny nose, sore throat, coughs and sneezes are often present. When these symptoms last for 3–4 days and are accompanied by a temperature of 38–39 °C (100.5–102 °F), the cause is likely to be a virus. Resting quietly at home for the duration of the illness is recommended. Fever can be controlled with the help of an aspirin (acetylsalicylic acid) or paracetamol (acetaminophen) preparation and plenty of fluids. Sporting activities should not be resumed until the temperature has been normal for a week.

A *doctor* should be consulted if:
- symptoms and fever persist for more than about 4 days;
- the temperature rises again after it had settled;
- the patient has chest pain or difficulty in breathing;
- a productive cough develops;
- pain is felt in the sinuses, ears, etc.

Any of these symptoms suggests that a bacterial infection may have occurred and that antibiotics may be necessary. A doctor's advice and antibiotic prescription may similarly be needed if tonsillitis occurs. This is likely to be indicated by red, swollen tonsils (sometimes covered or spotted with white exudate) and tender, enlarged glands in the neck.

Some upper respiratory infections are so mild that they pass almost unnoticed and neither athlete nor coach feels the need to discontinue training. It should never be forgotten, however, that any feverish illness can be complicated by the development of myocarditis (inflammation of cardiac muscle) which may have serious consequences, including sudden death. It may, however, pass with insignificant symptoms which are the same as those of a general infection—fatigue, a feeling of discomfort, and so on. Chest pains and palpitations may also occur.

Urinary tract

Urinary tract infections include infections of the urethra, bladder, ureters, renal pelvis, and kidneys. The symptoms include pain on urination, frequent urgent urination, and sometimes fever (fever occurs particularly when the renal pelvis is inflamed, in which case it is also likely to be accompanied by pain in the lower back). Anyone who suspects a urinary tract infection should consult a doctor as soon as possible for diagnosis and treatment.

In men, the prostate gland may become inflamed, causing vague discomfort over the bladder, an urge to pass water frequently, pain on urination, and sometimes a fever. Again, a doctor should be consulted for diagnosis and treatment.

The same rules apply to urinary tract infections as to other feverish illnesses.

No sporting activity should be resumed until all symptoms have resolved and the temperature has been normal for at least a week after infection. There is no place, in this respect, for acts of heroism.

Female athlete triad

Exercise and sports have many beneficial effects on women as well as men. However, some women suffer from a syndrome called the 'female athlete triad'. This is syndrome comprises three interrelated disorders: eating disorder, amenorrhea, and osteoporosis. The female athlete is most at risk of developing this syndrome during adolescence. It may occur in many sports, but is especially common in endurance runners and 'appearance' sports such as gymnastics, diving, figure-skating, and ballet. It is associated with the age at onset of training, the sport concerned, diet, and stress.

Eating disorders

There is a tendency in the modern world to feel pressure to lose weight. Some women feel this pressure more than others. For athletic women, the pressure may come from coaches who aim to improve performance or appearance in sports such as figure-skating, gymnastics, swimming, and running. This pressure may force women into a wide spectrum of harmful eating practices, which may be called 'disordered' eating. These range from voluntary starvation, purging, use of diet pills and diuretics, to the full-blown eating disorders such as anorexia and bulimia. The syndrome is also seen in long-distance runners who fail to meet the high energy needs of their demanding activity.

Amenorrhea

Amenorrhea can be defined as the absence of three to six consecutive menstrual cycles. It may be caused by impaired nutrition, and can lead to an increased incidence of musculoskeletal problems. If the athlete has been amenorrheic for longer than 6 months and pregnancy has been excluded, hormonal studies should be carried out, as well as bone mineral density assessment.

Osteoporosis

Osteoporosis is defined as having a reduction in bone mineral density due to an imbalance between resorption and formation; the bone most frequently affected is the trabecular bone found in the distal end of the radius of the wrist, vertebral bodies of the spine, and the neck of the femur. The risk for primary osteoporosis may be genetic, hormonal, or associated with nutrition or lifestyle (such as exercise). Secondary osteoporosis may be caused by underlying disease or drugs. Athletic amenorrhea and a subsequent reduction of ovarian hormones can result in osteoporosis. Bone loss in young women with amenorrhea may equal the 2–6% loss that occurs in postmenopausal osteoporosis and it can be irreversible. Women with amenorrhea need intake of 1500 mg of calcium to stay in calcium balance. Calcium intake alone will, however, not prevent bone loss. The goal is the resumption of spontaneous menstruation; otherwise replacement doses of ovarian hormones should be prescribed to prevent further bone loss in the group of amenorrheic athletes. Increasing body weight by 2–3% recommended. Extreme activities should be avoided, but moderate exercise is desirable (p. 12).

Amenorrhea is reported to occur in 40% of female athletes in the USA and eating disorders in up to 60% of collegiate gymnasts. Long-standing amenorrhea should require a consultation with a physician. The disorders of the triad are chronic conditions with high morbidity rates due dehydration, electrolyte abnormalities, cardiac arrhythmias (irregular heart rhythm), depression, and increased risk of injury including stress fractures. As these disorders are often hidden or denied, they may not be easily recognized. Early recognition and referral for treatment can improve the prognosis.

If a female athlete has a stress fracture, the female athlete triad should be suspected.

Bibliography

Snow-Harter C. (1994) Bone health and prevention of osteoporosis active and athletic women. In: Agostini R (ed.) *The Athletic Woman. Clinics in Sports Medicine*, 13/2, pp. 389–404. Philadelphia: W Saunders.

Yeager KK et al. (1993) The female athlete triad. *Medicine & Science Sports and Exercise* 25: 775.

Pregnancy

Physical activity has no adverse effect on a normal pregnancy, but should be moderated as the pregnancy develops. Physical fitness can make both pregnancy and delivery easier. Most active sportswomen stop competing in the fourth or fifth month of pregnancy and are content with only a limited training program. Caution, however, is advisable particularly in contact sports and in sports where a large increase in core body temperature may occur.

After delivery, sporting activity should not be resumed for 6–8 weeks when any discharge has ceased and the uterus has returned to its normal size. During the 8 weeks after delivery pelvic muscle exercises will help to prevent possible future problems such as uterine prolapse. Other training and competitive sporting activities can then be resumed gradually.

Many women breast-feed their babies, and milk production adversely affected by heavy physical training. During the breast-feed period the breasts are also relatively enlarged and thus more easily damaged by physical activity.

Lifestyle factors

Doping

Doping increases the risk of injuries and endangers health. It is also illegal, and cheating. Regulations have been developed by the International Olympic Committee and others, and must be followed.

Alcohol

Consumption of alcohol impairs performance and causes a marked increase in the risk of injury. The breakdown of alcohol in the body occurs at a constant speed and is not influenced by such measures as physical exercise or sauna baths. *Sport and alcohol do not mix.*

Overweight and obesity

The overweight are usually less physically active than their lighter fellows and hence tend to have a less robust musculoskeletal system. This, combined with the greater load they have to support, increases the risk of injury and can accelerate joint degeneration.

Obesity is a significant, though probably comparatively minor, risk factor for the development of cardiovascular disease. Its main cause is a surplus of unused food energy; an underlying physical disorder is the exception rather than the rule. The energy surplus is converted into fatty tissue.

A man who has a sedentary job and does no physical exercise in his spare time requires 8000–10 000 kJ (2000–2500 kcal) every 24 hours. Most people's diets, however, are not ideal, so that in order to ensure a sufficient intake of important nutrients, they have to consume the equivalent of 10 000–12 000 kJ (2500–3000 kcal) daily, which for many people is far more than they need. The problem can be solved by:
– eating smaller quantities of food, but making sure that the diet is well-balanced;
– increasing the rate of metabolism by exercise or other physical activity.

A combination of these two methods is more likely to be successful than one used in isolation.

Fluids

Sweating and fluid supply

During physical exertion the body's core temperature increases. The cooling effects of wind and heat loss by radiation are insufficient to

prevent it rising dangerously; they are supplemented by the productio
and evaporation of sweat. Sweating begins after 1½–3 minutes of wor
and increases steadily before leveling out after 10–15 minutes, or long
in a humid environment.

70% of the human body is composed of water, most of which
contained inside the cells. When sweating, fluid is drawn mainly fro
this intracellular supply with a resulting adverse effect on cell metabo
lism. Fluid loss therefore causes impaired performance, which become
apparent when 1–2% of the body weight has been lost as sweat. Whe
the fluid loss amounts to 4–5% of the body weight the capacity fo
hard physical work is reduced by nearly 50%. Further fluid losses a
likely to lead to collapse, and this does occasionally happen durin
sporting competitions, especially long events conducted in war
weather.

Fluid replacement

In order to maintain physical performance, especially during prolong
training sessions or competition, an adequate fluid supply is essenti
When a match or competition continues over a long period in a war
environment and the resulting fluid losses are considerable, it is almo
impossible to replace all the lost fluid during the session itself. It
important, therefore, to ensure fluid balance the day before the comp
tition and during the preliminary warm-up so that hydration is adequa
from the outset. If the period of competition lasts for less than
minutes it is generally unnecessary to break for fluid intake.

The sensation of thirst is not an accurate guide when it comes
replacing fluid lost by sweat. Slaking one's thirst generally provides on
about half the amount of fluid required, and anyone who indulges
strenuous physical activity would be well advised to drink considerab
more than he thinks he needs. Checking body weight on an accura
balance is advised.

The fluid used for replacement should be of an appropriate compos
tion to replace those substances lost by the body during strenuous phys
cal exercise. Water is the most important component but sugar too
needed. Sugar is absorbed from the intestinal tract into the bloodstrea
and transported to the muscles, brain and nervous system. If the blo
sugar level is markedly reduced, performance deteriorates. Sensations
faintness, dizziness and hunger are likely to occur and collapse can ensu
Judgment and reaction time may be affected so that the risk of injury
increased.

Although some sugar is necessary in the replacement fluid, too mu
(< 6–8%) should be avoided as the fluid is retained in the stoma
(sometimes causing discomfort).

Except at very intense levels of exercise, the absorption of fluid i
the body is independent of intensity of activity, so that it is immater
whether the body is at rest or hard at work. The rate at which
stomach empties is, however, reduced by strenuous physical activi
Thus if fluid high in sugar content is ingested, emptying of the stoma

virtually stops and the fluid is no longer transferred into the intestinal tract. Athletes should therefore take their fluid replacement during the less strenuous parts of competitions. Plain water should be considered when exercising in very warm environments.

The replacement fluid chosen should be palatable (flavored with lemon, for example) and at a temperature of 25–30°C (77–80°F). As it is difficult to drink more than 300–400 ml (12–15 fl oz) of liquid in one go, this amount should be supplied at frequent intervals (for example, 15–25 minutes) and, consistently, every 5–6.5 km (3–4 miles) in, for example, orienteering, crosscountry running and skiing. The hotter the weather, the more fluid is required, even during training sessions. Fluid intake during training should be partly to establish the habit of taking frequent fluid level before the competition itself and partly to keep up a good pace, which is at least as important. In all training lasting more than 40 minutes, water with or without sugar solution should be drunk fequently.

A suitable solution can be made by dissolving 25–75 g (¾–2½ oz) of granulated sugar or glucose in 1l (1.76 pt) of water. This constitutes a sugar content of 2.5–7.5 per cent, which is as high as that of most of the sports drinks at present on the market.

- *During warm-up periods* 250–500 ml (½–1 pt) of fluid should be ingested.
- *During sporting activities* sugar solution should be taken regularly and often. In winter its sugar content can be 5–15%, and in summer 2.5–7.5%.
- *After sporting activities* large quantities of fluid should be consumed, including sugar and electrolytes (e.g. juice), in good time before retiring to bed.
- Weight can be checked every morning as changes are most often due to alterations in fluid level.

Nutrition

Muscles need energy in order to work. At rest, energy supplied by the metabolism of substances within the body is used primarily to maintain a temperature of 37°C (98.6°F) and to fuel the vital functions of the internal organs. During exercise energy production in the musculature is 50–100 times greater than during rest.

Fatty tissue, of which an average man has 8–10 kg (22–33 lb) distributed in various parts of the body, is the largest of our fuel stores and provides 36 kJ/g (9 kcal/g) of energy.

The carbohydrates that we eat (for example, bread, rice and potatoes) are stored as glycogen in the muscles and liver. Normally muscle contains 10–15 g/kg (¼–½ oz/lb) of glycogen, and combined muscle and liver glycogen totals 400–500 g (14–17 oz). Glycogen provides 17 kJ/g (4.1 kcal/g) of energy, or 6,600–8,300 kJ (1,500–2,000 kcal) in total. This is approximately the amount of energy used by a top-level skier or cyclist during 1½ hours of hard competition. Thus glycogen is a limited energy reserve.

Choice of fuel

When pure carbohydrate is metabolized, 21 kJ (5.1 kcal) of energy are released for each litre of oxygen consumed, and the corresponding figure for fat is 20 kJ (4.7 kcal). In competitions in which the pace is so fast that the athlete's oxygen absorption is maximum or nearly maximum, carbohydrate is the fuel consumed first. Fatty acids, however, provide an equally good fuel source, and the more highly trained the muscles, the more fat is metabolized.

At rest and during moderate muscular work with minimal load on oxygen-transporting mechanisms, the body chooses fat as its principal fuel. When the pace of muscular work increases to more than 70% of the maximum oxygen uptake, carbohydrates become the predominant energy source.

Carbohydrate (glycogen) is the most important fuel for athletes during competition, whether of long or short duration. As the glycogen is depleted, the body gradually begins to burn fat and as it does the pace is reduced. The results of a competition may be directly influenced by lack of glycogen.

Under normal circumstances, the body's glycogen stores are sufficient to supply energy for competitions lasting up to 1–½ hours. Before more prolonged efforts, some dietary loading of carbohydrate is recommended.

Short competitive period

Before competitions that last for up to 1 hour, no particular dietary adjustment is necessary, since the body's normal glycogen stores are sufficient. An unnecessarily high carbohydrate intake results in a weight increase as considerable quantities of fluid are bound in muscles and liver during glycogen storage (1 g of sugar binds 2–3 ml of water).

3–4 hours before every competition a light meal should be eaten.

Long competitive period

Before competitions of 1–3 hours' duration, some consideration should be given to dietary preparations. Sports such as walking, running, orienteering, cycling, skiing and canoeing, which depend upon physical fitness, are liable to use up the available glycogen during the course of the competition. Therefore in the days leading up to the competition, meals should include food rich in carbohydrates. As it takes about 48 hours for glycogen stores to be built up, no prolonged or hard training that would deplete the stores should take place in the 48 hours prior to the competition.

Prolonged competitive periods

In competitions that last for over 3 hours (for example, marathon races) the final result is to some extent dependent on the glycogen content of the body at the outset.

Depleted glycogen stores and low blood sugar levels impair physical as well as mental performance and increase the risk of injury.

Training and competition abroad

In order to maximize the benefits of training and competition in another country, certain aspects of foreign travel should be considered before departure.

When a journey abroad is planned, information should be obtained about the local weather and humidity at the time in question. Details about the height above sea level, time differences, and so on should also be ascertained. On the basis of this information the flight and time of departure can be arranged to minimize the effect of jet lag, so that the need to acclimatize on arrival can be accommodated. Other important factors to be aware of before arrival are the standard of living and sanitation of the areas to be visited, the prevalent diseases and the medical care available. Before major competitions the team doctor should visit the place of competition well ahead of the date of the event, to prepare for the team visit (ideally at the same time of year as the competition will take place).

Changes in daily rhythm

Time differences between home and destination can disrupt the daily rhythm of the body, affecting sleep, body temperature, cardiovascular functions, mental performance, appetite, bowel activity, and certain hormone levels.

- *Sleep disturbances* result in lack of initiative and in lethargy. If the flight goes westwards, e.g. from Europe to the USA, the time changes by 5–8 hours, and it will be 2–4 days before sleep patterns return to normal. The time needed for adjustment is shorter in younger people and in extrovert, fit, 'evening' types. Some people have great difficulty adjusting.
- *Changes in body temperature* influence metabolism and may affect performance.
- The *ability to concentrate* is impaired and can sometimes be reduced for 4–6 days.
- A *change in eating habits* and *reduced appetite* can also affect bowel activity, with resultant diarrhea or constipation.
- *Hormone balance* takes longer than temperature to be restored to normal, during which time performance is probably impaired. In women there can be changes in the menstrual cycle and menstruation may either fail to occur, or do so earlier or later than expected.

In general terms, one day's physical disturbance occurs for ever
hour's time difference.

The complaints that result from disruption of the daily rhythm can b
prevented by adjusting the rhythm by 2 hours per 24 hours during th
week preceding departure. Alternatively, if adjustment is to start at th
destination, departure should be timed so that arrival is well before th
competition (at least 6–10 days before, if the Atlantic or Pacific
crossed).

Disease prophylaxis

Before travelling abroad it is essential to find out in good time whic
vaccinations are compulsory for the countries in question and which a
recommended. Vaccinations against certain diseases, such as typho
fever and cholera, must be given well before departure so that the boc
will have time to build up the necessary resistance. As far as malaria
concerned, it is necessary to take precautions, in the form of tablet
against the disease before, during, and after visits to an area where the
is a risk of infection. An immunoglobulin injection given a few da
before departure provides some protection against hepatitis for 4–6 wee
and is particularly desirable for travel to less developed areas. Freque
travellers should be immunized against hepatitis.

Travellers abroad come in contact with a different bacterial and vir
environment from that at home, and may therefore be more susceptib
to infections including stomach, bowel complaints, and colds. Meticulo
personal hygiene is therefore essential. In many countries ordinary t
water is unsuitable for drinking and bottled mineral water should be us
instead. If there are doubts about the standard of hygiene, hot cooked
fried dishes should be ordered, and cold dishes, salads, pastries, a
desserts—in some places even ice cream—should be avoided. All fr
should be peeled before being eaten. If this is not possible the fr
should be rinsed in mineral water. Drinks accompanying meals shou
be mineral water, bottled soft drinks, pasteurized milk, or boiled beve
ages such as coffee and tea.

It is important to find out whether the local water supply is cle
enough for bathing, and in hotels of doubtful standards it is preferab
to shower rather than to bath. A team member who falls ill while abro
should be isolated and a doctor consulted.

20

Training and exercising

Preparation for activity and competition

Only a complete training program leads to good results, enabling athletes to build up their muscles, strengthen their joints and bone structure, and improve coordination with minimal risk. Active training will eventually produce enhanced performance, provided it is accompanied by a generally healthy life style, balanced nutrition and adequate time for recovery.

It is important that body parts that are loaded during training should be given the opportunity to rest and recover. The harder the training, the longer the break needed for full recovery. Exercising repetitively with a heavy load, for example, would require 1–5 days of recuperation before the next session. Less strenuous forms of training, can be practiced daily. Daily training, however, is of little benefit to those who have either had a long break from training or are physically unfit. Instead they should break themselves in gently, starting with 2 or 3 days' training per week.

Athletes should analyze the demands of their chosen sport before deciding on a training program. Apart from the specialized techniques of individual sports, there are other factors that influence performance, and each athlete needs to consider the following questions:
1. What factors influence performance in my chosen sport?
2. Which of these factors can I influence and improve by training?
3. How should I train in order to influence each of these factors to best effect?
4. How much time should I devote to training in order to influence each specific factor and when should the training be carried out?
5. Considering all these factors, how should I train in order to reduce the risk of injury to a minimum?

Training intensity, load and recovery time should be adapted by the athlete to correspond to the level of physical fitness achieved.

Basic physical fitness

Good physical fitness is of the utmost importance in avoiding injury. Those whose basic fitness is below normal are more prone to injury both from trauma and from overuse.

479

After a period of inactivity, the ability of the body tissues to utiliz
oxygen decreases noticeably. In one experiment, five healthy test subject
stayed in bed for 20 days without any physical activity whatsoever. Thi
relatively short period of inactivity reduced their capacity to utiliz
oxygen by 20–45%. This and similar experiments demonstrate hov
quickly the body adapts to the physical demands made on it. When th
demands are reduced there is a corresponding decrease in the cardia
output, muscle mass diminishes (hypotrophy), and blood volum
decreases. The body is less efficient in transporting oxygen from th
lungs to the tissues, and as a result the capacity of the muscles to conver
nutrients into energy is reduced.

Basic physical fitness can be achieved by exercises and general physica
activity continued throughout the year. All training aimed at achieving goo
basic physical fitness should progress gradually, and this applies above a
to those who are no longer young. During a period of rehabilitation follow
ing illness, injury, or a break in training, it is important that a reasonabl
level of basic physical fitness is reached before competition is resumed.

The warm-up period

Warm-up exercises are designed to prepare the body for the ensuin
sporting activity. They have two functions: to prevent injury, and t
enhance performance.

In a body at rest the blood flow to the muscles is low, and most c
the small blood vessels supplying them are closed. When activity begin
the blood flow to the muscles increases as the vessels open. At res
15–20% of the blood flow supplies muscles, while the correspondin
figure after 10–12 minutes of exercise can be 70-90%. A muscle ca
achieve maximum performance only when all its blood vessels ar
functional. Physical work increases the potential energy output and th
temperature of the muscles, and this in turn leads to improved coord
nation with less likelihood of injury.

A progressive warm-up leads to a marked decrease in the risk of injur
and an enhanced performance, while at the same time providing som
psychological preparation for the task to come. *Warm-up exercises shou
begin with movements of the large muscle groups*, as these are the main are
to which blood is redistributed. After this general warm-up, mor
specialized exercises can begin. Runners, for example, should concentra
their warm-up on the muscles and joints of the lower limbs. Stretchir
of muscles and joints is essential, but heavy loads at the outer limits c
joint movement should be avoided (Figure 20.1). The final stage c
warm-up concentrates on technique, perhaps checking a run-up c
practicing a sport-specific movement. The pace of the exercises can k
gradually increased, and the warm-up sessions should last for at lea
10–30 minutes, depending on the sport involved.

Depending on the circumstances surrounding the activity in questic
(such as temperature and humidity) it may be advantageous to put on
fresh shirt after a warm-up, to prevent the muscles from cooling tc
quickly as sweat evaporates. A tracksuit may also be advisable fc

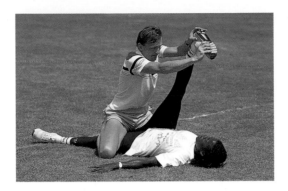

Figure 20.1
Stretching muscles
and joints is an
essential part of
warm-up to activity.
Passive stretching
requires an
experienced physical
therapist (by courtesy
of All Sport:
photographer, Gray
Mortimore.)

warmth. The effect of the warm-up soon starts to wear off and ideally the time delay before competition should be no longer than 10 minutes. Warm-up exercises should be completed before both training and competition, and clearly represent a major factor in preventing injury and enhancing performance.

After training or competition, cooling-down exercises, such as gentle jogging, are desirable. Stretching should also be part of the cooling-down process if maximum benefit is to be achieved.

Effects of inactivity and training on tissues

The musculoskeletal system, comprising the bones and their associated joints, ligaments, muscles, tendons, nerves and blood vessels, undergoes qualitative changes in response to levels of physical activity.

Effects on bone

The bone structure of athletes who have been immobilized for some time or who have not exercised becomes decalcified. This weakens the bone, with increased risk for fracture. Immobilization stimulates bone resorption and depresses bone formation, resulting in osteoporosis. Of the total bone loss, 30% is due to increased bone resorption and about 70% to decreased bone formation. If weightbearing is allowed despite immobilization, bone loss is less than in non-weightbearing conditions. If the bone structure is exercised regularly by physical training, it adapts to increased demands and becomes more robust, though those parts that are subject to decreased stress may still undergo some weakening and degeneration. These changes take place slowly during the rehabilitation period after injury and—most importantly—during prolonged, unbalanced training of children and young people (see Chapter 16). These changes can be permanent.

There is a relationship between the different states of loading and tissue quality: during training, the lower the initial loading state, the faster and better the adaptation; during immobilization, the higher the initial loading state, the faster and more severe the demineralization. The reverse is true for both situations.

Effects on cartilage

There are early histological changes in articular cartilage after loss of motion and weightbearing. The content of water and proteoglycan (p 18) decreases, and there is increased metabolic activity, especially in the areas that are subjected to compressive loading. The cartilage surface becomes soft and fragmented, the chondrocytes (cartilage cells) die in increasing numbers, the collagen fibers split, disintegrate and fibrillate and the bone under the cartilage demineralizes. These early changes are probably reversible. It has, however, been suggested that after 8 weeks of complete immobilization, the changes may become permanent and start a vicious cycle leading to osteoarthritis.

The central parts of the joint surfaces are least susceptible to strain. Overloading the joint at the peripheral areas should be avoided. For example, any attempt to hop, squat, or do the splits should be delayed until these extreme positions have been incorporated gradually into the regular training program. The best way of keeping articular cartilage in good condition is by gentle exercise, as any repetitive, unbalanced extreme load can damage it.

Effects on muscle

Muscle tissue hypotrophy begins after as little as 1–2 weeks of immobilization and disuse. The degree of hypotrophy depends on factors such as:

– the duration of immobilization—the longer the immobilization, the greater the hypotrophy;
– the position of immobilization—tissue immobilized under tension hypotrophies significantly less than in the relaxed position;
– the preinjury condition—as trained athletes appear to suffer greater relative losses after immobilization than the untrained;
– slow and fast twitch fibers may react differently to immobilization;
– sex and age may affect the degree of hypotrophy.

The proportion of functional loss is greater than the loss in muscle mass or volume, both of which are greater than the loss in extremity circumference. Most typically, after complete immobilization for 6 weeks the isometric or concentric strength of human quadriceps muscle decreases by approximately 30–40%, while the cross-sectional area of the muscle as measured by a CT or MRI scan decreases by 20–30%, and thigh circumference measured by tape decreases by 10–20%. The main reason for the greater decrease in muscle function compared with the cross-sectional area may be due to nerve factors, i.e. deterioration neural activity of the muscle. Immobilization also damages the mechanical properties of the muscle–tendon unit, especially breaking strength and elasticity.

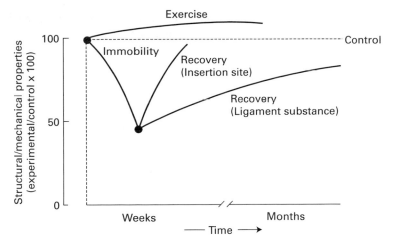

Figure 20.2 Musculoskeletal tissues improve and maintain their structural and mechanical properties if they are continually exercised; immobilization has the opposite effect (by permission of the International Society of Biorheology and IOS Press).

With regular exercise, the muscle increases in size (hypertrophies). With aging the total mass is more or less maintained, but the muscle strength diminishes as some of the muscle fiber volume is replaced by fat. Hypotrophy is delayed and can be reversed by exercise. A healthy, active muscle structure can help to protect the joints from injuries by improving the way forces are distributed.

Effects on tendons

Inactivity and immobilization cause tendon hypotrophy, although at a slower rate than that of muscle. The tensile strength, elastic stiffness, and total weight of the tendon tissue decrease; the collagen fibers that compose the tendon become thinner and disoriented; and the crosslinks between the tendon fibrils may become smaller and reduce in number.

Regular exercise can preserve the strength of the connective tissue and delay the degeneration that normally occurs with age. It also improves the mechanical properties (material composition) and the structural properties (breaking strength) of the tendon (Figure 20.2)

Effects on ligaments

Inactivity weakens the ligament and joint capsule. Ligaments have been known to shrivel and shrink, impairing mobility and putting inappropriate strain on the joints. There is a decrease in total collagen mass overall. The anterior cruciate ligament decreased in tensile strength by one quarter and elastic stiffness by one quarter in animal studies. Regular exercise improves the mechanical properties (material composition) and also the structural properties (cross-sectional mass or size) of the ligaments. The joint capsule is very susceptible to overuse and irritation and reacts by secreting more synovial fluid than usual, resulting in effusion in the joint.

The effects of inactivity and immobilization can be devastating. More research and education are needed on ways of limiting these harmful effects.

Rehabilitation and remobilization

The effects of rehabilitation and remobilization vary from tissue to tissue. In general, the positive effects of rehabilitation and remobilization occur much more slowly than the negative effects of immobilization. The functional properties of skeletal muscles can be significantly impaired even years after the injury and following immobilization. It is still unknown whether the marked structural changes in muscles are permanent, and if they are, what their effect is on functional recovery during remobilization.

Bone responds well to remobilization and loading if the immobilization period does not exceed 6 months, after which osteoporosis becomes more or less irreversible.

Bibliography

Kannus P, Jozsa L, Renström P et al (1992) The effects of training, immobilization and remobilization on musculoskeletal tissue. 1. Training and immobilization. *Scandinavian Journal of Medicine and Science in Sports* 2: 100–118.

Kannus P, Jozsa L, Renström P et al (1992) The effects of training, immobilization and remobilization on musculoskeletal tissue. Remobilization and prevention of immobilization hypotrophy. *Scandinavian Journal of Medicine and Science in Sports* 2: 164–176.

Woo SL, Gomez MA, Wood YK, Akeson WH (1982) Mechanical properties of tendons and ligaments. II. *Biorheology* 19: 397–408.

21 Rehabilitation

Movement therapy and physical therapy

General exercises are part of the athlete's warm-up before training sessions and competition and have an essential function in preventing injuries.

The role of athletic trainers and physical therapists in sports medicine is one of participation in both prevention and treatment. As far as prevention is concerned each sport has its own pattern of movements which subjects various muscle groups to different types of load. A knowledge of these patterns is vital to the athletic trainers and physical therapists, whose tasks are to emphasize the importance of warm-up, make appropriate suggestions for strength and flexibility training with regard to the requirements of the sport in question, and recommend specific training based upon the needs of each individual athlete.

When an injury has healed, the aim is to restore original function to the affected part. The athletic trainer's instructions are of the utmost importance in ensuring that the correct muscle groups are trained with the appropriate movements and with a well-balanced load.

If surgery is contemplated, physical therapy can be valuable both before and afterwards. Prior to a meniscus operation, for example, it is essential for the patient to exercise the thigh muscles as they are responsible for stabilizing the knee, and if they are well trained before the operation, rehabilitation is facilitated.

Assessing an individual's functional state is part of the athletic trainer's and physical therapist's work. Analyzing the causes and consequences of a functional impairment enables a program to be drawn up for the treatment of muscles, joints, and ligaments. The treatment methods used are flexibility, strength, and coordination training in prescribed proportions, together with encouragement, rest, and use of modalities to reduce pain and swelling.

The treatment of functional disorders, e.g. joint immobility caused by muscle damage, is based on neuromuscular stimulation, an improvement in the interaction between nerves and muscles. This interaction is disordered when joints are immobilized, and there is increased tone in the muscles surrounding the joint. Treatment aims to relax the muscles to improve the range of movement. Stretching should be carried out slowly and smoothly, in order to prevent a rapid reflex muscle contraction (stretching exercises are described on p. 487).

In all strength training it is essential that the correct load is used. After an injury, training should be appropriate to the type and extent of the damage and to the stage of the healing process reached. No strength training should exceed the pain threshold. The first stage is usually isometric training without external load, after which the training frequency and subsequently the load can be increased gradually. When isometric training can be carried out without pain, dynamic training can be started. Hydrotherapy allows earlier and more aggressive intervention to help physiologic recovery. Muscle training may be supported with electrical muscle stimulation when conventional exercises cannot be carried out.

Exclusive training of an injured area should be avoided, and a comprehensive training program should be drawn up to include all the training elements relevant to the sporting activity concerned.

It is important to monitor the healing process so that the injured area is not overused and healing delayed. Athletes do not always have the patience to wait for an injury to heal, and it is common for intensive training to be started too early. This emphasizes the important role of the athletic trainer and physical therapist, who should oversee the training program to ensure that it is appropriate in both type and intensity.

Physical therapists and athletic trainers should be involved in the treatment of sports injuries to a far greater extent than is the case at present. This should include the functional and sports-specific training and tests needed before the athlete returns to sport.

Principles

The aim of rehabilitation is to limit the amount of scarring, and preserve strength, elasticity, and contractility of the tissue's components. The objective in training these muscles, tendons and joints after injury is to:
- regain normal mobility (range of motion) of the joints;
- stretch connective tissue fibers of the tendons and muscles to an optimal length;
- increase the strength and endurance of the muscles;
- increase the strength of muscle and tendon attachments;
- improve coordination and proprioception.

Biomechanical considerations

The range of movement of a joint is normally limited by the articular surfaces, the ligaments, and the joint capsule, and by the length and flexibility of muscles and tendons. The ligaments and joint capsule are comparatively inelastic and are responsible for maintaining passive stability, while muscles and tendons control active stability.

Muscles, tendons, and ligaments all contain collagen fibers. A tendon, for example, consists of 90% collagen fibers and 10% elastic fibers. The collagen fibers run parallel in tendons, in tendon attachments, and in the areas where they merge with muscles. They are under no tension at rest but are loaded and stretched during muscle contraction. Collagen tissue can be elastic (resilient) or plastic (pliable), and has a high viscosity (internal friction). The fact that it is both viscous and elastic means that the speed with which it is loaded is of importance. The faster a tendon is loaded, the stiffer (less elastic) and less pliable it becomes. During slow loading, on the other hand, there is an increase in its elastic and plastic properties.

The collagen in tendons must be subjected to extension for at least 6 seconds for its plastic properties to change. At temperatures of about 38 °C (100–101 °F) or just above normal body temperature, there is an increase in the elasticity and plasticity of collagen fibers, so a careful and thorough warm-up should be carried out before any flexibility training begins. Localized warming of tendons followed by slow stretching to the pain threshold results in extension of the collagen fibers of the tendons to their maximum length. The stretching should be carried out within 15–20 minutes of the application of local heat treatment, otherwise the warm-up effect will be lost.

Range of motion

Full, pain-free range of motion (ROM) is the goal of all rehabilitation programs. However, this need not be achieved completely before strengthening exercises are initiated as long as the exercises are pain-free. Range-of-motion exercises can be facilitated through the use of thermotherapy to limit pain and increase blood flow to the area, resulting in increased tissue extensibility. These exercises may be done passively or actively. Passive ROM exercises allow for early motion without the use of contractile tissues. Often in the early stages of rehabilitation, passive motion is indicated to allow for tissue healing; active motion may be painful. Active ROM exercises require muscular action for movement to occur. This is the method of choice as rehabilitation progresses and muscle activity is safe.

Flexibility

Flexibility, the ability to move a joint painlessly through its full range of motion, is an important goal of rehabilitation. Flexibility is believed to contribute to fluidity of movement patterns. Most agree that adequate flexibility is necessary for good performance and injury prevention, although this is based primarily on observation rather than research.

Flexibility exercises should be designed to improve joint ROM. They include static stretching, proprioceptive neuromuscular facilitation techniques, and ballistic stretching.

Static stretching is an extremely effective and popular technique. Thi method involves passively stretching a muscle and holding it in its extende position for a period of 10–60 seconds (most often, 20 seconds). Stati stretching is probably safer than ballistic stretching because the extensibil ity limits of involved muscles are less likely to be inadvertently exceedec Training with static stretching should be an integral part of the rehabilita tion program following an injury. In most cases, it can begin soon after th injury occurs, although in cases of muscle or tendon rupture, it should b postponed until a doctor gives approval. Generally, static stretching ca start when there is no local tenderness in the injured area and when stati muscle contractions can be performed without pain. However, stati stretching can be used to evaluate healing in an injured muscle or tendo by using the level of pain as a measure of the state of the healing proces

Proprioceptive neuromuscular facilitation (PNF) is a technique for us with flexibility exercises, involving a combination of alternating isome ric and isotonic contractions and subsequent relaxation of both th agonist and antagonist muscle groups. The exercises are often performe with a partner, and consist of 10 seconds of contraction followed by 1 seconds of relaxation and stretching.

Ballistic stretching involves repetitive, small-amplitude bouncing motion It is generally accepted as less safe because of the quick stretches ar somewhat uncontrolled forces within the muscle, which may exceed th limits of the muscle fiber. However, used correctly, it can be effective.

During any flexibility exercise, the involved muscles should be warm and stretched slowly, and controlled to the point of slight resistance tightness. In order to improve flexibility, each exercise should performed daily, for five or six repetitions, held for a minimum 20 seconds. Stretching should be included as part of a warm-up to prepa muscles for activity. Stretching after activity may prevent some musc soreness and help increase flexibility by stretching loose, warm muscle

Strengthening

The development of muscle strength is an essential component of a rehabilitation program. Strength is the ability of a muscle to genera force against some resistance. Muscle weakness or imbalance can resu in abnormal movement or impaired performance. Physiological improv ments occur only when an individual physically demands more of the tissues than is normally required—the 'overload principle'. The muscl and tendons must be stressed above the normal load in order effective to increase their performance and strength. Progressive resistive exerci (PRE) is the most common strengthening technique used for recond tioning the muscle after injury. It is important to allow the overload tissue to recover and to allow adequate time for recovery.

Muscle training after injury

Muscle strength is proportional to the cross-sectional area of the mus (i.e. to the diameter and number of muscle fibers). The larger t cross-sectional area, the greater the force that the muscle can generate. The degree of force generated varies inversely to the speed at which the muscle contracts. Maximum force is generated by isometric contractions in which a large number of motor units are used. The faster a muscle contracts, the less force it can generate, as fewer motor units are used.

Strength training increases the strength not only of the muscles but also of their attachments. The strength of tendons, ligaments, and the skeleton does not increase as quickly as that of the muscles since their metabolism is slower, and this fact should be borne in mind when training growing individuals. During rehabilitation after injury, strength training should be carried out to the pain threshold. In order to shorten recovery time, training of muscles in the injured area can begin along the following lines.

Muscle contraction is the basis for all movement and exercise. There are three kinds of muscle work: *isometric* (or static) work involves contraction without a change in the length of the muscle (for example, holding a weight stationary in an outstretched hand); *concentric* work implies the muscles contract and shorten in length simultaneously so that their attachments are drawn closer together (for example, the contraction of quadriceps muscles when climbing stairs); *eccentric* work implies that the muscles contract and lengthen simultaneously so their attachments are drawn apart (for example, the action of the quadriceps muscles when walking downstairs).

During activity that involves change from eccentric to concentric muscular work, or vice versa, there is a risk of tearing a muscle or tendon. Concentric work mainly accelerates a moving object, eccentric work decelerates it. Injuries often occur during deceleration.

Static (isometric) training

After many joint and muscle injuries, isometric training can start immediately (Figure 21.1). For best results the muscle contractions should be as strong as the pain allows. A slow isometric contraction increases the load on the injured tissue gradually, with no movement of the joint or limb where the contraction occurs. It is then easier to avoid exceeding the pain threshold and the strength limit. The training starts with relatively few muscle contractions per day and increases gradually.

An increase in the number of muscle contractions should precede an increase in the load.

Rest should be taken between successive isometric muscle contractions so that the lactic acid formed in the tissue can be dissipated. If possible, a physical therapist should check constantly that no further problems develop as a result of the training. If there are no other medical or structural contraindications, once isometric training can be carried out without pain, supervised dynamic training can start. Training of this type is suitable for the extensors and flexors of the knee joint, for example.

Dynamic training

After bandaging has been removed and medical permission has been given to move the joint, dynamic training can start, at first using only

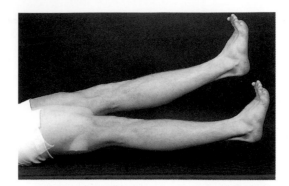

Figure 21.1 An example of isometric or static muscle training of the extensors of the knee joint.

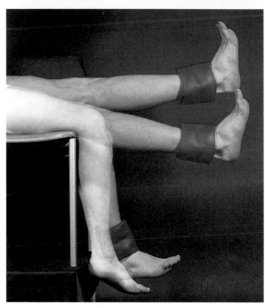

Figure 21.2 An example of dynamic isotonic muscle training of the flexors and extensors of the knee joint.

body weight or the weight of the limb as the load (Figure 21.2). Subse quently the load can be increased gradually by the addition of extern resistance such as weights. In dynamic training with weights (isoton training) maximum loading of a joint can only be achieved during pa of the range of motion. This leads to the risk of overloading the joint its weaker points. This risk is much reduced in isokinetic trainin although this requires the use of special apparatus (Figure 21.3). Isok netic training involves working at a constant speed, usually expressed degrees/second. The speed is determined by the trainer or therapist. Th resistance throughout the range of motion is determined by the effort the person being treated. This makes it possible to train at the maximu level of pain-free resistance at all points in the motion. The risk overloading injured tissues is limited to the extent that the person trai ing is able to keep their effort level beneath their pain level.

Dynamic training should start with a low load, and in the early stages t training program should be expanded by increasing the frequency of t exercise rather than the load. This enables the stamina and the blood flo of the muscle to improve before it is stressed further. When load is increase

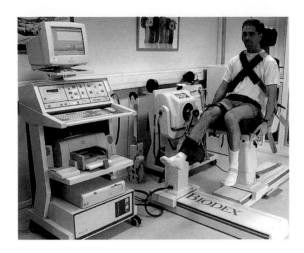

Figure 21.3
Special apparatus
for dynamic
eccentric isokinetic
training.

it is important to remember that the force to which a joint is subjected can be great. Placing a weight over the ankle joint during training of the knee, for example, increases the load on the knee joint by 10 times.

Dynamic training has a limited effect on the isometric strength of a muscle, except when it is carried out at low speed, in which case it resembles static training. Similarly, static training has only a limited effect on the dynamic strength of a muscle. In other words, all training should be relevant and designed specifically to work on those elements used in the sport in question.

Summary

To sum up, isometric (static) training is used particularly in the early stages of rehabilitation of muscle–tendon injuries or when an injured limb is immobilized. Dynamic isotonic training is used in the later stages of rehabilitation but can also be used to increase and maintain a certain level of strength in preventive training of some risk areas. Dynamic isokinetic training is less arduous since, by choosing a higher speed of motion, provision can be made for reducing resistance at any points which are painful in one range. In addition, isokinetics induce a marked increase in strength, whether performed at high speed or at low speed with maximum resistance. Training with a variable but not adjustable resistance allows particular muscle groups to be isolated for individual training and facilitates eccentric muscular work and mobility training.

After an initial period of rehabilitation the pain limit can be exceeded during the final few contractions in the exercise program in order to increase the pain threshold.

It is important to consider the following points before commencing strength training after an injury:
- All strength training should begin with warm-up exercises.
- All training should begin without load and should not exceed the pain threshold.
- There should be a gradual increase in load but it is better to increase the number of repetitions with one load before proceeding to greater loads.
- Asymmetrical exercises should usually be avoided.
- Rest and recovery are important in all types of strength training.

- Strength training should be combined with flexibility training.
- At the end of rehabilitation the strength training should be as sport specific as possible.

Open and closed kinetic chain exercises

An injury and subsequent disuse has a negative effect upon the proprioceptive sense in the joints, tendons, and skeletal muscle. Different types of exercise should be used in order to re-establish normal strength and proprioceptive function. Two of these types of exercise are known as open and closed kinetic chain exercises.

Open kinetic chain exercises are those involving a fixed proximal body segment and a distal segment that exerts effort through a relatively free range of motion. Examples of open kinetic chain exercises include overhead pressing or seated throwing exercises for the upper body, and the seated knee extension or cable pulls for the lower extremity. Open kinetic chain exercises can produce great gains in peak force production, but some of the most commonly used open chain exercises are limited to single joint or single plane motions. This can limit the extent to which they resemble useful, functional activities, and thus reduce their ability to improve proprioceptive ability along with strength.

Closed kinetic chain exercises involve a fixed distal segment and a relatively free proximal segment. Examples of closed kinetic chain exercises include pull-ups and push-ups for the upper body and squats and lunges for the lower body. A physical therapy ball allows many different and sport specific closed kinetic chain exercises. These exercises commonly use the subject's body weight to create some or all of the resistance, and involve movement of the subject's body in relation to a fixed hand or foot position. Closed chain exercises commonly involve multiple joint segments moving through multiple simultaneous arcs of motion. Most closed kinetic chain exercises are weight bearing and stimulate at least some level of agonist/antagonist co-contraction. Both these factors contribute to a reduction in joint shear forces, increased proprioceptive activity in joints and tendons, and improved postural and stabilization mechanics.

Open and closed kinetic chain exercises can both play an important role in the process of rebuilding strength, proprioception, and functional ability.

Plyometrics

Success in most sports is dependent upon technical skill, speed, muscular strength and power, and a series of coordinated activities that are linked together to make up the sport. While conditioning and weight training can produce gains in strength and endurance, speed and coordinated movements need specialized training techniques. A form of training that attempts to combine speed of movement and neuromuscular coordination with strength is called 'plyometrics'.

Plyometrics heightens the excitability of the nervous system by engaging the inherent stretch–shortening cycle of skeletal muscle. Through rapid initial eccentric stretch of a muscle, tension is produced prior to initiating an explosive concentric contraction of the same muscle. This mechanism releases the prestretch energy in an equal and opposite reaction, producing a powerful response of the contracting muscle. Picture an athlete about to perform a standing broad jump. As a final step before jumping, the legs are bent at the knees and hips providing an eccentric stretch of the quadriceps. Then as the athlete recoils, a quick concentric contraction occurs in the same group of muscles to provide the power necessary to propel the athlete forward. In contrast, consider the same athlete performing the jump without the initial recoil or stretch of the quadriceps, and note the difference in length of the jump.

After an injury, this neuromuscular pathway is weakened from disuse. Retraining this mechanism is important for safe and successful return to sport. Caution should be used in plyometric programs as they are intense, explosive, and stressful to the tissues involved.. It is necessary that the athlete participating in this type of program has normal range of motion and flexibility of the affected part, and near-normal strength. The program should include a progressive approach, beginning with small movements on the spot, working up to jumping and bounding of high amplitude, including sport-specific drills. Recovery time between sessions of plyometric training should be 3–5 days to allow for muscle recovery. It is important to stress that this is an end-stage rehabilitation activity, since it requires good strength and produces high explosive force.

Proprioception and coordination

Proprioceptors are specialized sensory receptors located in tendons, joints, muscles, and ligaments, which are sensitive to stretch, tension, and pressure. These receptors detect changes in position and movement, and send immediate feedback to allow the athlete to modify the movement to prevent injury. Injury and subsequent immobilization or disuse alter the function of these proprioceptors, resulting in decreased reaction time, increased balance deficits, and slower motor control. This cycle may increase the risk of re-injury.

Coordination and proprioception are intricately linked. Movement requires muscular interaction to execute particular tasks utilizing this proprioceptive feedback. Injuries affect this timing, rhythm, and judgment for specific skills.

A comprehensive rehabilitation program must include the retraining of these proprioceptors. Activities should begin with balancing on a wobble board or walking heel to toe with eyes closed, progressing to sport-specific tasks such as running in zigzag patterns, backwards, and in figures of eight. Intensity levels should increase as the athlete is able to complete each skill efficiently and without pain. Additional agility and coordination skills may be added through the use of sports equipment such as a ball—throwing, catching, kicking, etc. Once the athlete can complete these tasks and demonstrate pain-free, smooth, fluid, controlled movements, then a return to sport may be considered.

Proprioceptive training is one of the most important aspects of rehabilitation.

Cardiovascular endurance

Cardiovascular endurance is a necessary component of fitness that must not be ignored during the rehabilitation process. Also commonly referred to as aerobic capacity, cardiovascular endurance is defined as the body's ability to sustain submaximal exercise over an extended period. This capacity depends largely on the efficiency of the pulmonary and cardiovascular systems. Detraining of this system begins quickly, usually within 1–2 weeks of cessation of training.

It is important that during the rehabilitation process aerobic exercise is begun as quickly as is safely possible to prevent detraining. Athletes with upper extremity injuries can often ride a stationary bicycle comfortably in the early stages of recovery. Lower extremity injuries can present a more difficult challenge, but there are many non-weightbearing endurance activities that may be safe early on. Swimming, stationary cycling, and even rowing may be included in a program. It is recommended in order to maintain cardiovascular fitness that the work-outs be scheduled 3–5 times per week for 20–30 minutes at 70–90% of the athlete's maximum heart rate.

Sport-specific skill conditioning

Sport-specific demands must be incorporated into all rehabilitation programs. Each sport imposes specific requirements on the athlete. A functional progression is a sequence or succession of activities that simulate actual sports skills, enabling the athlete to gradually re-establish the skills necessary to perform the sport safely and effectively. These functional exercises allow for sequential improvement in strength, endurance, mobility, coordination, and agility. This step in the rehabilitation process is essential in easing the athlete's anxiety and apprehension about returning to sport after injury.

Return to sport

The ultimate decision as to whether an athlete is fit to resume sport lies with the physician. Criteria for a safe return include full, pain-free range of motion; normal and equal strength bilaterally; and ability to meet the demands of the sport without substitution, pain, or swelling. Sport-specific tests should be carried out before a return to sport. Although not all injuries can be prevented, a well-conditioned, fit athlete has less risk of re-injury.

Shoulder and upper extremity

There are several common issues to be remembered when dealing with shoulder rehabilitation, despite the wide variety of injuries that may be sustained by the shoulder complex.

- The shoulder girdle is a series of complex joints and articulations that function together to provide smooth, rhythmic, and coordinated movement. The complexity of this combination of joints and its heavy reliance on soft tissues to provide both dynamic and static stability often make the shoulder a difficult rehabilitation challenge.
- The rotator cuff and the periscapular muscles must be rehabilitated together to maintain the dynamic stability of the shoulder girdle.
- Weakness in the stabilizers of the scapula changes the biomechanics of the shoulder girdle: there is abnormal stress in the anterior capsule, greater compression of the rotator cuff, and decreased activity of the rotator muscles.
- Normal range of motion of the shoulder girdle must be achieved to maintain rhythmic scapulothoracic and glenohumeral motion. This should include both capsular motions and muscular soft tissue flexibility Increased thoracic curvature (kyphosis) results in decreased glenohumeral mobility.
- An understanding of the biomechanics and joint kinematics of the shoulder movements and the demands of various sports and activities is necessary to provide important information about the injury and the rehabilitation needs.

Shoulder range-of-motion exercises

Pendulum exercises

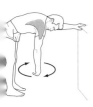

The goals of pendulum exercises are threefold: to improve muscular relaxation; to establish a limited arc of pain-free, relaxed motion; and to prepare the shoulder complex for additional activity. Stand, holding on to a stable object with the uninvolved arm. Bend over slightly at the waist and let the involved arm hang straight down, relaxing all the shoulder muscles.

Swing the arm gently (a) forward and back, (b) side to side, and (c) in circles, first clockwise and then counterclockwise, increasing the diameter of the circle. Using the momentum of the swing, keep the muscles as relaxed as possible. Repeat 10–15 times each way.

Their pain-relieving and relaxation-enhancing qualities make pendulum exercises a good choice also for 'cooling down' exercises.

Cane-assisted exercises

Using a cane, a stick or a broom handle, use the uninvolved arm to assist the involved arm in increasing the range of motion.

Forward flexion
Lying on your back, grasp the cane with both hands, shoulder width apart, palms down. Start with the cane resting across the hips. Lift the cane with straight arms out in front of you, as high as you can until a stretch is felt (assisting the involved arm with the uninvolved arm). Pause at the top for 5 seconds, then return to the starting position. Repeat 10 times.

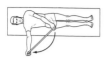

Abduction

Lying on your back, grasp the cane with both hands, palms down, shoulder-width apart. Start with the cane resting across the hips. Using the cane, push your involved arm out to the side, as high as you can. Pause at the top for 5 seconds, then return to the starting position. Repeat 10 times.

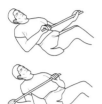

Internal/external rotation

Lying on your back, grasp the cane with both hands, elbows bent to 90°, hands shoulder-width apart. Using the cane, keep your elbows tucked in to your waist, and rotate the involved arm out to the side as far as you can. Hold for 5 seconds, then return to the starting position. Repeat 1 times. Repeat the exercise, rotating your arm across your body in the other direction.

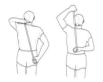

Internal rotation behind back

Hold the cane behind your back, with the uninvolved arm at the top. Use this arm to pull up the involved arm up your back as far as you can. Hold for 5 seconds, then return to the starting position. Repeat 1 times.

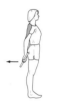

Extension

Stand with your arms at your side, elbows straight. Hold the cane behind your back with both hands, palms facing away from you. Slowly push the cane away from your body. Hold for 5 seconds, then return to the starting position. Repeat 10 times.

Upper extremity stretching

Latissimus and teres major stretch

Facing a doorway, hook the fingertips of the involved arm over the top of the door molding. Lean forward through the doorway. Feel the stretch along the underside of the arms. Hold 20 seconds, repeat 5 or 6 times.

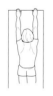

Pectoralis stretch

Stand in a doorway with elbows bent 90 ° and upper arms held parallel to the floor. Hold the elbows against the door jamb and lean forward. The arms stretch backwards as the body pushes forwards. The stretch should be felt across the front of your shoulders. Hold 20 seconds, repeat 5 or 6 times.

Pectoralis, biceps, deltoid stretch

Stand in a doorway with your hands behind you at shoulder level. Grab the door jamb with thumbs pointed upwards. Lean forward through the doorway keeping your elbows straight. The stretch should be felt across the front of your chest. Hold 20 seconds, repeat 5 or 6 times.

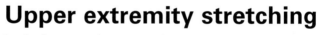

Deltoid/rhomboid stretch (posterior capsule)

Grasp the elbow of the involved arm with the uninvolved arm. Pull the involved arm across the chest at shoulder level. The stretch should be felt behind the involved shoulder and across the back of the upper arm. Hold 20 seconds, repeat 5 or 6 times.

Triceps stretch (inferior capsule)

Raise the involved arm overhead. Bend the elbow down behind the head. Using the other arm, gently pull the elbow of the involved arm behind your head. The stretch should be felt along the back of the upper arm. Hold 20 seconds, repeat 5 or 6 times.

Biceps stretch

Hold the involved arm straight out to the side at shoulder height. Start with the palm facing up, then turn the palm down toward the floor. Slowly bring the arm back behind you, keeping the elbow straight. Feel the stretch across your upper arm. Hold 20 seconds, repeat 5 or 6 times.

Latissimus dorsi

Repeat the triceps stretch and side-bend the trunk to the opposite side. Feel the stretch along the trunk. Hold 20 seconds, repeat 5 or 6 times.

Levator stretch

Sitting, lean your head forward on a diagonal, looking toward your right elbow. Feel the stretch down the left side of your neck, shoulder, and upper back. Repeat to the other side. Hold 20 seconds, repeat 5 or 6 times.

Wrist flexor stretch

Straighten your elbow completely and, with palm downward, grasp your hand with the other hand. Pull wrist back as far as possible. The stretch should be felt along the bottom of your forearm. Hold for 15–20 seconds, repeat 5–6 times.

Wrist extensor stretch

Straighten your elbow completely and, with palm downward, grasp your hand with the other hand. Push wrist down as far as possible. The stretch should be felt across the top of your forearm. Hold for 15–20 seconds, repeat 5–6 times.

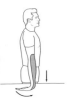

'Tennis elbow' stretch (wrist extension/pronation stretch)

Stand with the back of the involved hand resting on a table, while keeping the elbow straight. Exert a downward force toward the table. Grasp the involved hand with the other hand and rotate the wrist and hand of the involved side to the outside, while maintaining a bent wrist. The stretch should be felt across the top of the forearm and top of the wrist. Hold for 15–20 seconds, repeat 5–6 times.

Shoulder strengthening

Rubber tubing exercises

Fasten a piece of rubber tubing to a stable object such as a door or heavy piece of equipment or furniture. Tie a knot in the other end, to hold. Each exercise should be performed in a slow, controlled manner to minimize momentum. Perform 2 or 3 sets of 10–15 repetitions. The trunk must be kept stable throughout exercises.

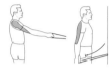

Shoulder extension (latissimus dorsi, triceps, teres major)
Stand facing the tubing, with the involved arm fully extended. Pull the tubing straight back, keeping the arm straight. Slowly return to the starting position. Repeat.

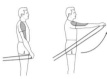

Forward flexion (anterior deltoid, biceps, infraspinatus)
Stand facing away from the tubing, involved arm extended and down by your side. Keeping the arm straight, lift it forward to shoulder height. Slowly return to the starting position. Repeat.

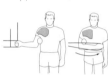

Internal rotation (subscapularis, pectoralis)
Stand sideways with the involved shoulder closest to the tubing, elbow bent to 90°. Squeeze a rolled-up towel between your side and elbow. Grasp the tubing in your involved hand, and by rotating your arm from the shoulder, pull the band across the front of your body, keeping your elbow tucked into your side. Slowly return to the starting position. Repeat.

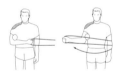

External rotation (teres minor, infraspinatus)
Stand sideways with the uninvolved shoulder closest to the tubing, elbow bent to 90°. Squeeze a rolled-up towel between your side and your elbow. Grasp the tubing with your involved hand, and by rotating your arm from the shoulder, pull the tubing away from your body, keeping your elbow tucked into your side. Do not pull far enough to create pain in the shoulder. Slowly return to the starting position. Repeat.

Abduction (deltoid, supraspinatus)
Stand sideways with the uninvolved shoulder closest to the tubing, arm straight at your side. Lift the tubing away from your body to shoulder height while turning your thumb up. Slowly return to the starting position. Repeat.

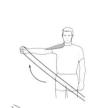

Diagonal patterns
(1) Stand sideways with the involved shoulder closest to the tubing and the arm out straight with palm facing forward. Pull the arm down and across your body towards opposite hip. Slowly return to the starting position. Repeat.

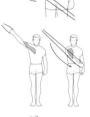

(2) Stand sideways with the involved shoulder away from the tubing. Position your arm diagonally across your body with the palm facing backwards. Pull the arm up and across your body as shown. Slowly return to the starting position. Repeat.

Isolated shoulder exercises

Exercises of the shoulder should train for both acceleration and deceleration. The following exercises isolate specific musculature surrounding the shoulder. They are vital to the proper functioning of the rhythmic movement of the shoulder complex. They should be performed precisely and with small weights (0.5–1.5 kg, 1–3 lb) held in the hand. The weights should be light enough that the motion can be completed without any pain. Perform 2 or 3 sets of 10–15 repetitions (depending upon the sport).

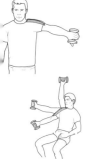

'Empty can' exercise (supraspinatus)
Stand with the elbow straight and thumb rotated inwards. Raise your arm diagonally out to the side to 45° from the body, keeping your thumb pointing downwards. Stop at shoulder height. Hold for 3 seconds and slowly lower. Repeat.

Elevation in the scapular plane (scapular stabilizers)
Standing with elbow straight and thumb rotated upwards, raise your arm overhead diagonally away from your body to 45°. Hold for 3 seconds and slowly lower. Repeat.

Prone shoulder extension (rhomboid, latissimus, teres major)
Lie face down on a table or the edge of a bed, with your involved arm hanging straight down. Keeping the elbow straight, with the thumb rotated inwards, raise your arm backwards to the level of the table. Hold for 3 seconds and slowly lower. Repeat.

Side-lying external rotation (teres minor, infraspinatus)
Lie on your uninvolved side with the involved arm resting on your body, elbow bent to 90°. Keeping the elbow of the involved arm fixed to your side, rotate your arm, from the shoulder, outwards. Hold for 3 seconds and slowly lower. Repeat. This exercise should not be taken to the point of pain, and in certain cases should be limited in range.

Prone internal/external rotation (infraspinatus, subscapularis, scapular stabilization)
Lie face down on a table with your shoulder out to the side at 90°, your elbow bent to 90°, and your palm facing the floor. Keeping your upper arm supported by the table, slowly rotate your shoulder outwards and then inwards as far as possible. Hold for 3 seconds at each position and slowly lower. Repeat.

Prone rowing (scapula stabilizers, triceps, posterior deltoid, teres major)
Lie face down on a table, arm hanging straight down. Lift your arm, leading with your elbow towards the ceiling, pinching your shoulder blades together as you lift. Hold for 3 seconds and slowly lower. Repeat.

Hands off back (rhomboids, suprascapularis)
Lie face down, place your involved arm behind your back on your buttocks, elbow slightly bent. Lift your arm towards the ceiling, trying not to straighten your elbow. Make sure to lift from the shoulder as you lift your whole arm towards the ceiling. Hold for 3 seconds and slowly lower. Repeat.

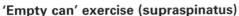

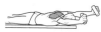

Lift over head (lower trapezius)

Lie face down, arms straight out overhead, elbows straight. Raise your arms up off the floor as far as possible. Be sure to keep your head and scapulae down. Hold for 3 seconds and slowly lower. Repeat. Alternatively use diagonal movements of the arms (one up, one down) and alternate.

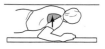

Lift off arm (middle trapezius)

Lie face down with your arm out to the side at 90°, your elbow bent to 90°, and your palm facing the floor. Lift your entire arm as one unit towards the ceiling, pinching your shoulder blades together as you lift. Be sure to keep your head down. Hold for 3 seconds and slowly lower. Repeat.

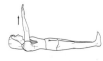

Scapular protraction (serratus anterior)

Lying on your back, raise your involved arm straight toward the ceiling keeping the shoulder at 90° to the floor, elbow straight. Lift your arm towards the ceiling as one unit (your shoulder blade should lift off the floor). Hold for 3 seconds and slowly lower. Repeat.

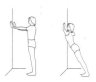

Wall push-ups (scapula stabilizers)

Stand in a corner, with your feet about one pace back from the wall. Place your hands on the wall(s) at shoulder height. Slowly lean into the corner, then push back out. Repeat. Alternatively, fall forward into the corner with raised hands.

Push-ups with a plus (scapula stabilizers)

Perform a standard push-up. Once elbows are straight, try to 'push-up' further by rounding your shoulders. Hold for 3 seconds and slowly lower. Repeat.

Rehabilitation protocols

Rehabilitation protocols for specific injuries are set out in the following tables:
- impingement syndrome: Table 21.1;
- anterior glenohumeral dislocation: Table 21.2.

Elbow, wrist and hand

Elbow rehabilitation

Whatever the injury, the rehabilitation program must address inflammation, restricted mobility, pain, weakness, and functional disability. The dangers of elbow joint immobilization, arthrofibrosis, and adhesive capsulitis (joint stiffness) have been well documented. It is imperative that early range-of motion exercises be initiated to minimize the degenerative effects of immobility. As with all rehabilitation, strength is important for proper function. The initiation of muscle activity early in the process is important

contd p. 51

Table 21.1 Rehabilitation protocol for impingement syndrome (see p. 134)

	Early phase	Intermediate phase	Late phase	Return to activity
Goal	Decrease pain and inflammation Restore joint and capsular motion	Develop strength of rotator cuff and periscapular muscles Full AROM pain-free	Refine strength imbalances Increase muscular endurance	Functional progression into activity
Manual therapy	Posterior capsular stretching	Continue capsular stretching	Continue capsular stretching	
ROM	Cane-assisted exercises: – IR/ER – IR behind back – Extension – Forward flexion	Continue if deficits remain	Continue if deficits remain	
Strengthening	Isometrics: IR, ER, abduction, extension, flexion Isolated shoulder exercises: – prone extension – prone rowing – serratus anterior – side-lying ER	Continue previous program Add isolated shoulder exercises: – 'empty can', 'filled can' – lower trapezius – middle trapezius – rhomboid – prone IR/ER	Continue previous program Add: – rubber tubing exercises – diagonal rubber tubing exercises – push-ups with a plus – wall push-ups Isotonic upper extremity strengthening machines	Continue isotonic upper extremity strengthening machines Continue comprehensive strengthening program focusing on periscapular and rotator cuff muscles Include eccentric exercises
Stretching	Deltoid/rhomboid stretch Pectoralis stretch	Abduction, flexion in doorway Biceps stretch	Continue stretching Pectoralis stretch	Continue upper extremity stretching
Functional/ proprioceptive	Neuromuscular firing patterns	Light sports activity below the horizontal plane if painless (exercises with physical therapy balls)	Simulated sport activity with rubber tubing, weighted balls; deceleration exercises (catching balls)	Return to sport if full pain-free motion, full strength

AROM, active range of motion; ER, external rotation; IR, internal rotation; ROM, range of motion.

Table 21.2 Rehabilitation protocol for anterior glenohumeral dislocation (see p. 125)

	Immobilization phase (0–3 weeks)	Early phase (3–6 weeks)	Intermediate phase (6 weeks–3 months)	Late phase (over 3 months)	Return to activity
Goal	Heal joint capsule, trauma; Reduce/control pain	Initiate and maintain ROM	Normalize ROM; Aggressive strengthening	Normalize strength; Functional progression of activities	Prepare for return to activity
ROM	In sling full-time; Pendulum exercises; AROM of elbow, wrist, hand	Pendulum exercises; Cane-assisted exercises: flexion, extension, abduction; *Avoid combined abduction and ER*	Continue ROM exercises; *Avoid combined abduction and ER*	Abduction with ER allowed	
Stretching	None			Upper extremity stretching program	Upper extremity stretching program
Strengthening	Isometric strength training; Scapula stabilization	Isolated shoulder exercises: – DNF – prone shoulder extension – prone rowing – serratus anterior – side-lying ER, limited ROM – rhomboid; Rubber tubing exercises: IR/ER, limited ROM, flexion, extension	Continue previous exercises; Add isolated shoulder exercises: – lower trapezius – middle trapezius – prone IR/ER – Scaption; Push-ups with a plus; Isotonic upper extremity strengthening machines	Continue previous program; Add: – multiplane exercises – diagonal strengthening – push-ups with a plus – wall push-ups	Continue previous program
Functional/ proprioceptive	None		Light sport-specific exercises	Simulated sport activity with rubber tubing, weighted balls	Return to sport when ROM and strength are normal

AROM, active range of motion; ER, external rotation; IR, internal rotation; PNF, proprioceptive neuromuscular facilitation; ROM, range of motion.

to prevent tissue hypotrophy, and to re-educate muscle. Athletes whose sports involve throwing should include scapular stabilization exercises along with strengthening exercises for the whole shoulder–elbow complex.

Wrist and hand rehabilitation

Because the function of the wrist and hand is essential to daily activities, special care is needed to avoid compromising the functional integrity of these structures. In addition to range-of-motion and strengthening exercises, attention should be paid to dexterity exercises and to tactile senses. The wrist and hand are a series of complex joints which work together to give great mobility and range of function. Immobilization can result in joint contractures and stiffness, therefore active range-of-motion exercises should begin as soon as safely possible. A thorough understanding of the action of the hand musculature is necessary to isolate joint movement. Mobility of the metacarpal bones should be checked manually by the therapist. The elbow and forearm should be stabilized for rehabilitative exercises to minimize compensatory movements.

Range-of-motion exercises

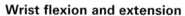

Elbow flexion and extension
Standing with your arms down at your side, slowly bend and straighten your elbow as far as possible. Hold each position 5 seconds, repeat 10 times.

Wrist flexion and extension
Resting your forearm on a table, with your hand over the edge, palm facing upwards, slowly curl your wrist up and down as far as possible. Be sure not to lift the forearm off the table. Hold each position 5 seconds, repeat 10 times.

Wrist pronation and supination
Rest your forearm on a table, with your hand over the edge. Begin with the palm facing upwards, then rotate your hand all the way outwards (supination) and all the way inwards (pronation). Hold each position 5 seconds, repeat 10 times.

Wrist radial and ulnar deviation
Resting your forearm and hand on a table, palm facing downwards, move your hand from side to side, keeping it flat on the table. Hold each position 5 seconds, repeat 10 times.

Elbow, wrist and hand strengthening

Use a small dumb-bell or rubber tubing for resistance. Perform 2 or 3 sets of 10–15 repetitions.

Biceps curl

Support the involved arm at the elbow with the opposite hand. Slowly bend your elbow as far as possible, and then extend the elbow as far as possible. Hold for 3 seconds at the end of each motion. Repeat.

Triceps curl

Raise the involved arm overhead. Provide support at the elbow with the opposite hand. Straighten the elbow overhead, then slowly return. Hold for 3 seconds at the end of each motion. Repeat.

Wrist extension

Rest your forearm on a table, hand over the edge, palm facing down. Slowly raise the wrist up and down as far as possible, being sure not to lift the forearm off the table. Hold each position 3 seconds. Repeat.

Wrist flexion

Rest your forearm on a table, hand over the edge, palm facing up. Slowly raise the wrist up and down as far as possible, being sure not to lift the forearm off the table. Hold each position 3 seconds. Repeat.

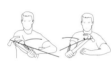

Pronation/supination

Rest your forearm on a table, with your hand over the edge. Beginning with the palm facing upwards, rotate your hand all the way outward (supination) and all the way inwards (pronation) against the resistance of rubber tubing. Hold each position 3 seconds. Repeat.

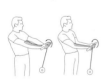

Curl ups

This exercise requires a 30–60 cm (1–2 ft) cane, broom handle or stick with a 1.2–1.5 m (4–5 ft) cord attached in the middle. Attach 0.5–2.25 kg (1–5 lb) weight on the other end of the cord.

– Extensors: grip the stick on either side of the cord, palms down. Curl the cord up by rotating the stick toward you; lower it slowly.
– Flexors: same as for extensors, but with the palms facing upwards.
Note: Use this exercise with caution if the patient has shoulder impingement symptoms.

Hand and finger strengthening

Elastic band exercise

Hold your fingertips together and put an elastic band around them. Spread your fingers out against the resistance of the band.

Ball squeeze

Hold a tennis ball or racket ball in your hand and squeeze it repeatedly at a rapid pace.

Neck

The neck should be examined very carefully by a physician before any exercise commences, because of the many sensitive structures it contains.

Range-of-motion exercises

Before the program starts a check-up with a physical therapist or an athletic trainer is advisable. Before performing each motion, align your head so your ears are over your shoulders. All motions should be slow and gentle, with no sudden or bouncing movements. Perform 3–5 repetitions.

Chin tuck

Use the muscles on the front of your neck to tuck your chin in. Hold for 5 seconds.

Side bending

Tilt your head over with your ear towards your shoulder. Be sure not to elevate your shoulder to your ear. Hold for 10–15 seconds. Return to center, and repeat to the opposite side.

Rotations

Slowly turn your head to look over your shoulder; hold for 10–15 seconds. Return to center, and repeat to the opposite side.

Flexion

Slowly tuck your chin towards your chest, and tilt your head forwards. Feel the stretch at the back of your neck. Hold for 10–15 seconds. Repeat.

Neck strengthening

Use your hand to apply resistance when performing these exercises. The resistance should be gentle and steady and there should be no head movement. Hold each for 5–10 seconds, 5–10 repetitions. Be careful with neck stretching.

Resisted side bends

In a sitting position, apply the palm of your right hand just above your right ear. While tilting your head to the right, use your right hand to apply resistance to the motion.

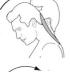

Resisted flexion

In a sitting position, apply the palm of your hand to the center of your forehead. Tilt your head forward while applying resistive pressure with your hand.

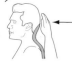

Resisted extension

In a sitting position, apply the palm of your hand to the back of your head. Tilt your head backwards while applying resistive pressure with your hand.

Lower back

Rehabilitation programs for the lower back must be based on individual assessments to address the specific needs of the patient. The first requirement is a thorough physical examination, which should include postural assessment, strength and range-of-motion measurements, also pain description and location details. Based on this evaluation, a rehabilitation program is then designed with additional focus on dynamic stabilization exercises of the lumbar spine, and education of the athlete about body mechanics, lifting, moving, and posture. The deep trunk muscles (transversus abdominis and lumbar multifidus) provided stability for the spine; muscle control leads to pain control.

Range-of-motion exercises

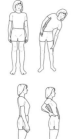

Standing side bends (lumbar/thoracic)

Standing up straight, bend to the side as you slide your hand down the outside of your leg as far as is comfortable. Repeat to the opposite side 10 times in each direction.

Standing back bends (lumbar/thoracic extension)

Standing up straight with your hands on your lower back, slowly bend backwards as far as is comfortable. Hold for 5 seconds and relax. Repeat 10 times.

'Cat–camel' (lumbar/thoracic flexion and extension)

On your hands and knees, slowly round up your back as far as is comfortable, then slowly let your back sink or sag down into a 'sway back' position. Repeat 10 times.

Lower back strengthening

Lower back strengthening is best done with professional guidance. Proper form is crucial to insure safety and effectiveness. These exercises can be done to the point of muscular fatigue, as long as proper form can be maintained. Proper balance between abdominal and back muscles is recommended. Physical therapy balls are good for strengthening the trunk (see Figure 9.10).

Pelvic tilt (multifidus, rotators, transversus abdominis)

Lie on your back with knees bent and feet flat. Tighten your abdominal muscles to tilt your hips backwards and flatten your lower back against the floor. Hold for 10 seconds, then relax. Repeat 10 times.

Partial sit-up (upper rectus abdominis)

Lying on your back with knees bent and feet flat, assume the pelvic tilt position. With your arms out in front of you, tuck your chin in and curl your upper body up until your shoulder blades are clear of the floor. Hold for 10 seconds, breathing normally, then relax. Repeat 10 times.

Diagonal sit-up (rectus abdominis, oblique muscles)

Lying on your back with knees bent and feet flat, assume the pelvic tilt position. Do a partial sit-up with your left hand reaching for the right knee. Hold for 10 seconds, breathing normally, and relax. Repeat in the opposite direction. Perform 10 repetitions in each direction.

Thoracic extension (erector spinae)

Lying face down with arms at your side, lift your upper body off the floor using your back muscles, keeping the chin tucked in. Hold for 5 seconds, breathing normally, then relax. Repeat 10 times. This exercise is not recommended for everybody.

Opposite arm and leg lifts (lumbar stabilization)

Lying face down with your arms reaching forwards, lift your left arm and your right leg. Hold them straight out for 3 seconds and relax. Repeat with the other arm and leg. Progress to the same exercise on all fours (hands and knees). Repeat 10 times.

Lower back stretching

Double knee to chest (lumbar flexion)

Lie on your back with knees bent and feet flat. Using both hands, bring first one knee to your chest and then the other. Hold for 10 seconds, then lower one leg at a time. Be sure to maintain a pelvic tilt while lowering your legs. Repeat 10 times.

Bent knee roll (lumbar rotation)

Lie on your back with knees bent and feet flat. Gently roll the knees to one side, hold for 10 seconds, and return to starting position. Roll to the opposite side, hold for 10 seconds. Repeat 10 times each direction.

Piriformis stretch (piriformis and gluteal muscles)

Lie on your back with knees bent and feet flat. With one hand, reach and grab the opposite knee. Pull your leg up and across chest toward the opposite shoulder. Hold for 20 seconds, then relax. Repeat with the opposite leg.

Hip and pelvis

Injuries to the pelvis, hip, and thigh involve the largest soft tissue structures in the body. Such injuries can be extremely disabling and often require a substantial amount of time for rehabilitation. The whole lower extremity must be considered, along with gait analysis and posture. When rehabilitating the hip and pelvis, proprioceptive and balance activities should be incorporated into the program at an early stage.

Range-of-motion exercises

Standing hip flexor stretch (iliopsoas)

While standing, bend one knee, grasping the ankle with the hand on th
same side. Gently pull your heel toward your buttock and extend you
hip. Be careful not to arch your back or bend forward at the waist. Slowl
continue to pull until a stretch is felt along the front of your thigh. Hol
for 20 seconds, repeat 5 or 6 times.

Alternatively, kneel on the right knee with the left foot on the floo
Rotate the right foot laterally while side-bending to the left.

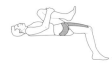

Thomas stretch (iliopsoas)

Sitting on the very edge of a bed or table, pull one knee up towards you
chest and hold it with both hands. Lie down, allowing the other leg t
hang over the edge. A stretch should be felt across the front of your hi
and thigh. Do not allow your back to arch off the bed. Hold for 2
seconds, repeat 5 or 6 times.

Modification: This stretch may also be done from a lunge positior
With one foot out in front of the other, lean forward with your uppe
body as you bend the knee in front to 90°. The back leg should b
stretched out with the knee resting on the floor. Lean forward and exten
the hip of the back leg. A stretch should be felt across the front of th
hip of the back leg. Hold for 20 seconds, 5 or 6 times.

Sideways lunge (adductors)

Stand with legs wide apart and upper body straight. Lean to th
uninvolved side, bending your knee, and keeping the involved leg straigh
out to the side as you lean. A stretch should be felt along the inside c
the involved leg. Hold 20 seconds, repeat 5 or 6 times.

Hip rotation stretch (gluteal muscles)

Sit with your right leg out straight and cross your left leg over your righ
leg, left knee bent, foot flat on the floor. Hook your right elbow aroun
your left knee and pull your left knee up towards your right shoulde
You should feel the stretch across your left buttock. Hold for 20 second
repeat 5 or 6 times. Repeat on the opposite side.

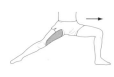

Modification (erector spinae, gluteal muscles): In the same positior
you may also push your left knee away from you and twist your body t
the left. This stretch is felt across your back. Hold for 20 seconds, repe
5 or 6 times for each side.

Piriformis stretch (piriformis, gluteal muscles)

Lie on your back with knees bent and feet flat. With one hand, reach an
grab the opposite knee. Pull your leg up and across the chest towards th
opposite shoulder. Hold for 20 seconds, then relax. Repeat with the other le

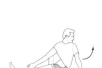

Iliotibial band stretch (tensor fasciae latae)

Standing, cross your right leg behind the left leg. Push your right hi
out to the right side as you reach and bend the upper body to the lef
You should feel the stretch along your outer right hip and thigh. Hol
for 20 seconds, repeat 5 or 6 times. Repeat for the other side.

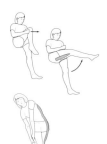

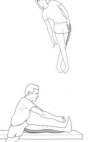

Modification (tensor fasciae latae, gluteus medius): Stand with your involved leg diagonally behind your uninvolved one. Press the side of your involved foot on the floor and lean to that side. A stretch should be felt along the outside of the involved hip. Hold for 20 seconds, repeat 5 or 6 times.

Sitting stretch (hamstrings)

Sit on the edge of an elevated surface, with one leg straight or bent and the other leg over the edge. Lean forward from the hips toward the toes until you feel a stretch behind your thigh. Be sure to keep your back straight. Hold for 20 seconds, repeat 5–6 times.

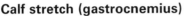

Wall stretch (hamstrings)

Lie on the floor, with one leg out straight through a doorway and the other leg up on the wall with your knee straight. Move your buttocks toward the wall until a stretch is felt behind your thigh. Be sure not to let your hips rotate or your knees bend. Hold for 20 seconds, repeat 5–6 times.

Calf stretch (gastrocnemius)

Stand facing a wall, one pace back from it. Place one foot in front of the other. Keep the back leg straight, heel on the floor, toes pointed forward. Place your hands on the wall and lean forward until you feel a stretch at the back of your knee. Hold for 20 seconds, repeat 5–6 times.

Soleus: Repeat this stretch bending the back leg slightly at the knee. You should feel the stretch lower in your calf. Hold for 20 seconds, repeat 5–6 times.

Hip strengthening

Each exercise should be performed in a slow and controlled manner. Resistance may be added by using cuff weights or rubber tubing. Perform 2 or 3 sets of 10–15 repetitions.

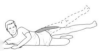

Hip abduction (gluteus minimus/maximus, tensor fasciae latae)

Lying on your uninvolved side, slowly lift the involved leg straight out to the side. Hold for 5 seconds, slowly lower. Repeat.

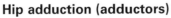

Hip adduction (adductors)

Lying on your involved side, bring your uninvolved leg behind you. Lift the involved leg 6 in (15 cm) straight up off the floor. Hold for 5 seconds, then slowly lower. Repeat.

Hip flexion (rectus femoris, iliopsoas)

In a seated position, slowly lift the entire involved leg from the hip. Hold for 5 seconds, then slowly lower. Repeat.

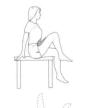

Gluteal extension (gluteus maximus)

Lying face down, bend the knee of the involved leg to 90°. Lift the entire leg from the hip, keeping your knee in the 90° position. Hold for 5 seconds, then slowly lower. Repeat.

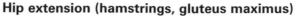

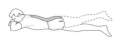

Hip extension (hamstrings, gluteus maximus)
Lie face down, legs out straight. Lift the entire involved leg from the hip, keeping the leg straight. Hold for 5 seconds, then slowly lower. Repeat.

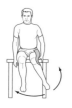

Hip internal/external rotation (internal/external rotator muscles)
Sitting on the edge of a table or a high chair with your upper legs supported and knees bent, rotate your leg from the hip to the outside, hold for 5 seconds. Slowly return and then rotate to the inside, hold for 5 seconds, then slowly lower. Repeat.

Sliding-board exercises have a beneficial effect on groin injuries.

Knee

Most recent trends in knee rehabilitation emphasize immediate motion, immediate weightbearing, early closed kinetic chain exercises (p. 492), strength exercises, and early return to activity. Effective rehabilitation programs require an understanding of any surgical procedures performed, the structure of the knee, and the nature of the injury. Strengthening should include both closed and open kinetic chain exercises, as appropriate to the particular needs of the patient. Assessment of patellofemoral alignment in both the static and dynamic modes, patella orientation, and patella tracking is essential to restoring the complete function of the knee and surrounding musculature.

Range-of-motion exercises

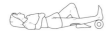

Gravity-assisted knee extension
Lying on your back, prop up the ankle on the involved side on a rolled-up towel. Be sure the entire leg is off the floor, especially the back of the knee. Relax the leg and allow gravity to pull the knee straight. Hold for 10–15 minutes. This stretch may also be combined with quadriceps setting and even straight leg raises (see below).

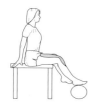

Gravity-assisted knee flexion
Sitting on the edge of a table or a high chair, rest the involved leg on a physical therapy ball. Bend the knee of the involved leg to a point of tightness. Maintain relaxation of the involved leg throughout the exercise. Hold for 20–30 seconds, relax, repeat 10 times.

Knee strengthening

Each exercise should be performed in a slow and controlled manner. Resistance may be added by using cuff weights or rubber tubing. Perform 2 or 3 sets of 10–15 repetitions.

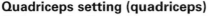

Quadriceps setting (quadriceps)

Sitting on the floor with your involved knee out straight, tighten the muscle on the top of your thigh as if trying to push your knee into the floor. Hold for 10 seconds, relax, repeat. This exercise may also be done sitting on the edge of a chair with the heel resting on the floor.

Short arc extension (quadriceps)

Sitting with your involved leg out in front of you and the other leg bent, place a rolled-up towel under the straight knee. Tighten your thigh muscle to extend the lower portion of your leg in a small arc. Keep the back of your knee in contact with the towel. Hold for 10 seconds, then slowly lower. Repeat.

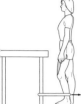

Terminal knee extension (vastus medialis obliquus, quadriceps)

Standing, loop one end of a piece of rubber tubing around an immovable object and the other end around the back of the involved knee. Step back, creating tension in the tubing. Keeping the other leg straight, allow the involved knee to flex slightly, then tighten the thigh muscle to pull the knee back into extension. Hold for 5 seconds, relax, repeat.

Full arc extension (quadriceps)

Sitting on the edge of a table or a high chair with your upper legs supported and your knees bent, slowly straighten your involved knee all the way into full extension. Hold for 5 seconds, then slowly lower. Repeat.

Full arc flexion (hamstrings)

Lying on your stomach, legs out straight, slowly bend your knee as far as possible using the muscles on the back of your thigh. Hold for 5 seconds, slowly lower. Repeat.

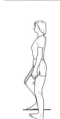

Step-up/down (quadriceps, hamstrings, gluteus)

Start with a 5 cm (2 in) step progressing to a 15 cm (6 in) step. Stand sideways, with the foot of involved leg on the step. Step up using the involved leg, then slowly lower down to the heel (not toes) of the other leg. Raise up again from the heel position and repeat. Be sure to keep the knee lined up over the ankle on the involved side, not too far forwards. Repeat.

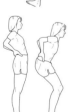

Double leg knee bends (quadriceps, hamstrings, gluteus)

Stand with your feet shoulder-width apart. Lean forward slightly and lower your body until your knees are at a 45° angle. Hold for 5–10 seconds, then stand back up, but do not lock your knees all the way straight. To accentuate this exercise, squeeze a rolled-up towel or a ball between your knees. Repeat.

This exercise can be made more challenging by going deeper than 45° of knee flexion, but it should remain challenging for the muscles rather than painful to the joint.

Closed kinetic chain exercises using a physical therapy ball are useful to stabilize the knee and the rest of the body. Eccentric exercises must be added at the end of such a program.

Rehabilitation protocols

Rehabilitation protocols for specific injuries are set out in the following tables:
- isolated MCL sprain: Table 21.3;
- patellofemoral pain syndrome: Table 21.4;
- partial meniscectomy or arthroscopy: Table 21.5;
- meniscus repair: Table 21.6;
- anterior cruciate reconstruction (patellar tendon): Table 21.7.

Ankle

The biomechanics of the ankle and foot are important for the normal function of the lower extremity. The foot is the terminal joint in the lower kinetic chain.

Range-of-motion exercises

Ankle dorsiflexion/plantar flexion
Sitting with your legs out straight, pull your whole foot and ankle up towards you as far as possible, keeping your knee straight. Hold for seconds, then push your foot and ankle away from you as far as possible. Hold for 5 seconds. Repeat.

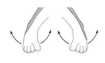

Ankle inversion/eversion
Sitting with your legs out straight, turn the sole of your foot inwards as far as possible. Be sure that the motion is coming from your foot and that your whole leg is not rotating. Hold for 5 seconds, then turn the sole of your foot outwards as far as possible. Hold for 5 seconds. Repeat.

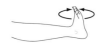

Ankle circles
Sitting with your legs out straight, turn your involved foot in small circles clockwise. Repeat counterclockwise. Start with small circles, then gradually increase the size of the circle. Repeat 10 times each way.

Ankle strengthening

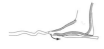

Towel curls (toe and foot flexors, extensors)
In a seated position, spread a towel out on the floor in front of you. Place the heel of the involved foot on the towel. Try to curl the towel up using your toes, keeping the rest of your foot still. Progress by placing a small weight or book on the end of the towel for more resistance. Repeat 5–10 times.

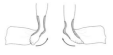

Towel inversion/eversion (ankle and foot inverters/everters)
From a seated position, spread a towel out to the side of the involved foot. Place the heel of the foot on the end of the towel and rotate your

foot inwards, pulling the towel with your toes and foot. Repeat until you reach the end of the towel. Spread it back out and repeat 5–10 times.

Repeat the above exercise with the towel spread to the inside of the involved ankle, and rotate the foot outwards, pulling on the towel. Repeat 5–10 times.

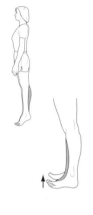

Heel raise (gastrocnemius, soleus)
Stand with equal weight on both feet. Slowly rise up on your toes as far as possible, then lower. Repeat 10–15 times. Progress to standing on your involved leg only and repeat the exercise. This may also be done with the heels hanging off the edge of a step for additional range of motion.

Toe raise (ankle dorsiflexors)
Stand with equal weight on both feet. Lift your toes and the front of your foot off the floor, keeping your heels in contact with the floor. Slowly lower. Repeat 10–15 times.

Exercises using rubber tubing
Secure a length of rubber tubing to a stable object low to the ground. Perform 2 or 3 sets of 10–15 repetitions.

Resisted dorsiflexion
Sitting on the floor with your legs out straight in front, loop the tubing around the top of your foot just below your toes. Slide back to place some tension on the tubing. Slowly pull your ankle towards you as far as possible against the tubing. Slowly lower. Repeat.

Resisted plantar flexion
This exercise can be done instead of standing heel raises if the patient is not ready for that level of loading.

Sitting on the floor with your legs out straight in front, loop the tubing around the ball of your foot, and hold the other end in your hand. Slowly point your foot downwards against the tubing, then slowly return to the starting position. Repeat.

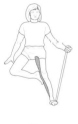

Resisted inversion
Sitting on the floor with your legs out straight in front, loop the tubing around the top of your foot just below the toes. The tubing should be to the outside of your involved leg. Slide your body to the side to place some tension on the tubing. Slowly turn the sole of your foot inwards, pulling against the tubing. Ensure the motion is coming from your foot and that your whole leg is not rotating. Slowly return to the starting position. Repeat.

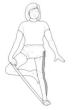

Resisted eversion
Sitting on the floor with your legs out straight in front, loop the tubing around the top of your foot just below your toes. The tubing should be to the inside of your involved leg. Slide your body to the side to place some tension on the tubing. Slowly turn the sole of your foot outwards, pulling against the tubing. Ensure the motion is coming from your foot and that your whole leg is not rotating. Slowly return to the starting position. Repeat.

contd p. 520   513

Table 21.3 Rehabilitation protocol for isolated medial collateral ligament (MCL) sprain (see p. 284)

	Early phase	Intermediate phase	Late phase	Return to activity
Goals	Reduce/control pain, swelling; Protect joint; Maintain ROM; Prevent quadriceps atrophy	Increase ROM; Protect joint; Restore strength; Increase function	Resolve remaining strength deficits; Functional progression of activities	Prepare for return to activity
Weightbearing status	To tolerance; Stabilizing brace of choice	Full weightbearing	Full weightbearing	Full weightbearing
ROM, flexibility	PROM/AROM knee flexion/extension; Hamstring stretching	Continue ROM exercises; Hamstring stretch; Standing hip flexor stretch	Continue if deficits remain	Continue previous strengthening
Open kinetic chain strengthening	Quadriceps sets; Straight leg raises; Short arc quads; Hip strengthening exercises	Continue previous strengthening; Isotonic quadriceps/hamstring strengthening through pain-free ROM	Full lower extremity isotonic/isokinetic program	
Closed kinetic chain strengthening	Double knee bends 0–45°; Terminal knee extension	Double knee bends 0–80°; Straight-ahead lunge, jump, hop; Step-up/down	Lateral lunges, hops, bounds; Quick feet (forward, back); Squats	Carioca, hop, skip drills, plyometric drills
Functional/proprioceptive	Maintain fitness: stationary cycling, swimming with flutter kick, deep water running	Double leg stance tiltboard; Stork stands, balance drills; Maintain fitness: cycling, swimming, stairclimbing, pool running	Single leg stance tiltboard; Slideboard, agility/balance exercises; Fitness activity: running, cycling, swimming	Functional running patterns; Jump rope; Sport-specific drills
Restrictions or recommendations	No jumping, cutting, or kicking sports; no frog kick in pool	No jumping, cutting, or kicking sports	Consider functional brace; Consider strength test	

AROM, active range of motion; PROM, passive range of motion.

Table 21.4 Rehabilitation protocol for patellofemoral pain syndrome (see p. 317)

	Early phase	Intermediate phase	Late phase	Return to activity
Goals	Reduce pain, inflammation Initiate medial quadriceps strengthening	Increase lower extremity flexibility Restore strength Improve patella tracking	Resolve remaining strength deficits Functional progression of activities	Prepare for return to activity
Weightbearing status	Full weightbearing	Full weightbearing	Full weightbearing	Full weightbearing
ROM, flexibility	Hamstring stretching Hip flexor stretching Quadriceps stretching	Continue aggressive lower extremity stretching	Continue if deficits remain	
Open kinetic chain strengthening	Quad sets Straight leg raises Short arc quadriceps Side-lying hip exercises	Continue previous exercises Isotonic short arc quadriceps/ hamstring strengthening if pain-free	Focused eccentric quadriceps strengthening Full arc isotonic quadriceps/hamstring strengthening if no pain	Continue previous strengthening
Closed kinetic chain strengthening	Double knee bends 0–45° Terminal knee extension	Step-up/down Double knee bends 0–45° Terminal knee extensions	Straight-ahead lunges, hops Quick feet (forward, back) Squats	Carioca, lateral lunges, hops Light plyometric drills
Functional/ proprioceptive	Maintain fitness: stationary cycling, swimming, deep water running	Double leg stance tiltboard Stork stands, balance drills Maintain fitness: cycling, swimming, stairclimbing, pool running	Single leg stance tiltboard Slideboard, agility/balance drills Running, cycling, swimming	Functional running patterns Jump rope Sport-specific drills
Restrictions or recommendations	Avoid exercises that increase patellar compression	Avoid exercises that increase patellar compression		Return to sport if pain-free

Table 21.5 Rehabilitation protocol after partial meniscectomy or arthroscopy (see p. 302)

	Early phase (0–2 weeks)	Intermediate phase (2–4 weeks)	Late phase (4–8 weeks) and return to activity
Goals	Reduce/control pain, swelling Increase ROM Quadriceps recruitment	Increase ROM Restore strength Increase function	Resolve remaining strength deficits Functional progression of activities Return to activity
Weightbearing status	To tolerance	Full weightbearing	Full weightbearing
ROM flexibility	PROM/AROM knee flexion/extension Hamstring stretching Patella mobilization	Continue ROM exercises Hamstring stretch Standing hip flexor stretch	Continue if deficits remain
Open kinetic chain strengthening	Quadriceps sets Straight-leg raises Short arc quads Hip strengthening exercises	Begin isotonic quadriceps/hamstring strengthening to tolerance	Full lower extremity isotonic/isokinetic program
Closed kinetic chain strengthening	Double knee bends 0–45° Terminal knee extension	Double knee bends 0–60° Step-up/down	Lateral lunges, hops, bounds Quick feet (forward, back) Squats, carioca, hopping drills Plyometric drills
Functional/proprioceptive	Maintain fitness: stationary cycling, swimming, deep water running (when incisions are healed)	Double leg stance tiltboard Stork stands, balance drills Maintain fitness: cycling, swimming, stairclimbing, pool running	Single leg stance tiltboard Slideboard, agility/balance drills Functional running patterns Jump rope Running, cycling, swimming
Restrictions or recommendations	No sports	No jumping, cutting sports	Return to sports if 85% strength

AROM, active range of motion; PROM, passive range of motion.

Table 21.6 Rehabilitation protocol after meniscus repair (see p. 304)

	Time elapsed since operation			
	1–7 days	7 days–4 weeks	4–12 weeks	12 weeks–4 months
Goals	Reduce/control pain, swelling Prevent quadriceps atrophy	Increase ROM Protect joint Increase function	Increase ROM Initiate strengthening	Resolve strength deficits Return to functional activities
Weightbearing status	Partial weightbearing in long leg brace locked at 0°	Full weightbearing in brace set to 0–30°	Full weightbearing Brace remains on for walking until 6 weeks, then gradually discontinued	Full weightbearing
ROM, flexibility	Patella mobilization, limited range AROM if allowed by surgeon	Patella mobilization At 2 weeks: – AROM exercises 0–90° only – hamstring stretching	AROM exercises 0–120° only Hamstring stretching	Progress ROM exercises Hamstring stretching
Open kinetic chain strengthening	Quadriceps sets Straight-leg raises Side-lying hip exercises	Brace remains on for exercises until 3 weeks: – quad sets – straight-leg raises – short arc quads – side-lying hip exercises – side-lying hip exercises with with no weight	Brace removed for exercises Continue previous strengthening up to 4.5 kg (10 lb)	Continue previous strengthening exercises—may use weights up to 14 kg (30 lb) Leg extension 0–60°, up to 14 kg (30 lb) Leg curl Hip strengthening
Closed kinetic chain strengthening	None	Toe raises, heel raises	At 8 weeks: – Double knee bends 0–60° only – step-up/down – straight-ahead lunges – double leg stance tiltboard – stork stand, balance drills	At 4 months: – carioca, hops, lateral lunges – plyometric drills
Functional proprioceptive	None	Standing balance on stable, flat surface	Gait training Fitness activity: swimming with flutter kick, cycling, nordic track, pool running At 8 weeks: stairclimbing	Jog, cycle At 4 months: – functional running patterns – jump rope – sport-specific drills Return to sport with doctor's permission
Restrictions or recommendations	No weight with exercises No sports	No weight with exercises	No jumping, cutting sports	

AROM, active range of motion.

517

Table 21.7 Standard rehabilitation protocol after anterior cruciate ligament (ACL) reconstruction (patellar tendon) (see p. 281)

(see p. 281)

	Rehabilitation phase/time frame		
	1. Preoperative	*2. Postoperative (first 7–10 days)*	*3. Return to weightbearing/full motion (up to 11 weeks)*
Goals	• Reduce pain/swelling • Improve range of motion (at least 0–120°) • Improve strength (muscle torque) as able • Maintain overall strength/aerobic capacity as able	• Full extension (compared to non-operative knee) • At least 90° of knee flexion • Reduce swelling and pain • Improve quadriceps/hamstring function	• Normal gait without brace • No swelling • Full range of motion • Improved strength (hip/knee/ankle musculature) • Improved proprioception/balance/postural stability • Maintain overall strength/aerobic capacity as able
Methods	*Prior to operation* *Measurements:* • IKDC score • Knee laxity measurement (KT 1000) • Isokinetic concentric/eccentric measurement of quadriceps and hamstring strength • Proprioception/postural stability test (KAT 2000) *Initial treatment:* • Cold and compression • Passive knee extension exercises • Active knee flexion exercises • Quadriceps control and straight leg raise exercises • Weightbearing as tolerated, brace and crutches as necessary	*Day of surgery, starting at the hospital* *Treatment:* • Cold and compression (cryo-cuff) • Passive knee extension exercises • Active knee flexion exercises • Quadriceps control and straight leg raise exercises • Weightbearing as tolerated with brace and crutches as necessary • Home program instruction *Notes:* • Outpatient therapy to be done 2–3 times a week • No high-intensity training for other body parts • Crutches are required until gait is	*Upon realization of phase 2 goals* *Treatment additions:* • Patellar mobilization (as needed) • Stretching of lower extremity (esp. hamstrings and gastrocnemius) • Gait training (with a mirror and/or therapist) • Closed kinetic chain exercises • Hamstring strengthening exercises • Proprioception, balance and coordination training • Exercise bicycle (when flexion >100°) • Pool exercises (avoid frog kick/breast stroke) *Exercises that may be added at week 5–6 (at the therapist's discretion):* • Active dynamic quadriceps training, 90–40° of knee flexion

Continued from previous page:

Note: Progress exercise and activity level, emphasizing painfree motion and strength and a gradual return to activities until a plateau is reached or surgery performed

- normal and painfree.
- Brace used for weightbearing activities during first 3 weeks.

- Functional exercises (jumprope, slideboard, etc.)
- Specific eccentric lower extremity training (walking downstairs, jumping down on a trampoline)
- Outdoor cycling
- Outdoor exercise walking, flat or uphill (uneven terrain–use poles)

Notes: Moderate intensity upper body/abdominal/opposite leg training

	Phase 4	Phase 5	Phase 6
Goals	*4. Return to straightline activities (3–4 months)* • Active quadriceps training against resistance without pain • Normal running gait • Maintain overall strength/aerobic capacity as able	*5. Return to cutting activities (4–6 months)* • >90% of normal muscle torque (measured isokinetically) • All types of running without pain and in full control • Jumping without pain and in full control	*6. Return to competition (6 months and beyond)* Return to full unrestricted activity approved upon: • Full range of motion and muscular flexibility as compared to the opposite leg • Isokinetic strength >90% of opposite leg • No pain or swelling as a result of training • Good results of all functional testing
Methods	*Upon realization of phase 3 goals* Treatment additions: • Submaximal isokinetic quadriceps training (open kinetic chain, concentric/eccentric, full range of motion) • Straightline jogging on even surface, flat or uphill only • Progress towards normal general and sport-specific training for all other body parts	*Upon realization of phase 4 goals* Treatment additions: • Jogging and running on uneven surfaces • Jogging with changes of direction (90°, 180°) • Zig-zag running with 45° cuts • Acceleration and deceleration training • Full-body sport-specific training with emphasis upon leg strength training	*Upon realization of phase 5 goals* Measurements: • IKDC score • Knee laxity testing (KT 1000) • Proprioception/postural stability test (KAT 2000) • Isokinetic concentric/eccentric measurement of quadriceps and hamstring strength • Objective functional testing, such as single leg hop, triple hop test, and/or stairs hopple (hopping) test • Full speed field or court drills as appropriate to sport(s) involved

Rehabilitation protocols

Rehabilitation protocols for specific injuries are set out in the following tables:
- ankle sprain: Table 21.8;
- lateral ankle reconstruction: Table 21.9;
- Achilles tendon repair: Table 21.10.

Lower extremity training

Proprioceptive balance and agility exercises

One foot balance

Holding on to a stable object (kitchen counter, table), practice balancing on your affected leg with:
- eyes open;
- eyes closed;
- standing on a book or pillow;
- gradually letting go of the support.

Time yourself; try to increase the length of time you are able to balance

Balance board

Holding on to a stable object (kitchen counter, table):
- Place feet on the edges of the board:
  1. Tilt board front to back, repeat 1–3 minutes.
  2. Tilt board side-to-side, repeat 1–3 minutes.
  3. Try to balance, keeping edges of board off the floor.
  4. Gradually try to reduce hold on stable object.
- Place one foot in middle of board. Repeat steps 1–3.
- Add ball toss (or sport-specific activity) while balancing on the board
- Try with eyes closed.

Directional walking and running (with or without sports cord

Begin at walking pace; progress to quarter speed, half speed, and then full speed (run):
- forwards;
- backwards;
- side-step (side shuffle)—lead with left foot, then lead with the right
- crossover step (carioca).

Jumping, hopping

Begin with both feet together. Place a line of tape on the floor to jump over; start with small jumps, then gradually increase speed and distance
- jump front to back;
- jump side to side.

contd p. 5

Table 21.8 Rehabilitation protocol for acute ankle sprain (see p. 368)

	Early phase	Intermediate phase	Late phase	Return to activity
Goals	Reduce/control pain, swelling Protect joint Maintain ROM	Increase A/PROM Protect joint Increase function Initiate strengthening	Resolve strength deficits Functional progression of activities	Prepare for return to activity
Weighbearing status	To tolerance with ankle stabilizing brace of choice	Full weightbearing with ankle support brace of choice	Full weightbearing	Full weightbearing
ROM, flexibility	Active PF/DF, toe extension	AROM IN/EV, PROM exercises: PF/DF, IN/EV Achilles towel stretch Standing calf stretch	Standing calf stretch	Continue previous program
Open kinetic chain strengthening	Isometric PF/DF; IN/EV Towel curls	Rubber tubing exercises: PF/DF, IN/EV Towel curls Towel IN/EV	Continue previous program Add: – rubber tubing exercises – multiaxial ankle exerciser	Continue previous strengthening Lower extremity strengthening
Closed kinetic chain strengthening	One-foot balance as tolerated	Heel raises Toe raises	Lunges, hops, bounds Quick feet (forward, back) Backward/forward running	Carioca, side-to-side hops, bounds Plyometric drills
Functional/proprioceptive	Maintain fitness: stationary cycling, swimming	Double leg stance tiltboard Balance drills, stork stands Maintain fitness: cycling, swimming, stairclimbing, pool running	Single leg stance tiltboard Slideboard, agility/balance drills Run, cycle, swim, stairclimbing	Functional running patterns Jump rope Box agility drills

AROM, active ROM; DF, dorsiflexion; EV, eversion; IN, inversion; PF, plantarflexion PROM, passive ROM.

Table 21.9 Rehabilitation protocol for lateral ankle reconstruction (anatomic) (see p. 378)

	Time elapsed since operation			
	0–3 weeks	3–6 weeks	6–12 weeks	12 weeks to 4–6 months
Goal	Reduce control/pain, swelling; Initiate ROM exercises	Normalize ROM; Initiate strengthening; Increase function	Normalize strength; Reduce functional deficits	Prepare for return to activity
Weightbearing status	Weightbearing to tolerance in ankle brace or walking boot	Full weightbearing in ankle stabilizer brace of choice	Full weightbearing; Ankle stabilizer brace for activity	Full weightbearing
ROM, flexibility	PROM DF/PF; Limited AROM toe flexion/extension	AROM DF/PF; *Avoid extreme IN/EV*; At 8 weeks: Achilles towel stretch	AROM, PROM exercises; Achilles tendon towel stretch	Continue ROM, stretching
Open kinetic chain strengthening	None	At 8 weeks: – isometrics: DF/PF, IN/EV – rubber tubing exercises: DF/PF	Full isotonic/isokinetic strengthening: all planes; Rubber tubing exercises: four planes	Continue previous strengthening
Closed kinetic chain strengthening	None	Heel raises; Toe raises	Straight-ahead lunges, hops, skip; Quick feet (forward, back)	Carioca, side-to-side hop, lunge, skip drills; Plyometric drills
Functional/proprioceptive	Maintain fitness: stationary cycling with walking boot on	Double leg stance tiltboard; Gait training; Fitness activity: cycling, swimming, deep water running	Single leg stance tiltboard; Slideboard; Fitness activity: cycling, swimming, stairclimbing	Functional running patterns; Jump rope; Sport-specific drills; Agility/balance drills; Jogging on flat surface at 4 months
Restrictions	No stretching or strengthening	No weightbearing sports	None	None

AROM, active range of motion; DF, dorsiflexion; EV, eversion; IN, inversion; PF, plantar flexion; PROM, passive range of motion.

Table 21.10 Rehabilitation protocol for Achilles tendon repair (see p. 352)

	Time elapsed since operation			
	0–4 weeks	4–12 weeks	12 weeks–6 months	6–8 months
Goal	Reduce/control pain, swelling Initiate ROM exercises	Begin to normalize ROM Increase function Initiate strengthening	Normalize strength Reduce functional deficits	Prepare for return to activity
Weightbearing status	Weightbearing as tolerable in walking boot or brace	Full weightbearing in ankle stabilizer brace and jogging shoes	Full weightbearing	Full weightbearing
ROM, flexibility	A/PROM PF 0–20° only Active toe flexion/extension	Careful A/PROM DF/PF; IN/EV *Avoid extreme DF* At 8 weeks: – Achilles towel stretch – standing calf stretch	AROM, PROM exercises Achilles towel stretch Standing calf stretch	Continue previous strengthening
Open kinetic chain strengthening	None	At 6 weeks: – isometrics: all directions At 8 weeks: – rubber tubing exercises – DF/PF, IN/EV	Full lower extremity isotonic/isokinetic strengthening: all directions	
Closed kinetic chain strengthening	None	At 8 weeks: – toe raises – heel raises	Straight-ahead lunges, skip Quick feet (forward, back)	Carioca, side-to-side hops, lunges Plyometric drills
Functional/proprioceptive	Maintain fitness: stationary cycling	Double leg stance tiltboard Gait training Fitness activity: cycling, swimming—no flip turns or diving	Single leg stance tiltboard Slideboard, agility/balance Fitness activity: cycling swimming, stairclimbing Jogging on flat surface at 4 months	Single leg toe/heel raises Functional running patterns Jump rope Sport-specific drills
Restrictions or recommendations	No stretching or strengthening Recommend scar mobilization as incision healing allows	No weightbearing sports	May return to non-contact sports at 4 months	None

AROM, active ROM; DF, dorsiflexion; EV, eversion; IN, inversion; PF, plantar flexion; PROM, passive ROM.

Practice jumping on both feet straight up, trying to increase the height each time.

Place pieces of tape on the floor, jump in random patterns to the tape marks.

Hopping on one foot, continue over a line:
- hop on one foot straight up;
- hop from front to back;
- hop from side to side.

Running activities

Begin on a flat, level surface:
- start at quarter speed, jog in a straight line only;
- progress to half speed on straights, quarter speed on curves;
- progress to three-quarter speed on straights, half speed on curves;
- progress to full sprint on straights, jog curves;
- add bouts of acceleration, then deceleration, then acceleration.

When you can complete the above drills, progress to other surfaces.

Zigzag running

Progress to this exercise when you are able to complete the previous running activities. Set up cones or obstacles in a straight line 60–90 cm (24–36 in) apart:
- begin at quarter speed, zigzagging through the cones;
- progress by increasing speed;
- progress by decreasing the distance between the cones.

Figures of eight

Begin by jogging in a large figure-of-eight pattern:
- jog in both clockwise and counterclockwise directions;
- progress by increasing speed;
- progress by decreasing the size of the figure of eight.

Box running

Set up cones or lines in the shape of a square:
- begin with a large square, run clockwise and counterclockwise while facing in the same direction;
- gradually decrease the size of the box;
- add other activities, such as jumping, hopping, side steps.

Pivots

Practice planting one foot and pivoting in different directions
- 90° pivot;
- 180° pivot.

Sport-specific drills

Add dribbling of a football, hockey ball, or basketball to the above running drills.

REMINDERS

1. Warm up before the drills by stretching and slow jogging.
2. Cool down afterwards by stretching and slow jogging.
3. Wear supportive court shoes for zigzag runs and figures of eight.
4. Wear any supportive braces (knee, ankle) as prescribed by your physical therapist, athletic trainer, or physician.
5. If you experience swelling, pain or a feeling of instability during or after your exercises, consult with your physical therapist or athletic trainer and apply ice and elevate for 15–20 minutes.

Power and speed drills

High knees
Run in place bringing your knees as high as you can. Concentrate on knee height, not speed. Perform one set of 15 seconds, one set of 20 seconds, one set of 15 seconds. Repeat with both eyes closed.

Quick skip
Skip as fast as you can, hardly lifting your feet off the ground. Use arms in a fast motion. Perform two sets of 55 m (50 yards). Repeat with eyes closed.

Bounding, power skip
Bring the right knee up with the left leg straight. Forcefully switch legs. Head and back should be straight. Concentrate on explosiveness and distance, use arms in fast motion. Perform two sets of 55 m (50 yards).

Single leg bounding
Bring your right leg from a hip and knee flexed position to a forceful hip and knee extension without touching the ground, landing on your left foot; forward progression should be from left leg hopping and force of right leg motion. Perform two sets of 55 m (50 yards).

Leaps
Forcefully bring one leg into hip and knee flexion causing your body to leap upwards. Concentration should be on vertical height rather than on speed or horizontal progression. Perform two sets of 55 m (50 yards).

Lunges
Bring your knee up high then extend the leg forwards in a lunge position. The opposite knee should bend until it is *not quite* touching the ground. Hold for 5 seconds then repeat. Do this drill slowly. Perform two sets of 55 m (50 yards).

Double leg speed jump, tuck jumps
Jump as high as possible, bending your knees as you land. Bring the knees high and forwards. Land, then jump again. Use your arms to help with lift. Do 2 or 3 sets of 10–15 repeats; resting 1 minute between sets.

Single leg speed hop
In the same position as for the double leg jumps, hop on one leg only, as high as possible. Do two sets of 10 repeats, resting 2 minutes between sets.

Squat jump

With your feet shoulder-width apart, interlock your fingers and put your hands behind your head. Drop into a half-squat position, then immediately explode upwards as high as possible. Do three sets of 20 repeats, resting 2 minutes between sets.

Quick feet

Place a line of tape on the floor and stand facing the line. As quickly as you can, step back and forth over the line, alternating feet. Perform timed intervals of 10, 20, 30 and 60 seconds. Repeat standing sideways to the line, and progress to jumping or hopping over the line.

Sport-specific rehabilitation in water

Hydrotherapy or aquatic training has many benefits (Figure 21.4). It allows for earlier and more aggressive training. The increased effects on circulation, respiration and metabolic rate are just as important as increases in range of motion, strength, power and endurance. Side-effects such as psychological well-being and relaxation are always welcome.

The therapist must understand the hydrodynamic principles of buoyancy, viscosity, hydrostatic pressure, refraction and temperature, as well as the biologic effects of immersion: the aim is to combine this knowledge with the requirements of the athlete's diagnosis, sport, and goals. Regulating the intensity is important so that the athlete gets the right level of training. To increase the intensity, the use of faster and bigger movements or of resistance equipment is recommended.

Healthy athletes can use water training as a complement to their usual training so that injuries from over-training may be avoided.

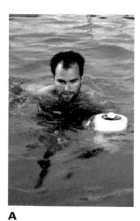

A

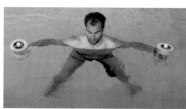

B

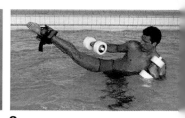

C

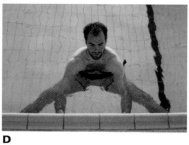

D

Figure 21.4 Hydrotherapy: (**A**) jogging; (**B**) strength training; (**C**) sport-specific exercises (here, for tae kwon do); (**D**) relaxation and stretching activities.

Index

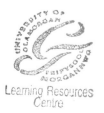

Learning Resources
Centre